ISBN 978-0-266-85601-6
PIBN 10899955

THE

HOMŒOPATHIC VADE MECUM

OF MODERN

MEDICINE AND SURGERY.

FOR THE USE OF

JUNIOR PRACTITIONERS, STUDENTS, ETC.

BY

E. HARRIS RUDDOCK, M.D.,

LICENTIATE OF THE ROYAL COLLEGE OF PHYSICIANS; MEMBER OF THE ROYAL COLLEGE OF SURGEONS; LICENTIATE IN MIDWIFERY, LONDON AND EDINBURGH, ETC.; PHYSICIAN TO THE READING AND BERKSHIRE HOMŒOPATHIC DISPENSARY.

Author of "The Stepping-Stone to Homœopathy & Health," "The Lady's Manual of Homœopathic Treatment," "On Consumption, its Symptoms, Causes, and Treatment," etc.; Editor of "The Homœopathic World."

THIRD EDITION, RE-CAST, RE-WRITTEN, AND GREATLY ENLARGED.

NEW YORK:
HENRY M. SMITH & BRO., 107, FOURTH AVENUE.
READING, ENGLAND:
SAMUEL COMPSTON, 145, CASTLE STREET.

And all Homœopathic Chemists and Booksellers.

1869.

[ENTERED AT STATIONERS' HALL.]

THE VADE MECUM OF MODERN MEDICINE AND SURGERY

MAY BE OBTAINED IN THE FOLLOWING FORMS:

(1) *Toned Paper, good Binding, with an extensive* CLINICAL DIRECTORY *and a Section on* POISONS, *now added for the first time* - - - - - 7s. 6d.

(2) *Ditto, ditto, in half-morocco Binding, marbled edges, with* 32 *pages of ruled paper, for Notes, etc.* - - 10s. 6d.

(3) *Cheap Edition, Cloth, without any of the above additions* - - - 5s. 0d.

Printed by Jarrold and Sons, London Street, Norwich.

ADE

SURGI

[redacted]

THE

HOMŒOPATHIC VADE MECUM

OF MODERN

MEDICINE AND SURGERY.

magnesia, antibilious pills, and even preparations of mercury and opium—*are* employed. We are not, then, *originators* of domestic medicine; but, finding drugs largely used by amateurs, we have laboured hard to *reform* the practice by substituting remedies and suggesting measures which, while harmless for evil, are powerful for good, if properly used. Simple and uncomplicated cases often arise that may be successfully met by the treatment herein prescribed. Cold, fever, dyspepsia, etc., may often be arrested at their outset, while, if neglected till the symptoms assumed proportions which seemed to justify the consultation of a doctor, might form the nucleus of serious or fatal disorders.

A fact which specially justifies the composition of this Manual is the necessity of meeting, as far as possible, the requirements of persons residing in localities where professional Homœopathic treatment is inaccessible. An extensive correspondence with persons in various parts of Great Britain, Europe, India, and the colonies, convinces the Author of the importance of making some provision for patients so circumstanced; at least, till professional men generally have been led to the study and practice of the discoveries of the illustrious Hahnemann. Information frequently reaches us showing the urgent need for the wider diffusion of Homœopathic knowledge, and also of the happy and often striking results of the application of that knowledge, even when derived from domestic publications.

While making these statements it is our duty to connect with them the recommendation that in every serious or doubtful case of illness, or when the treatment herein prescribed is insufficient to effect *improvement* in a reasonable time, a Homœopathic practitioner should be consulted. The vast and ever-accumulating resources at the disposal of a professional Homœopath, of which this manual represents but an inconsiderable fraction, places him on high vantage ground compared with a domestic practitioner. Cases are of daily occurrence which show that, equally for the Homœopathic and the Allopathic practitioner, it is impossible to act in the best way for the interests of patients without a knowledge of anatomy, physiology, and the general teaching of the medical schools. Apparently trifling symptoms which escape the non-professional observer, clever though he may be, immediately attract the attention of the informed eye and ear of the physician, and put him on the alert for further discovery. A trifling impediment in the speech, and a slight difference in the size of the pupils, so insignificant as to escape the observation of the patient or his friends, may be indicative of a grave organic disease when associated with some little strangeness in the conduct or defect in the memory. These, and a hundred other little points, the professional eye detects, and estimates according to their importance. And the doctor alone can do so, for a special education is necessary for the recognition, particularly the *early* recognition, of many important signs and symptoms. A trained medical observer, too, views disease from a higher stand-point, and often recognises a relationship between a local lesion and a constitutional condition. In many diseases described in the following pages we have pointed out that connection; but diseases occur under such widely differing circumstances, and vary so much in their effects, duration, and intensity in individual cases, that considerable modifications have to be pursued in treatment.

A great advantage arising from professional treatment is the amplitude of the resources of a Homœopathic doctor, not merely in the multitude of remedies at his command, but in the varieties of attenuations or dilutions which he can adapt to the constitutional peculiarities, age, sex, and habits of the patient. The writer is neither a low nor a high dilutionist, but ranges his doses from low tinctures or triturations to the higher attenuations. The question of dilution is one of greater importance than is usually attached to it. Thus, for example, *Nux Vomica*, extremely useful in many cases of indigestion, if given for constipation in the first or second dec. dil., frequently aggravates; while in a higher dilution it is a remedy of prime importance in the correction of this condition. On the other hand, we have often found low dilutions, and even the strong tinctures, efficacious in our practice after the high dilutions had been found inefficient.

In conclusion, the author trusts that the contribution he here makes to medical literature may serve as a faithful guide to the cure of disease, the preservation of health, and the prolongation of life to the allotted term of earthly existence. He has great confidence in the principles enunciated in the volume; and this confidence continually deepens as, year after year, his experience accumulates from the application of them in the exercise of his profession. He heartily thanks numerous correspondents for the unsolicited testimonies they have sent him of the success which has followed the adoption of the prescriptions contained in the former editions. He anticipates a yet larger amount of good, both in prevention and cure, from the publication in its present form.

E. HARRIS RUDDOCK.

12, *Victoria Square, Reading,*
October, 1869.

HINTS TO THE READER.

I.—When the work is consulted, the *whole* section devoted to the disease should be studied—the symptoms, causes, medicines, and accessory means—before deciding on the treatment. One portion of a section throws light upon another, and hesitation in the choice of a remedy may often be removed by considering the section in its entirety.

II.—Facility of reference may be secured by an acquaintance with the arrangement of the Manual; it is divided into Parts, Chapters, and Sections; the headings on the top of the left-hand pages mark the general subject or class of diseases under consideration, and those on the right, the particular topic or disease to which it is appropriated.

At the commencement of each Section in Part II., the principal designations by which a disease is known are given; the first, in thick type, being invariably the one adopted in the *New Nomenclature*, and that by which it is desirable that the disease be in future uniformly styled; the second, in italics and within parenthesis, is the Latin name; when other names follow, they are synonyms or common appellations. By noting the class of disease indicated in the left-hand page-heading, the reader may form an idea of the nature of any particular disease; thus, Diphtheria, Influenza, Hooping-cough, etc., occur amongst the *Blood* diseases—those in which the blood itself is affected; Rheumatism, Anæmia, Phthisis, etc., are classed with the *Constitutional* diseases—those in which the whole system is involved. The recognition of these points will often be most suggestive to the initiated reader, and influence the prognosis and treatment of the case. Medical terms are occasionally used, but they are either explained in the text, or in the index at the end of the volume; this index is very copious, and every point of importance may be found by it. Consultation is further made easy by a table of contents at the commencement.

III.—Occasionally, remedies are prescribed without describing in detail the symptoms, by which their use is indicated. Under such circumstances, and whenever hesitating in the choice of a remedy, the reader is referred to the MATERIA MEDICA; a comparison should be made between the symptoms of the case under consideration, and the essential features peculiar to each remedy. The Materia Medica forms a very important part of the volume, and an attentive study of it will give a broad and tolerably exact knowledge of many valuable remedial agents, and a measure of skill in using them.

IV.—Persons desirous of being able to act wisely and promptly for the prevention or removal of disease should *read this Manual through, from the first page to the last.* The first Part is devoted to Hygiene; the second to Diseases and their Treatment; the third to Materia Medica; and the fourth to

Accessory Measures. All should be attentively studied. The fifth Part—the Clinical Directory—is chiefly valuable for the initiated, or for references to the Materia Medica. Many important practical points are scattered through the various Sections, but which, to economise space, are not repeated, and so may be lost to those who only read detached portions. Even after having read the Manual through, an occasional half-hour spent in perusing it will facilitate its consultation in cases of urgency. The *novice* in Homœopathy may first read *The Stepping-Stone to Homœopathy and Health*, especially the introductory chapters.

V.—Lastly, the author will be glad to receive notes of the experiences of persons using the Manual. These, and friendly criticisms, will always be acceptable.

CONTENTS.

PART I.

Introductory.

CHAPTER I.

PAGES

OBSERVATIONS PERTAINING TO HEALTH *(Hygiene)* - 25–58

§ 1.—Plan of General Dietary.
2.—Comparative Value of White and Brown Bread.
3.—Cooking.
4.—Water.
5.—Pure Air.
6.—Light.
7.—Healthy Dwellings.
8.—Exercise.
9.—Clothing.
10.—Bathing.
11.—Influence of Professions and Occupations on Health.

CHAPTER II.

SIGNS AND SYMPTOMS OF DISEASE - - 58–68

§ 1.—The Pulse.
2.—Temperature and the Clinical Thermometer.
3.—Breathing.
4.—The Tongue.
5.—Pain.
6.—The Skin.
7.—The Urine.

CHAPTER III.

PAGES

THE MEDICINES, ETC. - - - - - 68–74

Directions for taking the Medicines. The Dose. Repetition of the Dose. Alternation of Medicines. List of upwards of Fifty Remedies.

PART II.

Medical and Surgical Diseases, and their Homœopathic and General Treatment.

CHAPTER I.

GENERAL DISEASES:—*A.* BLOOD DISEASES - 75–164

§ 1.—Small-pox.
2.—Cow-pox and Vaccination.
3.—Chicken-pox.
4.—Measles.
5.—Scarlet-Fever—Scarlatina.
6.—Typhus-Fever.
7.—Enteric-Fever—Typhoid-Fever.
8.—Relapsing-Fever.
9.—Simple Continued Fever and Febricula.
10.—Yellow-Fever.
11.—Intermittent Fever—Ague.
12.—Remittent Fever.
13.—Simple Cholera—English Cholera—Sporadic Cholera.
14.—Malignant Cholera—Asiatic Cholera—Cholera Morbus; and Choleraic Diarrhœa—Cholerine.
15.—Diphtheria.
16.—Hooping-Cough.
17.—Mumps.
18.—Influenza.
19.—Erysipelas—St. Anthony's Fire—Rose.
20.—Puerperal-Fever and Puerperal Ephemera.

CHAPTER II.

PAGES

GENERAL DISEASES *(continued)*:—*B.* CONSTITUTIONAL DISEASES - - - - - - 165–233

§ 21.—Acute Rheumatism—Rheumatic Fever.
22.—Muscular Rheumatism.
23.—Chronic Rheumatism.
24.—Acute Gout.
25.—Chronic Gout.
26.—Syphilis.
27.—Cancer—Malignant Disease.
28.—Lupus.
29.—Scrofula.
30.—Tubercular Meningitis—Acute Hydrocephalus.
31.—Scrofulous Ophthalmia.
32.—Scrofulous Disease of Glands.
33.—Phthisis Pulmonalis—Pulmonary Consumption.
34.—Tabes Mesenterica—Consumption of the Bowels.
35.—Rickets.
36.—Diabetes—Diabetes Mellitus.
37.—Purpura—Land-Scurvy.
38.—Scurvy.
39.—Anæmia.
40.—Chlorosis.
41.—General Dropsy.

CHAPTER III.

DISEASES OF THE NERVOUS SYSTEM - - 234–272

§ 42.—Encephalitis, Meningitis, and Inflammation of the Brain.
43.—Apoplexy.
44.—Sun-stroke—Insolation—Sun-fever—Coup-de-Soleil.
45.—Chronic Hydrocephalus—Dropsy of the Brain—Water in the Head.
46.—Paralysis—Paralytic Stroke.
47.—Tetanus—Lockjaw.
48.—Hydrophobia—Rabies.
49.—Infantile Convulsions—Fits of Infants.

DISEASES OF THE NERVOUS SYSTEM *(continued)*.

PAGES

§ 50.—Epilepsy—Falling-Sickness—Fits.
51.—Chorea—St. Vitus's Dance.
52.—Hysteria.
53.—Neuralgia.
54.—Hypochondriasis.

CHAPTER IV.

DISEASES OF THE EYE - - 273–292

§ 55.—Catarrhal Ophthalmia.
56.—Purulent Ophthalmia.
57.—Purulent Ophthalmia of Infants—Ophthalmia Neonatorum.
58.—Gonorrhœal Ophthalmia.
59.—Iritis.
60.—Amaurosis—Weak Sight—Blindness.
61.—Muscæ Volitantes—Spots before the Eyes.
62.—Cataract.
63.—Inflammation of the Eyelids—Sore Eyes.
64.—Hordeolum—Stye on the Eyelid.
65.—Entropium—Inversion of the Eyelid; and Ectropium—Eversion of the Eyelid.
66.—Tarsal Ophthalmia—Granular Eyelid.
67.—Strabismus—Squinting.

CHAPTER V.

DISEASES OF THE EAR - - - 293–299

§ 68.—Inflammation of the Ear—Ear-ache.
69.—Disease of the Mucous Membrane of the Ear—Otorrhœa—Running from the Ears.
70.—Deafness.

CHAPTER VI.

PAGES

DISEASES OF THE NOSE - - 300–303

§ 71.—Ozæna.
72.—Epistaxis—Bleeding from the Nose.
73.—Polypus Nasi—Polypus of the Nose.
74.—Loss or Perversion of the Sense of Smell.

CHAPTER VII.

DISEASES OF THE CIRCULATORY SYSTEM - 304–317

§ 75.—Diseases of the Heart and its Membranes.
76.—Angina Pectoris—Breast-pang.
77.—Syncope—Fainting-Fit—Swooning.
78.—Palpitation and Irregularity of the Action of the Heart.
79.—Aneurism.
80.—Phlebitis—Inflammation of the Veins.
81.—Varicose Veins.
82.—[Goitre—Derbyshire-Neck].

CHAPTER VIII.

DISEASES OF THE RESPIRATORY SYSTEM - - 318–344

§ 83.—Hay-Asthma—Hay-Fever—Summer-Catarrh.
84.—Croup—Inflammatory Croup; and Laryngismus Stridulus —Spasmodic Croup—Child-crowing.
85.—Coryza—Catarrh—Cold in the Head; and Bronchial Catarrh.
86.—Aphonia—Loss of Voice—Hoarseness.
87.—Bronchitis.
88.—Asthma.
89.—Pneumonia—Inflammation of the Lungs.
90.—Pleurisy.

CHAPTER IX.

PAGES

DISEASES OF THE DIGESTIVE SYSTEM - - 345–429

§ 91.—Stomatitis—Inflammation of the Mouth.
92.—Thrush—Frog—Sore Mouth.
93.—Cancrum Oris—Canker of the Mouth.
94.—Teething.
95.—Toothache.
96.—Gumboil.
97.—Glossitis—Inflammation of the Tongue.
98.—Ulcer on the Tongue.
99.—Sore Throat.
100.—Relaxed Throat; Ulcerated Throat; and Pharyngitis—Clergyman's Sore Throat.
101.—Quinsy.
102.—Gastritis—Inflammation of the Stomach.
103.—Chronic Ulcer of the Stomach.
104.—Hæmatemesis—Vomiting of Blood.
105.—Dyspepsia—Indigestion.
106.—Gastrodynia—Pain or Spasms in the Stomach.
107.—Pyrosis—Water-brash.
108.—Vomiting—Sickness.
109.—Sea-Sickness.
110.—Dysentery—Bloody-Flux.
111.—Hernia—Rupture.
112.—Parasitic Disease of the Intestines—Worms.
113.—Diarrhœa—Purging.
114.—Colic—Spasms of the Bowels.
115.—Constipation—Confined Bowels.
116.—Fistula in Ano.
117.—Hæmorrhoids—Piles.
118.—Pruritus Ani—Itching of the Anus.
119.—Prolapsus Ani—Falling of the Bowel.
120.—Hepatitis—Inflammation of the Liver.
121.—Simple Enlargement of the Liver—Congestion of the Liver—Liver-Complaint—Biliousness.
122.—Jaundice—the Yellows.
123.—Peritonitis—Inflammation of the Peritonæum.

CHAPTER X.

PAGES
DISEASES OF THE URINARY SYSTEM - - 430–450

§ 124.—Bright's Disease—Albuminuria.
125.—Cystitis—Inflammation or Catarrh of the Bladder.
126.—Calculus—Stone—Gravel.
127.—Irritability of the Bladder; and Spasm of the Bladder—Stranguary—Difficulty in Passing Water.
128.—Incontinence of Urine—Wetting the Bed.
129.—Retention of Urine.
130.—Gonorrhœa—Venereal Disease.
131.—Spermatorrhœa—Involuntary Emissions.

CHAPTER XI.

DISEASES OF THE CUTANEOUS SYSTEM - - 451–491

§ 132.—Erythema—Inflammatory Redness of the Skin.
133.—Intertrigo—Chafing—Soreness of Infants.
134.—Roseola—Rose-rash—False Measles.
135.—Urticaria—Nettle-rash.
136.—Prurigo—Itching of the Skin.
137.—Lichen.
138.—Pityriasis—Branny Tetter—Dandriff.
139.—Psoriasis—Lepra—Dry Tetter.
140.—Herpes—Shingles—Tetter.
141.—Eczema—Catarrhal Inflammation of the Skin—Scalled-Head—Milk-crust.
142.—Acne—Pimples.
143.—Sycosis—Mentagra—Barber's Itch—Chin-whelk.
144.—Chilblain.
145.—Ulcer.
146.—Boil.
147.—Carbuncle—Anthrax.
148.—Whitlow—Gathered Finger.
149.—Corn.
150.—Bunion.
151.—Nævus—Port-Wine-Stain—Mother's Mark; and Nævus Pilaris—Mole.

DISEASES OF THE CUTANEOUS SYSTEM (continued).

PAGES

§ 152.—Sebaceous Tumour—Wen.
153.—Warts.
154.—Parasitic Diseases of the Skin.
155.—Scabies—Itch.
156.—Irritation caused by Stinging-Insects and Plants.
157.—Poisoned Wounds.

CHAPTER XII.

MISCELLANEOUS DISEASES - 492–508

§ 158.—Morbus Coxæ—Scrofulous Disease of the Hip-Joint.
159.—Abscess.
160.—Obesity—Corpulence.
161.—Old Age and Senile Decay.

CHAPTER XIII.

INJURIES - 509–523

§ 162.—Asphyxia—Apnœa (from Drowning).
163.—Concussion of the Brain.
164.—Burns and Scalds.
165.—Contusion—Bruise.
166.—Wound.
167.—Foreign Bodies.
168.—Fracture—Broken Bone.
169.—Sprain—Strain.
170.—Exhaustion of the Muscles—Fatigue—Over-exertion.
171.—Poisons.

PART III.

Materia Medica.

		Page
1.	Aconitum Napellus	525
2.	Aloe Socotrina	529
3.	Antimonium Crudum	529
4.	Antimonium Tartaricum	530
5.	Apis Mellifica	531
6.	Arnica Montana	532
7.	Arsenicum Album	535
8.	Aurum Metallicum	538
9.	Baptisia Tinctoria	539
10.	Baryta Carbonica	540
11.	Belladonna	540
12.	Bryonia Alba	544
13.	Cactus Grandiflorus	546
14.	Camphora	547
15.	Cannabis Sativa	549
16.	Cantharis Vesicatoria	549
17.	Carbo Vegetabilis	551
18.	Causticum	552
19.	Chamomilla	552
20.	Calcarea (*including* C. Carbonica and C. Phosphorica)	554
21.	Calendula	556
22.	China Officinalis (*including* Quinine)	557
23.	Cimicifuga *or* Actæa Racemosa	559
24.	Cina Anthelmintica	563
25.	Cocculus Indicus	564
26.	Coffea Cruda	565
27.	Colchicum Autumnale	566
28.	Collinsonia Canadensis	567
29.	Colocynthis	568
30.	Conium Maculatum	568
31.	Cuprum	569
32.	Digitalis Purpurea	570
33.	Drosera Rotundifolia	571
34.	Dulcamara	571
35.	Euphrasia Officinalis	572
36.	Ferrum (*including* F. Metallicum *and* F. Phosphoricum)	573
37.	Gelseminum Sempervirens	574
38.	Glonoine	577
39.	Graphites	578
40.	Hamamelis Virginica	578
41.	Helleborus Niger	579
42.	Hepar Sulphuris	580
43.	Hydrastis Canadensis	581
44.	Hyoscyamus Niger	582
45.	Ignatia Amara	583
46.	Iodium	584
47.	Ipecacuanha	586
48.	Iris Versicolor	588
49.	Kali Bichromicum	589
50.	Kali Hydriodicum	591
51.	Kreasotum	591
52.	Lachesis	592
53.	Lycopodium Clavatum	593
54.	Mercurius (*including* M. Solubilis, M. Vivus, M. Bin-iodidum, M. Corrosivus, *and* M. Sulphuratus Rubrum *or* Cinnabaris)	594
55.	Muriatis Acidum	600
56.	Nitri Acidum	601
57.	Nux Vomica (*including* Strychnia)	601
58.	Opium	604
59.	Phosphorus	606
60.	Phosphori Acidum	609
61.	Phytolacca Decandra	610
62.	Platina	612
63.	Plumbum	612
64.	Podophyllum	613
65.	Pulsatilla	613
66.	Rhus Toxicodendron	616
67.	Ruta Graveolens	618
68.	Sepia Succus	619
69.	Silicea	619
70.	Spigelia Anthelmia	620
71.	Spongia Marina Tosta	621
72.	Staphysagria	622
73.	Sulphur	622
74.	Sulphurosum Acidum	627
75.	Terebinthina	628
76.	Veratrum Album	629
77.	Veratrum Viride	630
78.	Zincum	632

or a little home-fed, cold, boiled bacon, chicken, or game, may be substituted, for those who take much bodily exertion. A breakfast-cupful of cocoa, deprived of its excess of oil, such as is sold by most Homœopathic chemists, or black tea, with milk, may be substituted; but the latter is less nutritious.

Breakfast is an important meal, and its digestion ought never to be endangered by taking it too hurriedly, or commencing a quick walk immediately after it. It would be an immense gain to the active man of business to make it a uniform habit to rise sufficiently early to give himself ample time to enjoy a quiet breakfast, and sufficient time after it for its digestion to have made some progress before again taxing the physical or mental powers.

Dinner. *Dinner* at one, p.m. Wholesome fresh meat and vegetables carefully proportioned, plainly cooked, served hot, and properly masticated. These should be varied from day to day, with occasional additions, in moderate quantities, of fruit or farinaceous puddings; and fish substituted once or twice a week for animal food. Highly-seasoned dishes, pickles, salt and dried meats, rich or heavy pastry, and cheese, should be excluded from tables aiming at wholesomeness. Weakly persons who are obliged to take much exercise, may drink a small quantity of malt liquor, never exceeding half a pint, if they are benefitted by it; but in by far the majority of cases, fermented liquors had better be avoided altogether at dinner, and a few sips of filtered water, or a wine-glass of claret diluted with an equal quantity of water, substituted. Too much cold water lowers the temperature of the stomach, and so interrupts digestion. The habit of taking wine after dinner is one of luxury, not of health; and all that can be said of it, from a hygienic point of view, is, *the less the better*. An occasional slight dessert of wholesome fruit is not objectionable,—apples, oranges, grapes, strawberries, gooseberries,

Tea. *Tea* may be taken at six or half-past, and include one or two cups of black tea, bread or dry-toast, with butter, fruit, or marmalade, as may be found most digestible or agreeable. If it be the last meal in the day, and the person is not plethoric, and takes a great amount of physical exercise, the meal may include a little light meat, chicken, or white fish.

Late Dinners. A different arrangement is necessary for those who dine late—say at six, p.m.—as then a *luncheon* should be taken at about one, p.m., which may consist of a small basin of good beef soup, with vermicelli, rice, or toasted bread in it. But if meat have been taken at breakfast, bread-and-butter, biscuits, or a sandwich may suffice; wine and malt liquors are better avoided at this time. At six, dinner may be taken, and include the dishes already mentioned. The custom of taking tea, or a simple warm liquid meal three or four hours after dinner, is a very salutary one, as the warm liquid assists the separation and absorption of the chyle from the chyme, which is effected at this period. But the introduction of solid food, especially large quantities of buttered-toast or rich cake, would seriously interfere with this process. Two moderate-sized cups of black tea, with a little milk and sugar, or a slice of lemon, form a useful and agreeable beverage, and serve to remove all acrid materials left undissolved by digestion, and which, if not carried off, might disturb that rest for which the appropriate hour now approaches.

When convenient, the dinner-hour may be advantageously deferred until six or seven, p.m., so that sufficient time may be devoted to it, and that rest taken after it which the principal meal requires, but which it is often impossible to give to it in the middle of the day. Persons much occupied should not eat full meals during the hours of toil; for such, a light repast is best in the middle of the day, and the principal meal taken in the evening, when the work of the day is finished. Heavy meals taken during the hours of physical labour, without sufficient rest, are almost certain, eventually, to lead to derangement of the digestive organs. The chapter on "Indigestion," to which the reader is referred, contains almost every other remark necessary to be made on the general subject of diet.

2.—Comparative Value of White and Brown Bread.

The importance of bread, aptly termed the "staff of life," the common food of all classes, and its abundance being properly regarded as one of our greatest national blessings, seems to justify a brief inquiry into the kind most conducive to health. We may at once state that our object is to impress upon the reader that no single constituent part of our food is capable of acting by itself alone, and that one missing element may make the others wholly inefficient. This applies forcibly to the subject of this section. Wheat contains the following principles, which slightly vary in different samples:—

Water	11 per cent.	Gum	4 per cent.
Gluten	13 "	Oil	2 "
Starch	60 "	Bran (the thin external husk)	2 "
Sugar	8 "		

It is important to remark that these elements are not *uniformly* distributed throughout a kernel of wheat. Immediately beneath the thin external covering is a layer of darkish-coloured matter, most rich in gluten, and in which the chief of the oil in the wheat exists in minute drops enclosed in its cells. In the ordinary course of grinding and dressing, a large portion of this is removed from the superfine flour, as it is not so readily reduced to a fine powder, and hence is rejected with the middlings and bran. Beneath this dark layer is the heart of the kernel, which is very white and chiefly composed of starch, and from it the best looking and finest flour is made. This portion is not absolutely destitute of gluten, nor is the dark portion free from starch; but they exist in excess in the parts indicated.

The mineral ingredients of a kernel of wheat are also unequally distributed. They are chiefly,—phosphoric acid, potash, soda, magnesia, oxide of iron, sulphuric acid, salt, and silica; and in superfine flour they exist in the proportion of a little over 1 per cent.; in the next quality, between 3 and 4 per cent.; still coarser flour, about 5 per cent.; and bran 7 per cent. Thus it will be seen that fine flour contains but a small portion of those mineral ingredients which are found in wheat before grinding, a large portion being cast off with the bran.

But the mineral constituents of the vegetables we consume are as indispensable to the human organization as any other; experiments upon the inferior animals prove that the withdrawal of these elements from vegetable food is prejudicial, and that animals so fed perish from starvation. Mineral ingredients form the nourishment for important parts of the animal economy, and, dissolved in the blood, are taken up at points where they are necessary to sustain local parts. Thus phosphate of lime is required by the bones, phosphates of magnesia and potash by the muscles, soda by the cartilages, phosphorus by the brain, silica by the hair and nails, and iron by the red globules of the blood and black colouring matter within the eye.

The dark portion, which chiefly contains the gluten, the most nutritious constituent of the wheat kernel, is almost entirely separated in the process of dressing; while the central is almost wholly starch, and of much less value to the body. In thus rejecting the dark portion which immediately underlies the bran, and is almost entirely removed with it, and used for the food of our cattle, we lose the most nutritious as well as the sweetest portion of the grain.

In the preparation of wheat for the purpose of food, it should be borne in mind that its value depends not upon the quantity of starch it contains, but upon the amount of gluten, and any process which diminishes this element is most objectionable.

The mere bran, without its underlying strata, may be partially removed without much detriment, for though useful in obstinate constipation, it is irritatng to the mucous membrane of the alimentary canal of some persons. In such cases the coarse portions of bran may be removed, but not to the extent of divesting it entirely of the bran and the darker portion referred to, and so sacrificing its nourishing properties for mere fineness or whiteness of bread.

Our supply of corn would suffice to sustain millions more if we could persuade the people in this and other countries, of the advantages, in wholesomeness, digestiveness, and flavour, which brown bread has over white. Liebig states that 1000 parts of wheat-corn contain 21 parts of the nutritive salts, but fine flour only 7 parts.

This difference is very great, and the value of the unbolted flour as compared with that ordinarily eaten, is not at all adequately appreciated.* Dr. Boudens, a French physician, states that during the Crimean war, the Russian prisoners, accustomed to a very coarse brown bread, were inadequately nourished by the French rations, and that it was found necessary to increase them. Magendie has proved by experiment, that a dog will die if fed on white bread, but if brown be given

* The necessity of the presence of the nutritive salts, in sufficient quantity, may be illustrated by the following fact:—It has been observed that when fodder is given to sheep, consisting of 2½ lbs. of winter straw and 3 lbs. of potatoes, a portion of the latter passes away undigested; but that if ½ lb. of peas be added, the starch is retained, and the animal rapidly gains in weight, which it did not before. Now peas are rich in nutritive salts, and they contributed, in the above instance, to render the starch available for the nutrition of the sheep.

him his health remains good. The subject merits the earnest consideration of the heads of households on whom the dietetic arrangements depend. In the case of the great working populations in whose diet bread is the chief constituent, they are sure to suffer from any deficiency in its nutritive properties, especially children and growing young people, who require suitable materials for the formation of the numerous parts of the animal frame. The subject is of less moment to those whose tables are daily supplied with edibles both abundant and varied, as they are less likely to suffer from the diminished nutritive value of any single article of food.

3.—Cooking.

Much depends, as to the digestibility and nourishing properties of animal food, on the mode in which it is prepared for the table. The following passage from Professor Johnstone's work contains the whole theory of the art of cooking meat, and we give it entire, as such knowledge cannot be too widely diffused:—

"In cooking animal food, plain boiling, roasting, and baking, are in most general favour in our islands. During these operations, fresh beef and mutton, when moderately fat, sustain loss as indicated below.

	In boiling.	In baking.	In roasting.
4 lbs. of beef lose ...	1 lb.	1 lb. 3 oz.	1 lb. 5 oz.
4 lbs. of mutton lose	14 oz.	1 lb. 4 oz.	1 lb. 6 oz.

The greater loss in baking and roasting arises chiefly from the greater quantity of water which is evaporated, and of fat which is melted out during these two methods of cooking. Two circumstances, however, to which it has not hitherto been necessary to advert, have much influence upon the successful result of these and some other modes of cooking.

"If we put moist flesh-meat into a press and squeeze it, a red liquid will flow out. This is water coloured by blood, and holding various saline and other substances in solution. Or if, after being cut very thin, or chopped very fine, the flesh be put into a limited quantity of clean water, the juices of the meat will be gradually extracted, and by subsequent pressure will be more completely removed from it than when pressure is applied to it in the natural state, and without any such mincing and steeping. The removal of these juices leaves the beef or mutton nearly tasteless. When the juice of the meat, extracted in either way, is heated nearly to boiling, it thickens or becomes muddy, and flakes of whitish matter separate, which resemble boiled white of egg. They are, in fact, white of egg or albumen; and they show that the juice of flesh contains a certain quantity of this substance, in the same liquid and soluble state in which it exists in the unboiled egg. Now, the presence of this albumen in the juice of butchers' meat is of much importance in connection with the skilful preparation of it for the table.

"The first effect of the application of a quick heat to a piece of fresh meat is to cause the fibres to contract, to squeeze out a little of the juice, and, to a certain extent, to close up the pores so as to prevent the escape of the remainder. The second is to coagulate the albumen, and thus effectually and completely to plug up the pores, and to retain within the meat the whole of the juice. Thereafter, the cooking goes on through the agency of the natural moisture of the flesh. Converted into vapour by the heat, a kind of steaming takes place, so that whether in the oven, on the spit, or in the midst of boiling water, the meat is in reality, cooked by its own steam.

"A well-cooked piece of meat should be full of its own juice or natural gravy. In roasting, therefore, it should be at first exposed to a quick fire, that the external surface may be made to contract at once, and the albumen to coagulate, before the juice has had time to escape from within. And so in boiling. When a piece of beef or mutton is plunged into boiling water, the outer part contracts, the albumen which is near the surface coagulates, and the internal juice is prevented either from escaping into the water by which it is surrounded, or from being diluted and weakened by the admission of water among it. When cut up, therefore, the meat yields much gravy, and is rich in flavour. Hence a beaf-steak or mutton-chop is done quickly, and over a quick fire, that the natural juices may be retained.

"On the other hand, if the meat be exposed to a slow fire, its pores remain open, the juice escapes, and the flesh pines and becomes dry, hard, and unsavoury. Or if it be put into cold or tepid water, which is afterwards gradually brought to a boil, much of the albumen is abstracted before it coagulates, the natural juices for the most part flow out, and the meat is served in a nearly tasteless state. Hence, to prepare good boiled meat, it should be put at once into water already brought to a boil. But to make beef-tea, mutton-broth, or other meat-soups, the flesh should be put into cold water, and this afterwards very slowly warmed, and finally boiled. The advantage derived from *simmering*, a term not unfrequent in cookery books, depends very much upon the effects of slow boiling as above explained."

It is a cause of regret to find how very extensively the principles expressed in the above quotation are disregarded. Even in well-informed circles, there exists lamentable ignorance or extreme carelessness as to the proper method of cooking animal food so as to utilize its most valuable constituents.

4.—Water.

There is no drink in the world so wholesome, or, to the unperverted taste, so agreeable, as pure water. It is the natural drink of man, is highly favourable to digestion, and may always be taken in moderation when thirst is present. It enters into the composition of the tissues of the body, forms a necessary part of its structure, and performs such important purposes in the animal economy as to be absolutely indispensable for life and health. Water enters largely into combination with our food, and articles that we take as food can only afford nourishment by being dissolved in it. It also acts as a vehicle to convey the more dense and less fluid substances from the stomach to their destination in the body. It gives fluidity to the blood, holding in suspension, or solution, the red globules, fibrine, albumen, and all the various substances which enter into the different structures; for the whole body is formed from the blood. Not only the soft parts of the body, but even the very bones, or the materials of which they are composed, have at one time flowed in the current of the blood, suspended or held in solution in water. To prove how essential water is for the development and maintenance of the animal body, we may here state that a calculation has been made which shows that a human body, weighing 154 lbs., contains 111 lbs. of water. Such a fact suggests the necessity for obtaining water pure, and taking it unpolluted by animal and mineral ingredients. When practicable, water for domestic purposes should be filtered.

Water may be obtained tolerably pure in rain or snow collected in suitable vessels in the open country, away from crowded dwellings and manufactories, where processes are constantly going on which tend to deteriorate the water. Spring-, river-, sea-, surface-, well-, and mineral-water, all contain various substances dissolved in them, which render them, without distillation or filtration, unsuitable for drinking, or even to be used in the preparation of articles of diet. The purest water is obtained from deep wells, bored through the earth and clay down to the chalk *(Artesian Wells)*. Even for cooking purposes and bathing, the purest water that can be obtained is the best.

It is a fallacy to suppose that surface well-water is purer than that obtained from deep wells because it is more sparkling and often cooler and clearer. The sparkling of these waters is due to the presence of carbonic acid gas, that acid being derived from the decomposition of animal and vegetable substances.

"The situation of these wells, especially in London, explains the origin of these impure matters. The water that supplies the surface wells of London is derived from the rain which falls upon the surface of the land, and which percolates through the gravel, and accumulates upon the clay. Now this gravel contains all the soakage of London filth; through it run all the drains and sewers of London, and its whole surface is riddled with innumerable cesspools. Here is the source of the organic matter of surface well-waters, and also the cause of their coolness, their sparkling, and their popularity. In most small towns there is a public pump, and, when this is near the churchyard, it is said to be always popular. The character of the water is no doubt owing to the same causes as that of London surface wells, the remains of humanity in the churchyard supply the nitrates and carbonic acid of the water.

"From this kind of impurity the water of deep wells in London, and of wells cut into rocks which bring their water from a distance from towns, are entirely free. They frequently contain inorganic salts in abundance, but they do not contain organic matters; hence, for drinking purposes, they are very preferable to the waters of surface-wells.

great number of these wells exist in London. There is one attached to almost every brewery in London; and manufacturers, who need pure water for their operations, sink these wells."—*Lancaster*.

Not one of the least important objects contemplated in the publication of this work is the removal of a foolish prejudice, which unhappily exists in the minds of many, against pure water, an element which God has provided for His creatures with the most lavish abundance; and of promoting, both for internal and external purposes, in health and sickness, a more regular use of this invaluable boon and blessing. Pure water has justly been regarded as an emblem of innocence, truth, and beauty. In a community in which this element shall be used as the chief beverage, and more abundantly for purposes of purification, we may hope to find in the morals of the people reflections of virtue of which water is so vivid a type. And, in a sense which more immediately bears on the subject of this manual, suffering will be more easily controlled by our remedies, and the development of those latent tendencies to disease which the habits and fashions of the present age seem to favour, most effectually prevented.

5.—Pure Air.

A proper supply of pure, fresh air is essential to the preservation of life and health. Although life may not be destroyed suddenly by breathing an impure atmosphere, still the vital energies are thereby slowly but surely impaired, and this is especially the case with growing children, and persons suffering from disease.

Air Spoiled by Breathing. It will be sufficient for our present purpose briefly to state, that in the process of breathing, the air loses a third part of its oxygen, the life-giving principle, and receives in exchange carbonic acid gas, a gas not only incapable of supporting life, but actually destructive to it. Such is the change effected by a solitary act of breathing; and if this process goes on in an ill-ventilated room where several human beings are gathered together, the carbonic acid gas accumulates, usurps the place of the oxygen consumed, and so renders the air less and less fit for the purposes of the renewal of life. Carbonic acid gas cannot support combustion; hence a lighted candle partially or completely surrounded by it, burns slowly or goes out; and so is it with human beings, when more or less completely enveloped in an atmosphere charged with this gas; all the functions of the body are tardily and imperfectly performed; the muscular tissues are enfeebled, the breathing becomes oppressed, the head aches, and, in extreme cases, life is extinguished amidst sufferings of the most distressing nature.

Airy Sleeping-Rooms. The fact that carbonic acid gas is inimical to health and life, shows the importance of making provision for its uninterrupted removal from our houses and places of assembly, and above all, from our sitting rooms and *sleeping rooms*, in which we pass so large a portion of our lives. *Airy, well-ventilated sleeping apartments should be ranked with the most important requirements of life, both in health and disease.* Bed-rooms, in which about one-third of human existence is passed, are generally too small, crowded, and badly ventilated. The doors, windows, and even chimneys are often closed, and every aperture carefully guarded so as to exclude fresh air. The consequence is, that, long before morning dawns, the atmosphere of the whole apartment becomes highly noxious from the consumption of its oxygen, the formation of carbonic acid, and the exhalations from the lungs and the relaxed skin. In an atmosphere thus loaded with effluvia, the sleep is heavy and unrefreshing, partaking more of the character of insensibility. Were due provision made for the uninterrupted admission of fresh air, and the free escape of impure air, the sleep would be lighter, shorter, and more invigorating. In nearly every instance the door of the bed-room may be left open, and the upper part of the window let down a few inches—a greater or less extent according to the state of the weather—with perfect safety. A current of air may be prevented from playing on the face of the occupant, by placing the bed in a proper situation, or by suspending a single curtain from the ceiling. We may be permitted to add, we always sleep with a portion of the top sash of the window down, except in very wet, windy, or foggy weather; and even then the door of communication with the adjoining room or landing remains open. During foggy weather, the apertures directly communicating with the external air may be closed.

The importance of the subject is very correctly and strikingly put by a medical writer of the last century. "If any person," he remarks, "will take the trouble to stand in the sun, and look at his own shadow on a white plastered wall, he will easily perceive that his whole body is a smoking mass of corruption, with a vapour exhaling from every part of it. This vapour is subtle, acrid, and offensive to the smell; if retained in the body it becomes morbid; but if re-absorbed, highly deleterious. If a number of persons, therefore, are long confined in any close place not properly ventilated, so as to inspire and swallow with their spittle the vapours of each other, they must soon feel its bad effects." Unpleasant as it is to dwell on such a subject, it is yet true that the exhalations from the human lungs and skin, if retained and undiluted with a continuous supply of oxygen, are the most repulsive with which we can come in contact. We shun the approach of the dirty and the diseased; we hide from view matters which are offensive to the sight and the smell; we carefully eschew impurities in our food and drink; and even refuse the glass that has been raised to the lips of a friend. At the same time, "we resort to places of assembly, and draw into our mouths air loaded with effluvia from the lungs and skin and clothing of every individual in the promiscuous crowd: exhalations, offensive to a certain extent, from the most healthy individuals, but which, rising from a living mass of skin and lung in a state of disease, and prevented by the walls and ceiling from escaping, are, when thus concentrated, in the highest degree deleterious and loathsome" *(Bernan)*.

Cautions as to badly-ventilated Churches, etc. The great practical inference is, that the only means of preventing people from poisoning themselves and others is to ensure their being constantly surrounded by fresh air; otherwise, low fevers may result, and such acute diseases as scarlatina, measles, small-pox, etc., may be excited in epidemic forms, marked by a class of symptoms described in medical terms as "typhoid" or malignant. The air of an apartment containing several human beings, if unchanged, not only becomes charged with carbonic acid gas, but also, as before stated, impregnated with animal particles which fly off from the skin and lungs, so minute as scarcely to be detected by the microscope, but capable of decomposition; and, taken by the breath into the lungs, may be absorbed, and develop the worst forms of scrofula and consumption. But if these particles are given off from bodies affected with, or recovering from, small-pox, scarlet-fever, hooping-cough, typhus, etc., they will exert a still more injurious influence upon the health, and probably generate in other bodies diseases like those from which they emanated. It is most important to bear in mind that the assembly in an ill-ventilated church, court of law, school-room, theatre, ball-room, or evening party, may include in its number some as yet unsafe convalescents from these or kindred diseases. The only security we can suggest is, as far as possible to avoid all places of public resort or private gatherings in which the most ample provision is not made for the admission of fresh air, and for the uninterrupted escape of air spoiled by carbonic acid gas or animal exhalations.*

6.—Light.

The importance of sunlight for physical development and preservation is not, it is believed, duly appreciated. Women and children, as well as men, in order to be healthy and well developed, should spend a portion of each day where the solar rays can reach them directly. Just as sprouts of potatoes in dark cellars seek the light and are colourless till they come under its influence, and as vegetation goes on but imperfectly in places where sunlight does not freely enter, so the cheeks of children and adults who live almost entirely in dark kitchens, dingy alleys, and badly-lighted workshops, are pale, and their bodies feeble. Houses are only fit to be occupied at night that have been purified by the solar rays during the day.

It has been pointed out by Dr. Ellis that women and children in the huts and even log cabins of America, which contain only one or two rooms, remain healthy and strong; but that, after the settler has built a house, and *furnished it with blinds and curtains*, the women and children become pale-faced, bloodless, nervous, and sickly; the daughters begin to die from consumption, and the wives from the same or some disease peculiar to women. At the same time, the adult males, who live chiefly out of doors, continue healthy.

* See an article by the author on "Ventilation in Cold Weather," in *The Homœopathic World*, Vol. 1.

The value of sunlight, with its accompanying influences, for animal development, may be illustrated by such facts as the following:—In decaying organic solutions, animalcules do not appear if light is excluded, but are readily organized when it is admitted. The tadpole, kept in the dark, does not pass on to development as a frog, but lives and dies a tadpole, and is incapable of propagating his species. In the deep and narrow valleys among the Alps, where the direct rays of the sun are but little felt, cretinism, or a state of idiocy, more or less complete, commonly accompanied by an enormous goitre, prevails, and is often hereditary. Rickets, or deformities, crookedness, and enlargement of the bones, are very common among children who are kept in dark alleys, cellars, factories, and mines.

During the prevalence of certain epidemic diseases, the inhabitants who occupy houses on the side of the street upon which the sun shines directly, are less subject to the prevailing disease than those who live on the shaded side. In all cities visited by the cholera, the greatest number of deaths took place in narrow streets, and on the sides of those having a northern exposure, where the salutary beams of the sun were excluded. It is stated that the number of patients cured in the hospitals of St. Petersburg was four times greater in apartments well lighted than among those confined in dark rooms. This discovery led to a complete reform in lighting the hospitals of Russia, and with the best results.

Except in severe inflammatory diseases of the eyes or brain, the very common practice of *darkening the sick-room* is a highly prejudicial one. The restorative influence of daylight is thus excluded, and also the grateful and natural succession of light and darkness, the two always making up the same period of twenty-four hours, which favours sleep at the appropriate time, and divests the period of sickness of the monotony and weariness of perpetual night.

7.—Healthy Dwellings.

To those who are able to choose their habitations we offer a few suggestions. The subject is especially important to delicate families, and to persons predisposed to consumption; it also deserves attention from those who are healthy, and desire to maintain that blessing unimpaired both in themselves and their children. We advise, if possible, a country residence, and the selection of a house so constructed as to secure dryness of the foundation, walls, and roof. The site should be dry,—a gentle slope, a gravel soil; and the aspect southerly or westerly; the bedrooms, especially those appropriated to cases of sickness, should have this aspect. It should also be a site *from* which there is thorough drainage, but *towards* which there is none. If the house is not upon a slope, the artificial *drainage* must be perfect. In towns and crowded places in which the accumulation of decomposing and decomposed animal and vegetable matter is great, artificial channels or drains must be so constructed that all noxious matters and vapours may be rapidly removed and carried to a distance, before they can impregnate the atmosphere and water. Every dwelling to be wholesome should be accessible to the free passage of currents of air, and provided with an unlimited supply of good water. In the choice of a site for a house, a locality should be avoided in which the water is impregnated with lead, iron, or other mineral substances, or in proximity to stagnant waters; the ground should be above the level of the mist or vapour which rises after sunset in marshy and other districts. This subject is of special importance to the Colonist who may have to select a site for his habitation. In short, the fundamental condition of healthy dwelling-places is—perfect purity of air and water; this must take precedence of all other considerations. The cause of the spread and fatality of the mediæval plagues was neglect of the conditions necessary to secure pure air and cleanliness.*

Other points of subordinate importance may be glanced at. The house should not be too closely surrounded by trees, or in immediate proximity to thick woods, as they both attract and retain moisture, while they exclude much of the valuable influence of sun-light, and thus render the climate damp and cold. A cheerful situation, at the same time commanding the sight of green trees, hedges, shrubs, etc., has a beneficial tendency. If compelled to live in a town, the house should face a park, square, or other open place, or at least be in a wide airy street, with a favourable aspect.

Some who read these pages may not have it in their power to carry out these hints fully, but be compelled to live where their occupations, families, or means determine; nevertheless even such may be benefitted by these suggestions, for although they cannot secure perfection in a house or situation, they may aim at an approximation to it.

* Whoever considers the record of the mediæval epidemics, and seeks to interpret them by our present knowledge of the causes of disease, will become convinced that one great reason why those epidemics were so frequent and so fatal was the compression of the population in faulty habitations. Ill-constructed and closely-packed houses, with narrow streets, a poor supply of water, and therefore a universal uncleanliness; a want of all appliances for the removal of excreta; a population of rude, careless, and gross habits, living often on innutritious food, and frequently exposed to famine from their imperfect system of tillage—such were the conditions which almost throughout the whole of Europe enabled disease to attain a range, and to display a virulence, of which we have now scarcely a conception. The more these matters are examined, the more shall we be convinced that we must look for their explanation, not to grand cosmical conditions, not to earthquakes, comets, or mysterious waves of an unseen and poisonous air; not to recondite epidemic constitutions, but to simple, familiar, and household conditions.—*Parkes' Practical Hygiene.*

7.—Exercise.

Exercise strengthens and invigorates every function of the body, and is essential to health and long life. No one in health should neglect to walk a moderate distance every day in the open air, and if possible in the country, where the pure and invigorating air can be freely inhaled. *Walking* is the healthiest as well as the most natural mode of exercise. Other things being equal, this will ensure the proper action of every organ of the body. The walk for health should be diversified, and if possible include ascents and descents, and varying scenery; and be alternated, when circumstances admit of it, with riding on horseback, active gardening, or similar pursuits; and with gymnastics and games of various kinds. Athletic sports and manly exercises should form a part of the education of youth, nor should they be neglected in after life, especially by persons of sedentary pursuits. Many aches and pains would rapidly vanish if the circulation were quickened by a judicious and regular use of the muscles. These modes of exercise, practised moderately and regularly, and varied from day to day, are much more advantageous than the exciting, immoderate, and irregular exertions which characterize the ball-room, the hunting-field, and even the cricket-ground or the rowing-match. These exercises are sometimes pursued so violently as to be followed by severe and permanent injury to the constitution. In the case of very feeble and infirm people, carriage-exercise, if it may be so called, and frictions, by means of towels and bath gloves, over the surface of the body and extremities, are the best substitutes for active exertion.

The best periods for exercises are,—when the system is not depressed by fasting or fatigue, or oppressed by the process of digestion. The robust may take exercise before breakfast;

but delicate persons, who often become faint from exercise at this time, and languid during the early part of the day, had better defer it till from one to three hours after breakfast. An evening walk in fine weather is also advantageous. Exercise prevents disease by giving vigour and energy to the body and its various organs and members, and thus enables them to ward off or overcome the influence of the causes which tend to impair their integrity. It cures many diseases by equalising the circulation and the distribution of nervous energy, thus invigorating and strengthening weak organs, and removing local torpor and congestion.

The philosophy of using the muscles is very correctly expressed in the following quotation from Dr. Chambers:—

"If an animal's limbs are duly employed, the muscles keep up their shape and their vigorous power of contraction, their flesh is of a rich bright red colour when the animal is fully grown, and is firm and elastic. Examine it under a microscope, and you find it made up of even parallel fibres, each fibre seeming to be engraved over with delicate equi-distant cross-markings, like a measuring tape, very minutely divided. The more the muscle has been used in a well-nourished frame, the more closely it conforms to the typical specimen of the physiologist:

'Use, use is life; and he most truly lives
Who uses best.'

But suppose this muscular fibre has been unworked, then the flesh is quite different in aspect; it is flabby and inelastic, of a pale, yellowish hue, and makes greasy streaks on the knife that cuts it. Sometimes even all traces of fibres have disappeared, and it is converted into an unhealthy fat. Sometimes you may trace fibres under the microscope, but their outline is bulging and irregular, the cross-markings are wanted, and you see instead, dark refracting globules of oily matter in them. In short, the muscle is degenerating into fat, retaining in a great measure its shape, but losing its substance. Such is, by God's law, the penalty of not using His gifts."

9.—Clothing.

The adoption of artificial clothing by man may be stated to serve three purposes,—the regulation of the temperature of the body; protection from friction, insects, and dirt; and ornament.

In this climate clothing is chiefly employed for warmth, which purpose it secures by moderating or restraining the escape of caloric from the body. Articles of clothing have no power in themselves of generating heat, and are designated as warm or cool just in proportion as they restrain or favour the escape of caloric. Thus a lady's muff and a marble floor are ordinarily of the same temperature; but the sensation produced by each is widely different, because the animal heat is retained by the muff, and rapidly carried off by the marble. Hence for clothing we select those substances which conduct heat least, such as the wool of sheep, and the silk produced by silk-worms, which are superior, as non-conductors, to cotton or linen. In this country we have recourse chiefly to the former in winter, and to the latter in summer, cotton and linen garments being coolest, the linen being cooler than the cotton.

There are several practical errors on the subject of clothing, committed perhaps by a majority of persons, to which we may briefly direct attention. "The first and most obvious of these," says Dr. Baikie, "is wearing too much clothing indoors or in bed, thereby both exhausting the natural powers of the skin, and exposing its action to a sudden check on going out into the cold air. This forms one of the principal objections to the almost universal use of flannel, *worn next the skin*, and kept on even during the night, as is the practice with many people. The skin is thus unnaturally excited, and in course of time loses its natural action; or, on the other hand, becomes so sensitive as to have its action checked on the slightest exposure. I venture to propose my own plan of clothing as suitable to elderly people and those of delicate constitutions in general.

"1. In summer as well as winter, I wear a cotton garment next the skin, thin in summer, stouter in winter; over this a very light silk shirt for summer, and a thicker one in winter. I also wear a narrow strip of flannel, lined with cotton, round the abdomen in summer, replacing it by a thicker one, made so as to double over the front of the belly in winter; my ordinary shirt is always of cotton.

"2. In the beginning of autumn I add a light-coloured flannel shirt *over* my ordinary one, leaving the front open, or wrapping it across according to circumstances. When the winter fairly sets in, I replace this by a stout flannel shirt: but in both cases, I take this off on dressing for dinner, so as to have the full benefit of it while exposed to cold in the *open air;* this I think of great importance, and I never use anything else than a light cotton shirt *to sleep in*, and strongly object to the common practice of sleeping in flannel."

Wearing Flannel next to the Skin. Having regard to the prevalence of this often-injurious habit, a few words on the subject may not be out of place here. It is well known that even in otherwise normal conditions, the skin of some persons is highly irritable and most unpleasantly excited by contact with flannel, and that when this exalted sensibility exists, the use of flannel next to the skin may develop decided physical alteration. It does this mechanically by increasing, or more correctly by retaining, the local heat, and intensifying reaction. Cases of skin disease often come before us in which pruritus is thus aggravated, and the affection prolonged, especially when combined with neglect of proper ablutions. In congested conditions of the skin, or in morbid states of the cutaneous nerves, flannel is inadmissible; or if necessary to guard against vicissitudes of the weather, it may be worn outside a linen garment, as before suggested. The diseases in which this advice is especially applicable are, according to Dr. Tilbury Fox,—erythemata, roseola, urticaria, certainly syphilodermata in their early stages, scabies, and prurigo. "A remembrance of this little practical fact," says the above author, "will sometimes give us the greatest cause to be thankful that we attended to it, trifling though it be."

The *colour* of clothing is not unimportant, light being preferable for the following and other reasons:—(1.) White reflects the rays of heat which the black absorbs; at the same time it impedes the transmission of heat from the body. Light-coloured clothes are therefore best both for winter and summer, retaining the heat in the former, and keeping it off in the latter. (2.) Particles which emanate from diseased bodies, as in miasmatic districts and unhealthy accumulations, are much more readily absorbed by dark than by light clothing. Therefore those who are exposed to contagious influences in the sick room, or in unhealthy neighbourhoods, should wear light clothing. Dark clothes favour the transmission of contagious disease from house to house much more readily than light.*

Another point deserving attention is, that of *frequent changing and cleansing of clothes.* The practice of adopting dark-coloured instead of light-coloured garments has frequently its origin in economy, dark clothes tolerating an amount of dirt inadmissible in light. It should be recollected, however, that dark garments contract dirt after being worn a little time as much as light, and if not changed and cleansed, may favour the production or spread of disease.

* We may mention as an illustration, that dark clothing imbibes odorous particles most readily, as,—the effluvia of the dissecting room; and even the peculiar odour of London smoke is at once detected in black clothing by country people.

In connection with this subject it may be well to advert to the inconvenience of heavy thick clothing, the tissues of which are close and firm. Materials for clothing should be chosen, the textures of which are loose and porous, and contain air in their interstices—air being a bad conductor of heat.

"The advantage of having numerous light instead of fewer heavy coverings to the skin are these—the stratum of air interposed between each layer of covering being a non-conductor, they are relatively much warmer than a much greater thickness in fewer pieces; 2ndly, they can be more easily laid aside to suit changing temperature; 3rdly, being lighter they are less apt to overheat the wearer, and thus lesson the chance of a consequent chill."*

Other points may be briefly referred to. Summer clothes should not be put on too soon, or winter ones too late. Thin-soled boots and shoes are destructive to health. So are *stays*. The body is strong enough to support itself; while stays often bring on diseases of the lungs and other important organs. The muscles of the body were intended to sustain it erect, but when stays are applied, they soon become indispensable, by superseding the action of the muscles; and, in accordance with a well-known law of the muscular system, when they cease to be used they cease to grow, and become insufficient for the discharge of their natural functions. Not only so, stays are directly injurious; and it is a well-ascertained fact, that cases of organic disease have arisen from, or at least were aggravated by, their use.

* In China, one of the most changeable climates in the world, the variation in one day being frequently 35 or 40 degrees, this is the mode adopted by the natives to protect themselves: a working man will often appear in the morning with 15 or 20 light jackets on, one over the other, which he gradually strips off, as the day gets warm, resuming them again towards night.

Finally, it may be stated that the clothing of children, whose feeble frames are less able to resist or endure cold than those of adults, is generally insufficient. When a baby is divested of its long clothes, it is in danger of being insufficiently clad, the danger increasing when it can run alone, and is more exposed to atmospheric influences. It cannot be too strongly impressed upon those who have the charge of children, that the practice of leaving those parts exposed, which when grown up we find it necessary to clothe warmly, especially the lower limbs and abdomen, is a frequent cause of retarded growth, inflammation, mesenteric disease, consumption, etc.

10.—Bathing.

The cold bath, often recommended in this work, when practised in a reasonable manner, is a most valuable aid to health. As a general rule, every person in health should bathe or sponge the whole body once a day with cold water, immediately following it by friction and exercise, to promote the reaction. This tends to health, just as opening the window lets fresh air into a room. Merely washing the hands, face, and neck, is by no means sufficient; the entire surface of the body requires the application of water, not only for the purpose of cleanliness, but as a means of invigorating the capillary circulation, and so fortifying the system as to enable it to resist atmospheric vicissitudes. The secret of attaining these ends consists in employing the cold in such a manner and degree, and in the body being in such a state before and after the application, as that the reaction or glow shall be most perfect. The cold sponge-bath may be adopted with safety by almost any one, the shock not being too great, and good friction rapidly causing agreeable warmth. The best period for a cold bath is on rising from bed, before the body has become chilled. The time the sponging should be continued must be regulated by the condition of the patient: if he be weak, the time should be brief, as from one to two minutes; for if continued too long, instead of tonic effects, depression will follow, and may continue during the whole of the day. If the weather and the water be very cold, the bath should be taken before a good fire. Very young children are benefitted by cold sponging or bathing, even during the winter months. Cold bathing should not, therefore, be practised when the body is cold or cooling, or when it is exhausted by exertion or fatigue, or is naturally too weak, or when the skin feels chilly, until this feeling has been removed by friction or exercise. A bath should not be taken too soon after a meal, for then the circulation should be undisturbed, as the stomach requires all its power to digest the food; nor should the time spent in the bath be too long; that may vary, according to circumstances, from about one to four minutes.

Temperature.—The water of the bath should not be colder than 59°, ranging from this to 64°, according to the season, and according to the temperature of the room. The temperature of the bath-room should be 64° or 65°; if lower than this the water should be a little warmer, and if the room is *cold*, then the water should be 68°, and the bathing process performed as quickly as possible. The temperature of the bath-room is a point of considerable importance, and it can only be accurately measured by a thermometer; one of these useful instruments should therefore be kept in every bath-room.

If the important conditions stated above are disregarded, the immediate depressing effects of the bath will be continued; there will be no glow of reaction, and subsequent chilliness and dulness will ensue. An occasional addition of sea-salt to the water, as recommended in the next paragraph, communicates a stimulating property favourable to reaction. A similar effect is likely to result from the force or shock with which the water is applied: probably a shower-bath is the most efficient, as it most excites those forcible and deep inspirations which are the most efficient cause of the reaction which follows. The reaction is further promoted by vigorous friction over the entire surface with coarse large towels, which operate both by stimulating the cutaneous vessels, and also by muscular exertion, which promotes the more energetic action of the heart. A brisk walk after the bath also tends to promote reaction.

Sea-Salt Baths. Patients who are unable to secure sea-bathing may enjoy, to a limited extent, its advantages, by adding a solution of *sea-salt* to the water of the bath. Sea-salt is the residuum of evaporated sea-water; and if it be added in proper quantity to a bath, so that the mineral ingredient approximates to that contained in sea-water, it will be very much more efficacious than a simple fresh-water bath, in consequence of the stimulating action of the water upon the skin imparted by the saline matter which it holds in solution. The addition of salt obviates the chill which fresh-water sometimes gives. It will often be found that consumptive patients, with feeble circulation and cold hands and feet, are much benefitted by a salt-water bath, who could not bear the shock of fresh-water. In the absence of sea-salt, a handful of bay-salt, or of common salt may be used.

Such a bath, taken regularly in the morning, is conducive to health in two ways:—It inures the body to a degree of cold greater than it is likely to be exposed to during the rest of the day, and so proves most serviceable in protecting it from atmospheric influences; and it tends to remove irregularities in the circulation, and, by exciting the healthy action of the skin, may aid that organ in removing disease.

It is not everyone, however, who can with safety practise bathing in the manner just now pointed out. Cold bathing would be very hazardous, not only to patients who are extremely weak, or who have any organic disease, especially of the heart or lungs, but there may be some idiosyncrasy or condition of the constitution peculiar to the individual which would render such a course the very reverse of beneficial. Patients who have any ground for doubt on the subject should consult their medical attendant. Caution is more particularly necessary in infancy and old age. The adaptation of the cold bath to individual cases may often be determined by the following criterion:—If, after a bath, the patient remains chilly, languid, and dejected, or suffers headache, it had better be discontinued; but if the sense of cold rapidly passes off, and a glow of warmth and animation of spirits succeed and continue for some time, the cold bath is almost sure to be productive of good.

The *warm bath*, to the feeble and exhausted frame, is often very beneficial, and a great luxury. The temperature may be varied according to the sensations of the patient, but as a rule should be that of the temperature of the blood—96° to 98°; if higher than 98°, the bath may be followed by a profuse perspiration, which weakens the system. Warm bathing, however, including the hot-air or Turkish-bath, except as a remedial agent, and prescribed by a medical man, is generally prejudicial.

For various forms of baths, and their admissibility to persons in disease, consult Part IV.

11.—The Influence of Professions and Occupations on Health.

Whatever may be the particular employment of an individual, it can rarely be divested of certain effects, more or less prejudicial to his general health. Occupations which permit of the free use of pure air and moderate muscular exercise, with exemption from want or anxiety, are those most conducive to a healthy, long life. Statistical tables afford evidence of the greater longevity of some pursuits as compared with others. The following table from Tarbell's "Sources of Health," published at Berlin in 1834, is on too limited a scale for general application, but is undoubtedly a close approximation to the truth.

Of 100	Clergymen	42	attained the age of 70 years and upwards.
"	Farmers	40	" "
"	Commercial Men	35	
"	Military Men	33	
"	Lawyers	29	
"	Artists	28	
"	Teachers	27	
"	Physicians	24	

The first half in the above list, with the exception of the clergymen, are necessarily much exposed to the air, and take physical exercise; but the other half, with the exception of the physicians, are chiefly confined in-doors, engaged in sedentary occupations. The difference between the longevity of the clergyman and the physician may no doubt be accounted for by the fact, that the literary pursuits of the former are not of so multifarious and unremitting a character as to prevent sufficient out-door exercise being taken; the nature of his studies may be regarded as favourable to a long life, by inspiring influences conducive to cheerfulness, hope, and serenity. The physician, on the other hand, is exposed to influences most adverse to health; he has frequently to encounter the poison of infectious disease, and is often unable to observe those rules and precautions which it is his duty to enforce in the practice of others; his responsibility often involves extreme mental anxiety; and his almost incessant occupation of both mind and body, no doubt account for his comparatively short life. There are, however, instances of medical men attaining an advanced age. Harvey reached the age of 81; Hoffman, 83; Hahnemann, 88; Heberden, 93; and Hippocrates, 109. The last, according to the best accounts, was much engaged in travelling, and passed a great deal more of his time in the country than in crowded cities.

Why Employments are Unhealthy. The circumstances which operate in rendering occupations unhealthy, are chiefly the following: deficiency of daylight and pure air; a bad posture of the body during employment; and the inhalation of mechanical or poisonous substances.

Abundance of sunlight is of great importance in workshops and offices, particularly where young people are employed. As already pointed out, patients make better and more rapid recoveries in well-lighted hospitals; and very serious cases are generally placed in the sunny side of such buildings. If, therefore, persons are more likely to regain health in such apartments, we may fairly conclude that health will be better preserved in a large, well-lighted workshop or office. Windows should be frequently cleaned, and the walls and ceilings whitewashed at least twice a year.

There is at present a general and just outcry about defective drainage; but the diseases and mortality from this source bear but a small proportion to that from over-crowding. Spacious, airy, and well-lighted offices and work-rooms for clerks, compositors, tailors, dressmakers, and others, would prevent a large amount of chronic disease; and, at the same time, work would be better done, and skilled labour rendered far more productive and valuable.

The influence of *posture* is not unimportant. The sedentary occupations, such as are followed by book-keepers, milliners, tailors, shoemakers, and many others, are often most unfavourable to health, as the sitting posture is generally combined with an inclination forwards, so as to compress the chest and stomach. To a limited extent, the hurtful consequences of such postures may be avoided by occasionally changing to a standing position when at work, and by taking out-door exercise during the hours of relaxation. Plenty of healthful recreation in the open air is the best corrective of the injurious consequences of sedentary employments.

Occupations, however, are only injurious accidentally, a certain amount of work being advantageous for man, both in regard to his mind and his body. Industry is necessary to preserve anything like a healthful contentment of the spirits, or to dispel melancholy from the mind; or remove those dissatisfied and restless cravings which prey upon the unemployed. Industry, moreover, is ordinarily followed by rewards such as are esteemed most desirable, even by the mere worldling; and when wealth accumulates or honour flows in upon a man, through God's blessing on his honest industry, it is immeasurably more precious to him than if ancestors had bequeathed it. We know there are districts of the earth where but little demand is made on the labours of the husbandman, the mountains and the valleys yielding almost spontaneously their rich produce. But the people of districts whose soil possesses the greatest fertility—Italy and Spain—are often sunk to the lowest condition in those mental, social, and moral qualities, which constitute the chief glory of a nation. Released from the necessity of industry, the body becomes enfeebled, the mind weak and vacillating, the sensuous passions preponderate over the intellectual powers; and man, in such circumstances, presents the humiliating spectacle of a mere stagnant humanity, excited into action only by the lowest instincts of his nature.

Having regard to the material frame of man, the point that comes especially within our province, we commend to all industrious employment, which, when followed under the conditions already indicated, is conducive to health and long life. The body was formed for active duties, and the performance of these is indispensable alike for perfect physical development, for health, and happiness. The muscles, the tendons, the ligaments, and even the bones, require exercise, and become feeble and deteriorated in structure from indolence. Hence, the *vertebræ* (backbones) of a carpenter, or of any one who has followed a similar occupation, are larger and also much heavier in proportion to size, than those of a shoemaker or tailor. It is stated of a person who, in consequence of a trifling lameness, took up the occupation of begging,—sitting almost wholly during the rest of his life, and using the limb as little as possible—that the thigh-bone of this limb was found to be considerably less in circumference, and shorter, than the other. From more than one point of view, then, it appears that the real good of life does not consist in being exempt from the necessity of daily toil, and that happiness is more equally distributed than would seem on a cursory glance on the surface of society. Providence, who has made industrious employment the heritage of man, confers at least daily bread, contentment, and physical well-being, as the reward of industry; while He would seem to have ordained that the carriage, the luxurious dwelling, and the rich and varied edibles, shall tend in a measure to deteriorate the health and blight the happiness of those possessing them. The man who has nothing to do is ever restless, and craving for a good not yet enjoyed; his pleasures lose their character as such by becoming the business of his life, and satiety produces disgust. In brief, the industrious man, if his labours are not too exhausting, or carried on in an unhealthy atmosphere, but relieved by daily out-door exercise and relaxation, will pass a happier life, and live longer than the indolent man; and though some occupations or professions may not be directly promotive of health, industry is man's best estate.

CHAPTER II.

Signs and Symptoms of Disease.

To recognise fully the various evidences of an unhealthy action of the system, a long course of study, including both healthy and morbid anatomy, is necessary. If the several points referred to in this chapter be carefully examined, with the different cases which come under our notice, they will aid us in arriving at a tolerably accurate idea of the nature and severity of the disease we have to treat. The following are several of the more common and well-known diagnostic signs.

1.—The Pulse.

The pulse is produced by the blood forced into the *aorta*, and thence into the various arteries of the body, by each contraction of the left ventricle of the heart; its character will consequently be modified by the condition of the heart, the blood-vessels, and the blood itself.

In feeling the pulse, great gentleness should be observed, and it should be done as easily as possible, so as not to excite the action of the heart, which would defeat the object in view. The pulse may be examined in any part where an artery is so close to the surface that its throb can be plainly felt; but in general the most convenient locality is at the wrist. While examining the pulse, there must be no pressure exerted upon the artery in any part of its course by tight sleeves, ligatures, etc. The examiner should place three fingers just above the root of the thumb and the joint of the wrist, with his thumb on the opposite side, so as to be able to regulate the pressure at will. Its frequency may thus be measured by the seconds-hand of a watch; but its peculiar characteristics, as indicative of various phases of disease, can only be appreciated by the educated hand of the medical man. By this method we can detect its rhythm, its fulness, or softness; whether by compression it may be rendered less perceptible; whether it is strong and bounding, forcing the fingers almost from the arm; or hard, or small and wiry, like the vibrations of a string; or intermittent, striking a few beats, and then apparently stopping for one or two beats; or whether the pulsations flow into each other, small and almost imperceptible.

HEALTHY PULSE.—The healthy pulse may be described as uniform, equal, moderately full, and swelling slowly under the fingers; it is smaller and quicker in women and children. In old age, the pulse becomes hard, owing to the increased firmness or structural change in the arterial coats. The average number of beats of the healthy pulse in the minute, at different ages, is as follows:—At birth, 140; during infancy, 120 to 130; in childhood, 100; in youth, 90; in adult age, 75; in old age, 65 to 70; decrepitude, 75 to 80.

The healthy pulse is influenced, however, by the following and other conditions, which should be considered in estimating the character of the pulse as a diagnostic sign. It is faster in the female than in the male, the former exceeding the latter by from six to fourteen beats; but this difference only occurs after about the eighth year. It is quickened by exertion or excitement; it is more frequent in the morning, and after taking food; it beats faster standing than sitting, and sitting than lying; but it is retarded by cold, sleep, fatigue, want of food, and by certain drugs, especially *Digitalis*.

PULSE IN DISEASE.—In estimating the differences of the pulse as signs of disease, allowances must be made for those sudden irregularities which are often observable under transient excitement or temporary depression.

The rapid pulse, especially if strong, full, and hard, indicates inflammation or fever; if small and very rapid, it points to a state of great debility, such as is often present in the last stage of typhoid fever.

The jerking pulse is marked by a quick and rather forcible beat, followed by a sudden, abrupt cessation, as if the direction of the wave of blood had been reversed, and is indicative of structural disease of the valves of the heart.

The intermittent pulse is that in which a pulsation is occasionally omitted, and is frequently owing to some obstruction in the circulation in the heart or lungs, or inflammation or softening of the brain, apoplexy, etc.; also in some forms of valvular disease of the heart; and where *Hernia*, or *Enteritis*, has proceeded to *Gangrene* of the intestine. In minor degrees, indigestion with flatulence may produce it.

The full pulse occurs in general plethora, or in the early stages of acute disease; while the *weak pulse* denotes impoverished blood, and an enfeebled condition of the system.

When the pulse resists compression, it is said to be *hard*, *firm*, or *resistant*; if it is small as well as hard, it is said to be *wiry*.

2.—Temperature and the Clinical Thermometer.

During the last few years considerable help has been derived in the diagnosis and treatment of disease by the use of the clinical thermometer. To count the pulse and the respirations, is not more important than to measure the heat, in all cases of illness. The thermometer aids the physician in arriving at definite and certain conclusions, and relieves him of much mental anxiety. In temperate regions the normal heat of the human body, at sheltered parts of its surface, is 98·4° Fahr., or a few tenths more or less; and a persistent rising above 99·5°, or a depression below 97·3° Fahr., are sure signs of some kind of disease. The maintenance of a normal temperature, within the limits above stated, gives a complete assurance of the absence of anything beyond local and trifling disturbances: but any acute disease elevates abnormally the temperature or animal heat, and many diseases are thus indicated some time before they could be detected by any other means.

The thermometer enables us to diagnose decisively between an inflammatory and a non-inflammatory disease; it also helps us to determine the severity of the inflammation by the number of degrees to which the thermometer is raised. *Hysteria*, it is well known, often simulates inflammatory disease; but the temperature of hysterical persons is *natural*, whereas that of persons suffering from inflammation is *always raised*. But the measurement of the temperature helps us also in the opposite direction. Thus, a case is recorded of a girl supposed to be suffering from hysteria simulating a case of inflammation of the membranes of the brain. The thermometer showed a temperature of 103·5°, proving the actual existence of a grave inflammatory disease, which evidence was afterwards confirmed by the fatality of the disease.

In *acute fevers*, the thermometer affords the best means of deciding in doubtful cases: it is often the best corrective of a too hasty conclusion, and is indispensable for prognosis; thus, in *typhoid fever*, the rise of temperature, or its abnormal fall, will indicate what is about to happen one or two days before any change in the pulse or other sign of mischief may be observed.

In *consumption* the thermometer affords us most valuable diagnostic information. The symptoms and signs are often obscure, or their true cause may be doubtful; especially in the early stage of the disease, when treatment is likely to be of greatest avail. The importance of the aid of the thermometer in this case will be recognized by the fact, that during the deposit of tubercle in the lungs, or in any organ of the body, the temperature of the patient is always raised from 98°, the normal temperature, to 102-3°, or even higher, the temperature increasing in proportion to the rapidity of the tubercular deposit. A persistent elevation of the general temperature of the body has often been found to exist for several weeks before loss of weight or physical signs indicating tubercle in the lungs could be appreciated. Hence an elevated temperature not only affords us certain information as to the existence of *phthisis*, but the degree of that elevation enables us to estimate the extent and progress of the disease; for a persistent rise shows that the disease is progressing, or that unfavourable complications are setting in.

In *ague*, several hours before the paroxysm, the temperature of the patient's body rises considerably.

In *acute rheumatism*, a temperature of 104° is always an alarming symptom, indicating grave complication, such as involvement of the valves of the heart. In short, a temperature of 104° to 105° in any disease, indicates that its progress is not checked, and that complications are liable to arise.

In all cases of convalescence, so long as the defervescence

proceeds regularly as measured by the temperature, no *relapses* need be feared; on the other hand, delayed defervescence in pneumonia, the persistence of a high evening temperature in typhus or typhoid fever, or in the exanthemata, and the incomplete attainment of normal temperature in convalescence, are signs of great significance. They indicate incomplete recovery, supervention of other diseases, unfavourable changes in the products of disease, or the continuance of other sources of disturbance requiring to be carefully examined into. The onset of even a slight elevation of temperature during convalescence is a warning to exercise careful watching over the patient, and especially for the maintenance of a due control over his diet and actions *(Aitken)*.

These remarks might easily be extended, and illustrations multiplied of the value of the thermometer as an aid to diagnosis; but beyond recommending a small, straight instrument, with a correct scale, and self-registering, and taking the observations regularly at the same hours daily throughout the disease, and noting at the same time the pulse and the breathing, we have not space for any further remarks here.

3.—Breathing.

Healthy inspiration is performed with great ease, by a nearly equal elevation of the ribs and enlargement of the chest; expiration is the natural return of the chest to its proportions during rest.

Dyspnœa, or difficult breathing, may result from spasm of the air passages, as in asthma; the presence of tumours, or false membranes, as in diphtheria and croup; or great swelling of the tonsils, or inflammation of the glottis; all of which obstruct the entrance of air to the lungs, and so occasion dyspnœa. Disease of the nerves which preside over the respiratory movements, or in that part of the nervous centres from which they proceed, may also produce serious difficulty of breathing. In pleurisy, fracture of the ribs, apoplexy, and cases of great exhaustion, when an insufficient supply of blood is sent to the great nervous centre—the brain—the respiratory movements are deranged, and otherwise greatly or even fatally obstructed.

The *odour of the breath* is also characteristic, and may be most disagreeable, as the result of want of attention to cleanliness of the mouth and teeth, indigestion, putrid sore throat, etc. During the eruptive fevers, and in typhoid and pestilential fevers, it is both offensive and infectious.

4.—The Tongue.

This organ affords important indications:—*Dryness* points to diminished secretion, and is common in acute and febrile diseases; *moisture* is generally a favourable sign, particularly when it succeeds a dry or furred condition. A *red tongue*, that is, preternaturally red, is common in the course of the eruptive fevers; in gastric and bilious fevers, and in bad cases of indigestion, the redness is often limited to the edges and tip. When the tongue is *livid* or *purple*, there is defective oxygenation of the blood. The *furred tongue*, is the most marked, and is common in inflammation and irritation of the mucous membranes, in diseases of the brain, in all varieties of fever, and in almost all acute and dangerous maladies. It should be added, some persons have usually a coated tongue on rising, without any other symptom of disease. A uniformly white-coated tongue is not very unfavourable; a yellow coat is indicative of disordered action of the liver; a brown or black, of a low state of the vital powers, and contamination of the blood. The gradual cleaning of the t[illegible] first from the tip and edges, shows a tendency to [illegible]d indicates much more than the disappearance of the coating that covered the organ, in short, the cleaning of the whole intestinal tract; in less fortunate cases, as the tongue gets browner, dirtier, and drier, each day, the nervous and muscular systems get weaker, and hope is gradually extinguished; when the fur separates in patches, leaving a red, glossy surface, it is also unfavourable; when the crust is rapidly removed, leaving a raw or dark-coloured appearance, the prognosis must still be unfavourable.

5.—Pain.

This is often a most important indication of the nature and seat of disease, pointing to an interruption of the harmony of the bodily organs; the severity and persistency of the pain being in proportion to the disorganizing violence of this interruption. When attended with a throbbing sensation, consequent upon the heart's action, it is called *pulsating pain;* when with a feeling of tightness, *tensive;* when with heat, *burning.* Inflammatory pain is continuous, grows gradually worse, and is aggravated by touch or pressure. *Nervous* pain may be recognised by its disposition to follow a certain course, without being rigidly limited to one particular part; by its being subject to perfect intermissions; and by the suddenness with which it comes and goes. *Spasmodic* pain is mitigated by pressure, by frictions, and by applications of heat; it comes on suddenly with greater or less severity, terminating abruptly. *Inflammatory* pain is constant, attended by heat, quickened pulse, is increased by movement of the affected part, and usually mitigated by rest. Frequently pain occurs, not in the part diseased, but in a distant one. Inflammation of the liver generally first shows itself by pain in the right shoulder; inflammation of the hip-joint, by pain in the knee; stone in the bladder, by pain at the end of the penis; disease of the heart, by pain down the left arm, etc.

6.—The Skin.

In health the skin imparts to the touch the sensation of an agreeable temperature, with just sufficient moisture to preserve its softness; it is also elastic, smooth, and neither too tense nor loose. A *harsh, dry, burning heat* of the skin is indicative of fever, and must ever be regarded as unfavourable, especially in inflammatory conditions of internal organs. If this condition be followed by *perspiration*, and at the same time by an improvement in the general symptoms of the patient, it is a favourable indication. Great relief is usually experienced on the supervention of the sweating stage in ague, rheumatism, and inflammatory fevers. On the other hand, complications may be feared if perspiration ensue without any amelioration of other symptoms.

Partial or local perspirations indicate a deranged condition of the nervous system, or an affection of the organs contained beneath the perspiring surface. If perspirations occur after trifling exertion, they point to excessive weakness. Night sweats, of frequent occurrence, not only show debility, but when preceded by chills and fever, indicate a hectic and consumptive state of the constitution.

The *colour* of the skin is also diagnostic. A bluish tint of the skin indicates structural disease of the heart. A yellow colour points to biliary affections. A rich blush of the cheeks, especially if it be circumscribed, and the surrounding parts pale, indicates an irritable condition of the nervous system, or a tuberculous cachexia.

7.—The Urine.

The urinary organs are,—the kidneys and bladder, with their appendages. The kidneys secrete the urine from the blood, and by this process the blood is relieved of many impurities, which if retained would give rise to disease in the whole system. The secretion of the kidneys reaches the bladder through little channels *(ureters)*, and when the bladder is filled, the urine is discharged, through the urinary canal *(urethra)*.

Healthy urine is of a brightish yellow or amber colour, a tint darker in the morning than in the afternoon, yielding a slight ammoniacal smell, devoid of unpleasant odour, and precipitating no deposit on standing, or only the merest trace of mucus, or of urates from a low temperature. In advanced age the urine becomes darker and slightly offensive; it is darker in persons who lead a very active life; different varieties of food also produce a marked effect both on the colour and odour of urine. The stream of urine should be round and large, and it should be passed about five or six times in twenty-four hours without any pain or straining.

The average *specific gravity* of healthy urine is 1,020, being in excess of water, which is the standard (1,000).

In disease, the urine presents many varieties, and furnishes valuable indications to the pathologist. Thus, it may be of a dark yellow or saffron colour, as in jaundice, or derangement of the liver; it may be red or high-coloured, and scanty, with quickened pulse, as in fever; it may be bloody or slimy, as in the affections of the kidneys or bladder; it may be pale and copious, when metamorphosis is checked, less urea excreted, and the unrenewed blood furnishes no colouring matter, as in nervous and hysterical ailments; it may be heavy, muddy, or of a purple colour, showing an unfavourable condition of the system; or it may be dark or black, indicating putridity. The urine may be passed too copiously or scantily, with pain, with effort, or it may be retained with difficulty. There may be a frequent or uncontrollable desire to micturate, with burning or scalding pain; or the pain may be only experienced in passing the last few drops.

When urine has to be examined, a little should be taken from the whole quantity that has been passed during twenty-four hours, as it varies greatly in its properties at different periods of the day.

The specific gravity of urine in Bright's disease, is 1,015 to 1,004; diabetic urine, 1,025 to 1,040.

CHAPTER III.

THE MEDICINES, ETC.

THE following brief description of the different forms of medicine used in Homœopathic practice, is given for the sake of the uninitiated. The preparations are of four kinds, viz., *Tinctures*, *Pilules*, *Globules*, and *Triturations*.

TINCTURES.—These contain the more active principles of the vegetable medicines, in a greater or less concentrated form, and are supposed to be quicker and more decided in their action, in acute diseases, than either pilules or globules. It is therefore advisable for those who reside at a distance from medical aid, to be furnished with such a selection of the tinctures as are adapted to sudden and acute diseases, in addition to a complete case of the pilules or globules. The selection recommended by the author may be found, page 73.

PILULES.—These are made of a porous, non-medicinal substance, and afterwards carefully saturated with the tinctures. They are very tangible; do not evaporate like tinctures; and retain their virtues for many years, if unexposed. They are probably the *best* form of medicine for domestic use.

GLOBULES.—In size, globules may be compared to poppy-seeds: they are, therefore, very portable, and, on this account, are often preferred by missionaries, emigrants, etc. They are prepared in the same manner as pilules.

TRITURATIONS.—These are in the form of powder, containing a portion of the original drug triturated with a given quantity of sugar-of-milk, and are necessary to the administration of the lower attenuations of *insoluble* medicines, such as *Calcarea*, *Carbo Vegetabilis*, *Hepar Sulphuris*, *Mercurius*, *Sepia*, *Silicea*, etc. Triturations are not generally used in domestic practice.

MEDICINE CHEST.—A case or chest to suit this manual should contain the medicines mentioned in the following list, should be constructed expressly, and used for no other purpose; it should also be protected from light and heat, and kept apart from substances which emit a strong odour. Immediately after using a vial it should be corked again, and the corks and vials never changed from one medicine to another.

CORKS.—If a cork decays, or becomes damaged, a new one should be at once substituted. Except for acids, good sound corks are preferable to glass stoppers, as they more effectually prevent evaporation, preserve the virtue of the medicine, and are easily replaced when broken. Missionaries, emigrants, etc., should take an extra supply of new ones.

If the above directions are observed, the medicines may be kept unimpared for years.

DIRECTIONS FOR TAKING THE MEDICINES.—*Tinctures* should be dropped into the bottom of a glass, and water, in the proportion of one tablespoonful to a drop, poured upon the medicine. It is desirable to drop the tinctures accurately; and to this end the bottle should be held in an oblique manner, with the lip resting against the cork: the bottle should then be carefully tilted (as shown in the accompanying drawing), when the tincture will drop from the lower edge of the cork. A little practice will enable a person to drop one

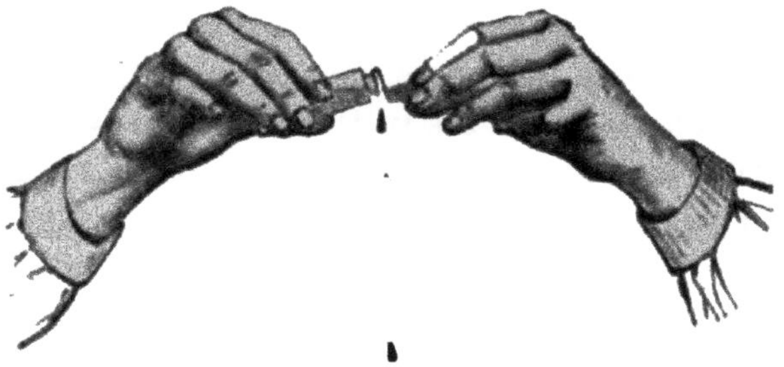

or any number of drops with great exactness. The vessel in which the mixture is made should be scrupulously clean, covered over, and the spoon not left *in* the medicine.* If it has to be kept several days, a *new* bottle and cork may be used.

Pilulos or *Globules* may be taken as they are; but it is better, if convenient, to dissolve them in pure soft water.

The *Triturations* should be placed dry on the tongue.

It is well before taking medicine, to rinse the mouth with water.

HOURS.—The most appropriate times for taking the medicines, as a rule, are,—on rising in the morning, and at bed-time; if oftener prescribed, about an hour before, or about two hours after, a meal. Under no circumstances should a patient be aroused from sleep to take medicine.

THE DOSE.—In determining the quantity and strength of doses, several circumstances must be taken into consideration, such as age, sex, habits, nature of the disease, etc. As a general rule, without reference to individual peculiarities, the following may be stated as the proper dose in domestic practice:—

* Glazed spoons, and graduated fine earthenware medicine-cups, with covers, numbered 1 and 2, specially made for this purpose, and sold by Homœopathic chemists, are the most suitable. These vessels are recommended, as they protect the medicines from light and dust, and distinguish them from other liquids. Mixtures prepared in glasses or other domestic vessels are often thrown away in mistake, sometimes causing great inconvenience.

FOR AN ADULT, one drop of the tincture, two pilules, four globules, or one grain of the trituration.

FOR A CHILD, about one half the quantity.

FOR AN INFANT, one third.

One drop, or a pilule, is easily divided into two doses by mixing it with two spoonsful of water, and giving one spoonful for a dose.

REPETITION OF DOSES.—The repetition of the dose must be determined by the character of the malady from which the patient is suffering, the urgency of the symptoms, and the effects produced by the medicines. In violent and dangerous diseases—such as cholera, croup, diphtheria, convulsions, etc.—the remedies may be repeated every ten, fifteen, or twenty minutes; in less urgent cases, every two, three, or four hours. In chronic maladies, every six, twelve, or twenty-four hours. When improvement takes place, the medicines should be administered less frequently, and gradually relinquished.

ALTERNATION OF MEDICINES.—To avoid the confusion resulting from mixing different remedies in one prescription, and to ascertain the pure effect of each drug, homœopaths do not mix several medicines together in one potion; but in acute diseases, when the symptoms of the malady are not met by a single remedy, and a second one is indicated, the two may be given in *alternation*; that is, one medicine may be followed by another at certain intervals of time, and in a regular order of succession. In croup, for example, *Acon.* and *Spongia*, or *Acon.* and *Iod.*; in pneumonia, *Acon.* and *Bry.*; etc. But the alternate use of medicines should, as much as possible, be avoided. Except in violent and rapid diseases, the author rarely prescribes medicines alternately, and strongly recommends the general discontinuance of that method, as one little calculated to yield exact and definite clinical experience.

LIST
OF THE
PRINCIPAL MEDICINES PRESCRIBED IN THIS MANUAL,

*With their English and Latin Names, their Abbreviations, and the Dilution recommended for general domestic use.**

	Latin.	English.	Abbrev.	Dil.
1.	**Aconitum Napellus**	Monk's Hood	*Acon.*	3
2.	**Antimonium Crudum**	Crude Antimony	*Ant. Crud.*	6
3.	**Antimonium Tartaricum**	Tartar Emetic	*Ant. Tart.*	6
4.	**Apis Mellifica**	Honey-Bee	*Apis M.*	3
5.	**Arnica Montana**	Leopard's Bane	*Arn.*	3
6.	**Arsenicum Album**	White Arsenic	*Ars.*	3
7.	**Aurum Metallicum**	Metallic Gold	*Aur.*	6
8.	**Belladonna**	Deadly Nightshade	*Bell.*	3
9.	**Bryonia Alba**	White Bryony	*Bry.*	3
10.	**Cactus Grandiflorus**	Midnight-blowing Cereus	*Cact.*	3
11.	**Calcarea Carbonica**	Carbonate of Lime	*Calc. C.*	6
12.	**Cantharis**	Spanish-fly	*Canth.*	3
13.	**Carbo Vegetabilis**	Vegetable Charcoal	*Carbo V.*	6
14.	**Chamomilla Vulgaris**	Wild Chamomile	*Cham.*	3
15.	**China**	Peruvian Bark	*Chin.*	1
16.	**Cimicifuga Racemosa**	Black Cohosh	*Cimic.*	3
17.	**Cina Anthelmintica**	Worm-seed	*Cin.*	3
18.	**Cocculus Indicus**	Indian Berries	*Cocc.*	3
19.	**Coffea**	Coffee	*Coff.*	3
20.	**Colocynthis**	Bitter Cucumber	*Coloc.*	3
21.	**Cuprum Aceticum**	Acetate of Copper	*Cup.*	3
22.	**Digitalis**	Foxglove	*Dig.*	3
23.	**Drosera Rotundifolia**	Round-leaved Sundew	*Dros.*	3
24.	**Dulcamara**	Bitter-Sweet	*Dulc.*	3
25.	**Ferrum Metallicum**	Metallic Iron	*Ferr.*	3
26.	**Gelseminum Sempervirens**	Yellow Jessamine	*Gels.*	3
27.	**Hepar Sulphuris**	Sulphuret of Lime	*Hep. S.*	6
28.	**Hyoscyamus Niger**	Black Henbane	*Hyos.*	3
29.	**Ignatia Amara**	St. Ignatius' Bean	*Ign.*	3

* For information respecting the properties and uses of the medicines in this list, their antidotes, etc., consult the Materia Medica at the end of the volume.

	Latin.	English.	Abbrev.	Dil.
30.	**Iodium**	Iodine	*Iod.*	3
31.	**Ipecacuanha**	Ipecacuanha	*Ipec.*	3
32.	**Kali Bichromicum**	Bichromate of Potash	*Kali B.*	3
33.	**Lycopodium Clavatum**	Wolf's Foot	*Lyc.*	6
34.	**Mercurius Corrosivus**	Bichloride of Mercury	*Merc. C.*	3
35.	**Mercurius Solubilis**	Black Oxide of Mercury	*Merc S.*	6
36.	**Nitri Acidum**	Nitric Acid	*Nit. Ac.*	3
37.	**Nux Vomica (Strychnos)**	Vomit Nut	*Nux V.*	3
38.	**Opium**	White Poppy	*Op.*	3
39.	**Phosphorus**	Phosphorus	*Phos.*	3
40.	**Phosphori Acidum**	Phosphoric Acid	*Phos. Ac.*	3
41.	**Platinum**	Platina	*Plat.*	6
42.	**Plumbum Metallicum**	Metallic Lead	*Plumb.*	6
43.	**Pulsatilla**	Pasque-Flower	*Puls.*	3
44.	**Rhus Toxicodendron**	Poison-Oak	*Rhus.*	3
45.	**Sepia Succus**	Inky Juice of Cuttlefish	*Sep.*	6
46.	**Silicea**	Silex	*Sil.*	6
47.	**Spigelia**	Indian Pink	*Spig.*	3
48.	**Spongia Tosta**	Roasted Sponge	*Spong.*	3
49.	**Sulphur**	Sublimed Sulphur	*Sulph.*	3
50.	**Veratrum Album**	White Hellebore	*Verat.*	3

Also the strong Tincture of Camphor, which must be kept by itself, or the saturated pilules; the latter may be kept, well corked, with the tinctures for external use.

In addition to the fifty remedies in the above list, some others are occasionally prescribed, a brief description of the general uses of which may be found in the Materia Medica.

Besides the medicines in pilules or globules, the following twelve tinctures for internal use, in acute cases, may be added, namely:—Nos. 1, 6, 8, 9, 14, 15, 30, 36, 38, 42, 43, and 47.

MATRIX TINCTURES, FOR EXTERNAL USE.

Arnica Montana	ϕ	Hamamelis Virginica	ϕ
Calendula Officinalis	ϕ	Rhus Tox. codendron	ϕ
Cantharis Vesicatoria	ϕ	(Camphor, as above)	

These are recommended to be kept, with Arnica-plaster, strapping-plaster, scissors, oiled-silk, etc., in a compartment separate from the medicines in the body of the chest.

Genuine Medicines. To obtain a beneficial action from the remedies herein prescribed, it is essential to procure them from a person of known character, who has been trained, and who is exclusively engaged as a Homœopathic chemist. Failures in Homœopathic practice, we doubt not, often arise from the inefficiency of the medicines employed. Inasmuch as any person has been hitherto allowed to assume the designation of "Homœopathic chemist," without submitting to any test of qualification, there is the greater need for exercising caution as to the source from whence the medicines prescribed are obtained. Persons who are in doubt on the subject, and in whose locality there is no such chemist as we have just indicated, should consult a Homœopathic medical man, who will inform them of trustworthy persons from whom the medicines may be procured. Homœopathic remedies should not be purchased from an Allopathic druggist's shop, unless a separate room is specially appropriated to them; otherwise the virtues of the medicines are liable to injury by close proximity to strong-smelling drugs: and, further, Homœopathy, with such associations is generally kept in the back-ground. Druggists, with few exceptions, are opposed to Homœopathy, often depreciate it, and when they can do so, recommend their own preparations in preference.

PART II.

Medical and Surgical Diseases, and their Homœopathic and General Treatment.

CHAPTER I.

General Diseases:—A. Blood Diseases.

The General Diseases are divided, in the new nomenclature, into two sections, A and B.

Section A comprehends those disorders which appear to involve a morbid condition of the blood, hence called *Blood diseases*; and which, for the *most part*, run a definite course, are attended with fever and eruptions on the skin, are more or less readily communicable from person to person, and possess the singular and important property of generally protecting persons from a second attack. They are apt to occur epidemically. Of these epidemic visitations Dr. Farr observes, that they distinguish one country from another, one year from another, have formed epochs in chronology, have decimated armies and disabled fleets, have influenced the fate of cities, nay, of empires.

Section B comprises, for the most part, disorders which are apt to invade different parts of the same body simultaneously or in succession. These are sometimes spoken of as *Constitutional diseases*, and they often manifest a tendency to transmission by inheritance.

Eruptive Fevers. The Exanthemata, or eruptive fevers, may be regarded as continued-fevers, having an eruption superadded. They have the following common characters: they arise from a specific contagious poison, between the reception of which and the occurrence of the symptoms a variable time elapses; run a definite course; are accompanied by a specific inflammation of the skin, called the eruption, which passes through a regular series of changes; affect some part of the mucous membrane as well as the skin; and, as a general rule, only attack an individual once.

The true *Exanthemata*, including all these characteristics, are,—the *small-pox*, *measles*, and *scarlet-fever;* but there are other less perfect forms, as *chicken-pox*, *nettle-rash*, and *rose-rash;* etc. These diseases are called by the Registrar-General, *Zymotic diseases*, a term implying their origin in a poison which acts like a *ferment* in the blood; but in the new nomenclature of the Royal College of Physicians, London, they are classed as *blood diseases*, and are regarded by sanitary reformers as preventible. In all of them a latent period intervenes between the reception of the poison and the accession of the fever, during which time the patient is, to all appearance, in good health.

The following table shows the latent period, or period of incubation, and the accession and disappearance of the eruption in the three chief eruptive fevers.

Diseases.	Period of Incubation.	Eruption appears.	Eruption fades.
Small-pox ..	12 days.	On 3rd day of fever.	Scabs form on 9th or 10th day of fever, and fall off about the 14th.
Measles	10 to 14 days.	On 4th day of fever.	On 7th day of fever.
Scarlet Fever	4 to 6 days.	On 2nd day of fever.	On 5th day of fever.

1.—Small-pox *(Variola)*.

This, the most marked of the eruptive fevers, is a disease of a highly contagious nature; but less common in this country, and far less disastrous and fatal in its results, than formerly.

Varieties of Small-pox. We may consider the disease as presenting two varieties: *Variola Discreta* and *Variola Confluens.* In the former, the pustules are comparatively few, remain distinct from each other, and may be easily counted. It is the simplest form of the disease, and, except during the first dentition, is rarely fatal. In confluent small-pox the pustules are numerous, their outline becoming irregular, or they run into each other forming large continuous suppurating surfaces, and it is attended with the greatest danger to life. This division of small-pox is of great importance, as the severity of the disease bears a direct proportion to the amount of the eruption, and danger in the confluent variety arises chiefly from the large quantity of pustulation. If the pustules are confluent *on the face*, whether they are so or not on other parts, we class it with the confluent kind. "The danger is always rendered greater, *cæteris paribus*, when the eruption is very full about the head, face, and neck" *(Mason)*. There is also a variety in which the pustules partially coalesce, termed *Variola Semi-confluens.*

Course.—In its course, small-pox runs through four stages:—The latent or *incubative period*, lasts about twelve days from the reception of the poison; the *primary* or initiatory *fever*, continues about forty-eight hours; the stage of *maturation*, of about nine days; and the *secondary fever* and decline of the eruption, vary in length according to the severity of the disease.

Symptoms.—As in most other fevers, the following

symptoms appear in the first stage:—chilliness, heat, headache, sometimes delirium; a *thickly-furred white tongue;* a deep flush upon the face; a hard and frequent pulse; a feeling of *bruised-pain* all over the body, but especially in the *back and loins;* more or less pain or *tenderness* at the *pit of the stomach,* and sometimes *vomiting.* When the pain in the *loins* and the *vomiting* are excessive and continuous, they may be regarded as the precursors of a severe form of the disease. On the third or fourth day, the *eruption,* often so minute as to escape observation, appears in the form of red spots, or small hard pimples, which feel like shot in the skin. It appears first on the face, neck, and wrists, then on the body, and finally on the lower extremities. If examined, the eruption may be seen upon the palate, and is often formed on the lining membrane of the larynx, trachea, and bronchi, giving rise to sore-throat, salivation, cough, painful expectoration, and hoarseness. The pimples gradually increase in size until about the eighth day from the commencement of the fever; the contents, at first watery and transparent, change to yellowish matter as the pimples become ripened into pustules. The pustules are *depressed in the centre,* and surrounded for a short distance by a rose-red areola. During the time the pustules are filling up, there is swelling of the eyelids and face, sometimes to such a degree as to obliterate the features. A peculiar, disagreeable odour now begins to emanate from the patient, which is so characteristic, that the disease at this stage might be known by this alone. On the first appearance of the eruption, the fever subsides; but when it is at its height, a fresh attack sets in, which, to distinguish it from the precursory fever, is called the *secondary* fever.

In about eight days from the first appearance of the eruption, the pustules break, and discharge their contents; scales then form, which dry up, and, in a healthy state of constitu-

, fall off in the course of four or five days. When this
e place, purplish red stains are left behind, which very
rly fade away; or indelible, depressed scars remain, which
called *pits*. In the latter case, the person so marked is
to be "pitted with the small-pox."

n *Variola confluens*, the secondary fever is often very
nse, and is the most dangerous period of the disease.
ere and even fatal results may arise from exhaustive
puration, erysipelatous inflammation, suffocative breathing,
, the most dreaded of all symptoms, a putrescent state of
blood.

IAGNOSIS.—An early recognition of this disease, both on
unt of the patient himself, and for the protection of
rs, is of great importance. It has been mistaken for
sles; but the eruption is more perceptible to the touch,
gives the sensation of shot under the skin. *Severe pain*,
ently not muscular, *in the small of the back*, is the most
acteristic symptom. The abruptness and severity of an
ck distinguishes it at once from the insidious invasion of
hoid fever. It differs from *chicken-pox* in the character of
eruption, that of the latter being vesicular, does not
eed to suppuration, and the fever is mild.

ANGERS.—The greatest danger arises from the *secondary*
in the confluent form of the disease, at about the ninth to
twelfth day, when the pustules are ripening; for then the
r is likely to return, the vital strength having already
much exhausted. Fatal chest symptoms may arise; or
e may be ulceration of the cornea, opacity, and loss of
t. An inflamed condition of the skin between the
ules, instead of the rose-red areola, is a bad sign.
ncy and advanced age are unfavourable periods; beyond
y years of age, Mr. Marson states, hardly any who take
scape death. Violent and uncontrollable delirium is
an attendant on the confluent variety, and if it occurs

early, in persons who have lived freely or irregularly, is an unfavourable symptom. "Draymen, barmen, potmen, tailors, and the women on the town, are very unfavourable subjects to be attacked with small-pox, owing to their habits of indulging freely, and almost daily, in strong drinks" *(Marson)*. A too plethoric habit, sleeplessness, irritability, the patient vexing himself about trifles, are unfavourable conditions. On the other hand, a quiet, contented, hopeful state of mind is favourable to recovery. Small, dark, and badly-ventilated dwellings, poor or scanty food, insufficient clothing, want of cleanliness, intoxicating beverages, and other similar influences, are also elements which determine the more severe form of this malady. It is worthy of remark, as Dr. Letheby states in one of his quarterly reports on the sanitary condition of London, as to an outbreak of small-pox and the increase of scarlatina, that "these sudden outbursts of zymotic disease show that the force of these maladies is not exhausted by sanitary measures, but only kept in check; and that, when occasion serves by neglect of proper precautions, the force manifests itself in all its original vigour."

CAUSE.—Contagion. It is supposed never to occur except from contagion; for large portions of the world have remained for centuries entirely free from it, until it was imported; and then it spread so rapidly, and often so fatally, as almost to depopulate whole countries. "There are some grounds for believing, however, that small-pox, in common with some other diseases, originated in the lower animals, and extended from them to the human species by infection or contagion" *(Aitken)*. "There is no contagion so strong and sure as that of small-pox; none that operates at so great a distance" *(Watson)*. The period during which the poison is most powerful, is probably when it is most perceived by the sense of smell.

Epitome of Treatment.—

1. *Primary fever.*—Acon., Bell.
2. *Eruptive stage.*—Ant. Tart.
3. *Suppurative stage.*—Ant. Tart., Merc.
4. *Retrocession of the eruption.*—Camph.
5. *Confluent and malignant cases.*—Sulph., Ars., Phos.
6. *Complications.*—Phos. (*Pneumonia*). Acon. (*Congestion of the Lungs*). Bry. or *Kali* Bich. (*Bronchitis*). Merc. (*Glandular Swellings*), Apis or Bell. (*Dropsical Swellings*). Bell. or Hyos. (*Delirium*).
7. *To prevent pitting.*—Smearing the parts with bacon fat, and protection from air and light.
8. *Desquamation.*—Sulph., with cleanliness and tepid sponging.
9. *Sequelæ.*—Sulph., Merc. Cor. (*Inflammation of the eyes*). Hep. S. (*Boils.*). See also the conditions and medicines under "*Complications*" above.

Aconitum.—This remedy is indicated, during the precursory fever, by shivering, heat, dryness of the skin, rapid pulse, swimming and pain in the head, nausea and vomiting, and pain in the back and loins; it may also be used during the course of the disease, whenever febrile symptoms are prominent. *Bell.* may alternate or follow *Acon.* if necessary.

Antimonium Tart.—This remedy is specific to small-pox, in consequence of its power of producing, in large doses, in healthy persons, an eruption so closely resembling it as to have been mistaken for it.* *Ant. Tart.* should, therefore, be administered as soon as the nature of the disease is ascertained; it is specially valuable during the eruptive stage; it is also useful in the primary fever, if nausea and vomiting, or convulsions should occur. During nearly the whole course of the disease, it may be given, either alone, or in alternation with any other remedy that is specially indicated. In favour-

* A striking illustration of the disease-producing effects of *Ant. Tart.* is recorded by Dr. Baikie in *The Homœopathic World*, vol. i., pp. 73-4.

able cases, if *Acon.* be given for the primary fever, and *Sulph.* during desquamation, to prevent after effects, *Ant. Tart.* is the only remedy required.

Belladonna.—If the *head symptoms* are severe,—delirium, intolerance of light, etc., a few doses of this remedy will generally afford relief.

Mercurius.—Ulcerated throat, salivation, or diarrhœa with bloody stools, especially during the process of suppuration.

Sulphur.—When the disease pursues an irregular course; when the eruption exhibits a tendency to disappear from the surface; when the pustules, instead of being transparent or yellow, are green, purple, or black; when the blood with which they are filled announces a decomposition of this fluid, it is not to *Arsenicum* that we should have recourse, but to *Sulphur* (*Teste*).

Coffea.—Great restlessness and inability to sleep. A few doses only will be required.

Camphor.—If the eruption *suddenly* disappears, or *suddenly* assumes a malignant type, with difficulty of breathing, coldness of the skin, and symptoms of paralysis of the brain; two or three drops in a little water, every ten or fifteen minutes, for several times, till the skin becomes warm, and the eruption reappears.

Opium.—Drowsiness or stupor and stertorous breathing.

Carbo Veg., *Nit. Acid.*, *or Arsenicum* may be administered under similar circumstances, or when *Sulph.* only partially succeeds.

Sulphur.—During the formation of the pustules, and when there is furious itching of the parts; it is the best when the disease is on the decline, and as a preventive to the usual sequelæ of the disease. It should be continued till complete recovery has taken place.

Vaccinine, *Sarracenia Purpurea*, *Verat. Vir.*, and some other remedies are said to have curative or prophylactic virtues in this disease, but with which we have not had sufficient experience further to recommend them.

ACCESSORY MEANS.—The patient should be kept cool; the sheets and linen be frequently changed, and ample provision made both for the *uninterrupted admission of fresh air*, and the *free escape of tainted air*. A small, ill-ventilated room, overheating, and hot cordials, interfere much with the tendency to recovery. In cold or cool weather a fire should be kept burning in the apartment, to maintain warmth and dryness, and to assist ventilation. During the entire course of the disease, especially when the skin becomes hot, painful, or irritable, the whole surface may be sponged with warm water, to which a few drops of *Carbolic Acid* have been added, and well dried with a soft towel. This generally affords great relief. The use of *Carbolic Acid* in the above manner, and a slight infusion of its vapour in the air of the apartment, tends both to mitigate small-pox, and to deprive it of its *contagious* character. In the early stage of the disease, great advantage may also be derived from the *wet-pack* (see Part IV), followed by a *sponge-bath*. If ulceration on the back or nates (*buttocks*) is threatened, the patient should be placed on a *water-bed*. When the pustules have burst, powdered starch, or any other dry powder, should be freely applied, to absorb the matter. Cleanliness and frequent tepid washings are especially necessary during the last stage of the disease. An occasional warm bath towards the end of the treatment is also very advantageous. To *prevent pitting*, when the eruption is out, the patient's room should be kept *dark*; as soon as the pustules have discharged, and begun to dry, they should be frequently smeared over with olive-oil, cold-cream, or a mixture of one-third of glycerine to two-thirds of water, to prevent permanent scars. Dr. Baikie states, in a letter to the author, when the eruption is thoroughly out, the heat and irritation may be materially alleviated by smearing the whole surface of the body with fresh-cured bacon fat. A piece is to be boiled with the skin on, and then cut horizontally, so as to leave about a quarter of an inch of fat adhering to the skin; this is to be scored across, and used to anoint the eruption, and may be repeated twice or thrice daily. It completely prevents pitting. If the patient be a child, his hands should be muffled to prevent scratching, which might lead to ulceration.

DIET.—Tea and dry toast, gruel, etc.; grapes, roasted apples, and wholesome ripe fruits in season. For drink, cold water is generally preferred; in addition, raspberry-vinegar-water, currant-jelly-water, and barley-water. For further hints as to diet and beverages, see Part IV.

2.—Cow-pox (*Vaccinia*) and Vaccination.*

Vaccinia (from *vacca*, a cow), is a specific disease of the cow, which, by inoculation, was accidentally discovered by Jenner, a hundred years ago, to be protective against small-pox in man. With cow-pox, therefore, we have nothing to do further, except in so far as it serves that purpose.

VACCINATION may be defined as the process by which the disease *vaccinia* is artificially introduced into the human system for the purpose of protecting it against small-pox.

The process of vaccination recognises the Homœopathic principle, as it is preventive of small-pox strictly in consequence of the Homœopathic relationship it bears to that disease. Its tendency is not only to prevent a fatal termination, and render the disease mild in its course, should it occur, but to keep off the disease altogether. The resident surgeon of

* It is stated that in Sweden, forty years *before* vaccination, out of every million persons, 2,050 died annually, *after* vaccination, 158 only. In Berlin, before vaccination, 3,422; after, 176.

the Small-pox and Vaccination Hospital at Highgate states, that in the course of his large experience, he found that when small-pox attacked persons who had not been vaccinated it killed 36 per cent. of them—that is, *one in every three died;* but that when vaccination had been performed, the death-rate of those attacked by the disease fell to *one in fifteen.* He also found that the protective power of vaccination was in proportion to the way in which it had been done; thus *one* permanent *cicacatrix* (scar) after the operation gives a mortality from the disease of nearly eight in the hundred; *two* scars of rather more than 4 per cent.; *three* scars less than 2 per cent.; and if four scars, not one in a hundred die when attacked by the disease.* This is a most important practical point to remember: if only one indifferent cicatrix remains after the operation, such persons, taking small-pox in after life, die at the rate of 12 in the 100; but if four or more cicatrices remain, only one in 200 will die of small-pox. Further, Mr. Marson states, of 370 persons treated in the Small-pox and Vaccination Hospital, London, who believed themselves vaccinated, but who had no cicatrix to show, and trusted to such vaccination for their protection, they died of small-pox at the rate of 23½ per cent. Persons, therefore, having no cicatrix remaining, are in a very unsafe condition.

In performing vaccination, the following are the chief points to be observed:—

1. The vaccine *lymph* used should be taken from a child free from scrofula, syphilis, or any constitutional *taint;* skin diseases, swollen glands, inflamed or sore eyes, are decided objections, and, if disregarded, might result in the transmission of disease to previously healthy children.

2. The vaccinator should employ *a clean lancet;* pyæmia, syphilis, and other kinds of blood-contamination, no doubt often follow from the use of a foul lancet.

* See the *Lancet*, August 15th, 1863.

3. The lymph should be taken on the eighth day, *unmixed with blood* or any other secretion. Attention to the above hints will afford ample security against any of the so-called *evils of vaccination.*

4. The matter should be inserted in four places in each arm, it having been found that the protective power of vaccination is in proportion to the number of the resulting *cicatrices* (scars), that being the most efficient which leaves the most and the best cicatrices.

5. When arm-to-arm vaccination cannot be practised, the lymph should be preserved in hermetically-sealed capillary tubes.

6. Vaccination should be performed not later than the third month; indeed its performance is now rendered compulsory during the first three months, which is perhaps the best period, as dentition has not then commenced.

7. *Treatment* is scarcely ever necessary, as the condition thus set up, described as *small-pox in miniature*, is very simple. Should, however, there be much inflammatory redness and swelling, a few doses of *Aconitum* or *Belladonna* will relieve the patient. Occasionally a poultice is necessary, or dusting the part with flour or finely-powdered starch. As the pock is declining, a few doses of *Sulphur* are usually recommended.

8. *Re-vaccination* should take place at the age of puberty; the great changes which occur in the system at this period of life rendering its repetition generally necessary. Persons at this period, especially if they are about to change their place of abode, should be examined, and if they have only one cicatrix, or if that is imperfect, or if there is no cicatrix at all, they should be re-vaccinated. Four good cicatrices are considered necessary to afford the necessary protection. "For just upon thirty years we have re-vaccinated all the nurses and servants who had not had small-pox, on their coming to live at the Small-pox Hospital, and not one of

them has contracted small-pox during their stay there" (*Marson*).

From the above observations it will be inferred that we think highly of the protection afforded by efficient vaccination. Evils indeed may have arisen from its careless performance; but they only tend to prove that this operation, like every other on the human body, should be performed with care and skill. But if small-pox do occur in vaccinated persons, it does so with a trifling mortality. The occurrence of the disease after one vaccination is not an argument for *non*-vaccination, but for *re*-vaccination. We fully endorse the following remarks:—

"It is thus clearly demonstrated how vaccination has thrown the *ægis* of protection over the world; and how ample, how great, and how efficient that protection may be. It has been shown to diminish mortality generally, and the mortality from small-pox in particular both in civil and military life, at home and abroad, and just in proportion as it is *efficiently* performed. It has been shown to diminish the epidemic influence; it has been shown to preserve the good looks of the people; it has been shown that it tends to render small-pox a mild disease compared with the same disease in the unprotected; it confers an almost absolute security against death from small-pox; and, lastly, it has been shown to exercise a protecting influence over the health of the community generally" (*Aitken*).

3.—Chicken-Pox (*Varicella*).

This is a pustular eruption, similar in its appearance to small-pox, for which it is at first often mistaken. It generally requires little medical assistance, but merely attention to diet, as in simple fever. It differs from small-pox in the slighter degree of fever which attends it, in the pustules becoming filled with a watery fluid about the second or third day, which is never converted into yellow matter, as in small-pox, and in its rapid course. Generally, on the third or fourth day, the pustules dry up, forming crusts or scabs, leaving no permanent scars.

TREATMENT.—If the fever is considerable, give *Aconitum* every four or six hours. When there is much headache, or other cerebral symptoms, flushing of the face, or sore throat, administer two or three doses of *Belladonna*. *Rhus Tox.* will generally be found one of the best remedies in this disease, and under its action it will soon disappear. *Apis*, if there be excessive itching with the eruption.

ACCESSORY MEANS.—Too early exposure to cold, and errors of diet, must be guarded against; the latter caution is more especially necessary if the digestive organs are at all impaired. A milk diet is generally best.

4.—Measles (*Morbilli*).

Formerly this disease was confounded with scarlatina; but there are well-marked differences, some of which are pointed out in this section. Measles, presenting symptoms varying according to constitutional or atmospheric peculiarities, is generally unattended with danger, unless improperly treated. Children are usually the subjects of its attack; but when adults succumb under its influence, it is often a severe disease. Like scarlatina and small-pox, it is highly contagious, often epidemic, and generally attacks the same person only once.

MODES OF PROPAGATION.—No susceptible person can remain in the same room or house with an infected person without risk of taking the disease; and it is almost impossible to isolate the disease in large establishments or schools. It is propagated by *fomites*. This is proved by the fact that children's clothes, sent home in boxes from schools where the disease has raged, communicate the disease; and also by the same circumstance resulting when susceptible children have lain in the same beds, or in the same room, shortly after it has been occupied by patients suffering from the disease *(Aitken)*. The contagion from *measles*, *scarlatina*, etc., only ceases when *desquamation* of the *cuticle* is complete.

SYMPTOMS.—Measles passes through its course by stages; there is its period of *incubation*, lasting from ten to fourteen days; its *precursory fever;* its *eruptive* stage; and its *decline*. The introductory fever is ushered in with lassitude and shivering, which are soon succeeded by heat of the skin, quickened pulse, loss of appetite, thirst, etc. But the peculiarity of the early symptoms is, their resemblance to those of a *common cold*, such as sneezing; red, swollen, and watery eyes; discharge from the nose; a hoarse, harsh cough; fever; and sometimes, diarrhœa and vomiting. The symptoms usually increase in intensity until, about the fourth day, the *eruption* appears, first on the face, then on the neck and breast, and soon after on the whole body. It is in the form of minute pimples, which multiply and coalesce into blotches of a more or less crescentic form, slightly raised above the surrounding skin, so as to be felt, particularly on the face, which is often a good deal swollen. An abundant eruption is more favourable than a scanty crop. The eruption is two or three days in coming out, and remains at least three days; the fever then abates, and the eruption declines, becoming browner as it fades, and the cuticle is afterwards thrown off in a fine bran-like scurf. As the rash declines, diarrhœa sometimes occurs: this, unless very troublesome, should not be interfered with, as it is often beneficial. The *temperature* rises rapidly towards the appearance of the eruption, and when that is reached is at its maximum degree. Except in severe cases a high temperature only lasts after the breaking out of the eruption beyond twelve to twenty-four hours. The temperature corresponds to that of most other fevers, and should be measured by a thermometer, by which severe and complicated cases may be distinguished.

TABLE SHEWING THE CHIEF DIFFERENCES BETWEEN
MEASLES AND SCARLET-FEVER.

MEASLES.	SCARLET-FEVER.
1.—*Catarrhal* symptoms are prominent—watery discharge from the eyes and nose, sneezing, harsh cough, etc.	1.—Catarrhal symptoms are usually absent, but there is great *heat of skin*, *sore throat*, and sometimes delirium.
2.—The rash is of a *pinkish-red* or *raspberry-colour*.	2.—The eruption is of a *bright scarlet-colour*.
3.—The eruption is somewhat *rough* so as to be felt by passing the hand over the skin, and is in groups or in rounded or *irregular-shaped masses*.	3.—The rash usually presents no *inequalities* to sight or touch, and is so minute and closely crowded as to give the skin a *uniform* red appearance.
4.—Liquid, tender, *watery* eye.	4.—A peculiar *brilliant stare*, as if the eyes were glistened by an ethereal lustre (*Duggan*).
5.—The cuticle is thrown off in minute portions, like *scales of fine bran*.	5.—Desquamation of the cuticle is in *large patches*, especially from the hands and feet.
6.—The most common *sequelæ* are diseases of the *lungs*, *eyes*, *ears*, and *skin*.	6.—The most frequent *sequelæ* are *anasarca*, especially after mild cases, and *glandular swellings*.

EPITOME OF TREATMENT:—

1. *Primary fever.*—Acon. and warm-bath.

2. *The rash and catarrhal derangement.*—Puls., Gelsem., Euph. *(copious watery discharge from the eyes and nose)*.

3. *Slow development of the eruption.*—Bell. *(drowsiness, startings, etc.)*, Puls. *(troublesome gastric symptoms)*, and the warm-bath (see Part IV).

4. *Retrocession of the eruption.*—Gelsem., Amon. Carb., Bry.

5. *Troublesome cough.*—Kali Bich., Spong., Bell., Ipec.

6. *Severe and complicated cases.*—Arsen., Mur. Ac., Phos., Bell., Rhus Tox.

7. *Secondary Diseases (sequelæ).* See page 92–3.

8. *Prevention of sequelæ.*—Sulph.

SPECIAL INDICATIONS.—*Aconitum.*—Well-marked febrile symptoms at the outset, or during the progress of the disease. Even after other remedies have heen administered, *Acon.* may have to be repeated, to control inflammatory action, which does not always subside on the appearance of the eruption. A dose every two, three, or four hours.

Pulsatilla.—Almost a specific in this disease, and may be given when the fever has been subdued by *Aconitum*, or in alternation with it, if both catarrhal and fever symptoms are present. *Puls.* is especially valuable for the following symptoms:—Cough, worse towards evening, or during the night, with rattling of mucus in the air passages, or expectoration of thick, yellowish or whitish mucus; thick, greenish or yellowish defluction from the nose; bleeding from the nose; catarrhal derangement of the stomach, and diarrhœa. A dose every three or four hours.

Ipecacuanha.—Retching, much vomiting.

Gelseminum—This remedy is useful in cases in which the eruption is slow in making its appearance, or in which it is imperfect, or too suddenly recedes. It may be given in frequently-repeated doses till improvement sets in.

Ammon. Carb.—This medicine is also strongly recommended for imperfect or retrocedent eruption.

Belladonna.—Sore throat, with painful and difficult swallowing; dry *spasmodic* cough; inflammation of the eyes; restlessness, and tendency to *delirium*. A few doses, at intervals of two or three hours.

Bryonia.—Imperfectly developed or suppressed eruption, with severe *chest symptoms*. A dose every two or three hours.

In addition to this remedy, a sudden recession of the eruption might necessitate a *warm-bath* (see Part IV).

Mercurius.—Glandular swellings in the neck, ulcers in the mouth and throat, bilious diarrhœa, dysenteric stools, etc.

Phosphorus.—Pale, imperfect, or irregular eruption; dry, hollow cough; pain in the chest; nervous or typhoid symptoms. In the latter condition, *Camph.*, *Ars.*, *Rhus*, *Mur. Ac.*, *Phos. Ac.*, or any other remedy indicated, should be given. If possible, however, such cases should always be under the care of a Homœopathic doctor.

Sulphur.—This remedy is required during the decline of the disease, as well as after the eruption has completed its natural course and the other medicines are discontinued, to prevent the usual after-effects, especially chest symptoms, and inflammation of the eyes and ears. A dose twice or thrice daily, for three or four days; afterwards once or twice for a a like period.

Diseases following Measles *(Sequelæ)*.—Measles is sometimes succeeded by diseases which are more difficult to treat, and more dangerous than the complaint itself; but, except in scrofulous or tuberculous children, they are generally the result of irrational treatment; under Homœopathic management patients usually recover rapidly and perfectly. If after the decline of the eruption, the patient retains a temperature above 100°, some complicating disturbance may be suspected. The following are some of the diseases liable to occur after measles, with the leading remedies to be used:—

Inflammatory affections of the eyelids.—Acon., Bell., Merc. Cor., Sulph.

Purulent discharge from the ear, or deafness.—Puls., Sulph., Merc.

Swelling of the glands.—Merc. Iod., Calc. Carb.

cough, hoarseness, or other affections of the chest.—
). Sulph., Spong.

s eruptions.—Sulph., Iod.

seases are described in other parts of this manual, be found by the index. Nearly all of them ofessional treatment. A more emphatic reference wing sequela may not be out of place.

s AND CONSUMPTION.—Tubercular disease of the more often, of the bowels, is by no means an sequelæ in delicate or strumous children. Cases ure are often under our care, and from long obser- ıave reason to believe that such a connexion is far nmon. Whenever, therefore, a child makes but a ıperfect recovery after an attack of measles, more r if there is tenderness, pain, or enlargement of en, diarrhœa or irregular action of the bowels, a titutional disease may be suspected, and no time lost in obtaining professional Homœopathic

RY MEASURES.—*Cold* water, gum-water, etc; no should be given. As the fever abates, milk-diet, eturning to a more nourishing kind of food. In the other eruptive fevers, the *Wet-pack*, described r, is of essential service. The patient should be ,, and the room sufficiently darkened to protect the the proper and constant circulation of pure air o means be interrupted. The temperature of the oom should be about 60° Fahr., and should be gainst rapid changes. Except during the very summer, a fire should be kept burning in the oid sponging, followed by careful drying, is neces- l *times* a day, also a frequent change of linen. isease has subsided, the patient should be warmly ken into the open air *frequently*, when the weather is fine. He must not, however, go out of doors too soon, or be in any way exposed to cold. Prevention of exposure to cold and wet is of great importance during convalescence, in consequence of the excessive susceptibility to inflammatory affections of the chest.

PREVENTIVE TREATMENT.—This is of little consequence, as the danger of measles under Homœopathic treatment is trifling. It may, however, be prevented or modified by giving children who have not had the disease a dose of *Pulsatilla* every morning, and one of *Aconitum* every evening, for a week or ten days, during its prevalence in the neighbourhood. *Puls.* has undoubtedly great influence, being to measles just what *Bell.* is to scarlatina.

5.—Scarlet-Fever—Scarlatina* (*Febris rubra*).

Like measles, scarlet-fever is an infectious and contagious, but much more to be dreaded disease, chiefly affecting children, and rarely occurring more than once in the same person. The second, third, fourth, and fifth years of life are those in which it most prevalent; after the tenth year its frequency rapidly declines. The opinion that the disease does not attack children under two years of age is very erroneous, as the following statistics prove. In 1862, the deaths from this disease in England were 14,834; out of this number 9,569 were children under five years of age, and of these 903 were infants, under twelve months old. Infancy therefore offers no exemption from severe attacks of scarlatina.

The increasing prevalence of scarlatina during the present century leads us to assign to it that pre-eminent rank among

* It is supposed by some persons that the two terms by which this disease is commonly known, signify different forms of the malady—*Scarlet-fever* being associated with the disease when it is severe, and *Scarlatina* with a mild attack. The terms are, however, strictly synonymous.

the causes of the mortality of childhood which was formerly occupied by small-pox, for it is second only to *Typhus*. In the year 1863, the mortality from scarlatina in London alone was 4,982, a year remarkable for the wide-spread character and fatality of this epidemic, for scarcely a town or district of England escaped. An excessively high rate of mortality also prevailed in London, Manchester, Leeds, and many other large towns, last year (1868), ranging from 100 to 120 deaths per week for many weeks.*

VARIETIES.—There are three forms of this disease, viz.:—1. *Scarlatina simplex*,—a scarlet rash, with redness of the throat, but without ulceration. It may be expected to terminate quite favourably under proper treatment. 2. *Scarlatina anginosa*,—a more severe form of the disease, with redness and ulceration of the throat, and a tendency to the formation of abscess in the neck. This has many points of danger, and in several ways may jeopardise the patient's life. 3. *Scarlatina maligna*,—extreme depression of the vital strength, and great cerebral disturbance, are superadded to the affection of the throat and skin, the fever soon assuming a malignant or typhoid character. The tongue is brown; there is low delirium; the throat is dark, livid, or even sloughy; the eruption comes out imperfectly or irregularly, or alternately appears and disappears, and is dark rather than scarlet. This form of the disease may terminate fatally on the third or fourth day, and is always one of such extreme danger that none survive it but patients of vigorous constitution, and when skilful treatment is commenced early.

Occasionally, however, scarlet-fever occurs without any rash or sore-throat being observed.

GENERAL SYMPTOMS.—Scarlatina commences with the ordinary precursors of fever—chills and shiverings, succeeded by

* See "Scarlatina: its Prevalence and Prevention," in *The Homœopathic World*, Vol. III., pp. 244–5.

hot skin, nausea, and sometimes vomiting, frequent pulse, thirst, and sore throat. In about forty-eight hours after the occurrence of these symptoms, a rash is perceptible, first on the neck and breast, which gradually extends over the great joints, limbs, and trunk, till the whole body is covered with it. The eruption is of a *bright-scarlet colour*, and consists of innumerable red points or spots, which have been compared to a boiled lobster-shell in appearance. These spots either run together, and diffuse themselves uniformly over the skin, or else appear in large irregular patches in different parts of the body. The appearance of the tongue, as afterwards described, is very characteristic of the disease. A diffused redness, sometimes of a dark claret-colour, covers the mouth, fauces, etc., which disappears as the febrile symptoms and rash subside. On about the fifth day, the *efflorescence* generally begins to decline and gradually goes off by desquamation of the cuticle, in the form of scurf, from the face and trunk; but from the hands and feet large flakes are separated, so that sometimes the scarf-skin comes away entire, like a glove or slipper. On about the eighth or ninth day the eruption has entirely disappeared, leaving the patient in a weak condition.

It is not always, however, that the disease pursues this uniform course. Sometimes the eruption is livid and partial, and is attended with prostration so extreme that the patient sinks in a few hours under its virulence. In puerperal and pregnant women, it is a most malignant disease, and nearly always leads to abortion and death.

Distinctive Features of Scarlet-Fever.—(1.) The *scarlet rash*, already described.—(2.) *The high temperature of the body.* The thermometer placed in the axilla *(arm-pit)* rises to 105° Fahr., sometimes to 106°; 98° being the normal standard.—(3.) The papillæ of the tongue are *red and prominent*, and may be first seen projecting through a white fur, or, as this fur clears away, on a red ground, and has been termed "the strawberry-tongue."—(4.) A peculiar brilliant glistening stare of the eye, easily distinguished from the liquid, tender eye of measles. (5) *The sore throat.* The throat is congested and swollen round the soft palate and tonsils, and the mucous membrane of the mouth and nostrils are generally affected.

Scarlet-Fever and Measles.—For the chief differences between these diseases, see the table in the section on *Measles.*

Cause and Modes of Propagation.—The poison of scarlet-fever is of a subtle nature, the earliest source of which is distinctly traceable to Arabia; and the disease has now spread over the whole world *(Aitken)*. Owing to the insanitary conditions of their dwellings, it spreads extensively, and with great fatality, among the poor. It may be transmitted by *fomites* —in the clothes, bedding, carpets, etc.; this is proved hy the fact that medical men have often carried the disease to their own families. The poison may be destroyed by a temperature of 205° Fahr., or by disinfection and ventilation. The infecting power probably commences with the primary fever, attains its maximum degree at the commencement of desquamation, and continues till the old cuticle is completely removed.

Prophylaxis—When scarlet-fever prevails in a family or neighbourhood, the administration of a dose of *Belladonna*, night and morning, to children who have not had the disease, will often entirely ward off an attack; should the disease occur, notwithstanding this treatment, it will, undoubtedly, greatly modify its severity.

Treatment.—It should be laid down as a maxim that in scarlet-fever medical advice ought always to be had recourse to; for the worst cases we meet with (as those in which mortification of the nose, cheek, or limbs, sometimes takes place) are those in which the disease has, from its apparently mild character, been left to itself *(Aitken)*.

EPITOME OF TREATMENT.—

1. *Scarlatina simplex.*—Acon. and Bell. alternately during the course of the affection, and Sulph. during its decline.

2. *Scarlatina anginosa.*—Acon. and Bell.; Gelsem., Apis *(great swelling of the throat)*; Mercurius *(ulceration)*; Nit. Ac. (internally, or as a gargle, or both).

3. *Scarlatina maligna.*—Ars., Mur. Ac., Cup. Ac., Nit. Ac., Hydrastis *(as a gargle, or the strong tincture as a paint to the tonsils)*.

4. *Secondary diseases (sequelæ).*—Mur. Ac., Apis, Merc. Iod., Phos., Sulph., etc. See pages 99–100.

5.—*Prophylactic Treatment.*—Bell. See previous page.

SPECIAL INDICATIONS.—*Belladonna.*—Immediately scarlatina is suspected, and especially when the *bright-red* rash appears; also if the swallowing is difficult, the throat and eyes are inflamed, and there is sleeplessness, with nervous excitement, starts and jerks. This medicine exerts a direct power over scarlet-fever, and should be administered every two to four or six hours, according to the urgency of the symptoms.

Aconitum.—Febrile symptoms. This medicine may precede *Bell.*, or be alternated with it.

Mercurius.—Inflamed, swollen, or ulcerated throat; acrid discharge from the nostrils; profuse secretion of saliva, or ulcers in the mouth. This remedy often suitably follows the administration of *Belladonna.* If swelling of the throat is very considerable, *Apis* should be given.

Coffæa.—Extreme *restlessness*, irritability, and a whining disposition, particularly at night.

Arsenicum.—Great prostration of strength, rapid emaciation, cold clammy sweats, frequent, weak pulse, nightly paroxysms of fever, with burning heat, and threatening *dropsical affections.*

Sulphur.—During the decline of the eruption, as a preventive of the secondary diseases so frequent after scarlet-fever.

Accessory Means.—As an invariable rule, the patient should remain in bed; the room should be well ventilated, at the same time that the patient is protected from direct currents of air. He must not go out too early, as secondary symptoms are of frequent occurrence from neglect of this precaution. His beverage may consist of cold water, gum-water, barley-water, weak lemonade, etc., in small quantities, as frequently as desired. The diet should be simple,—roast apple, toast, gruel, etc.; gradually returning, as the disease declines, to food of a more substantial kind. The fever being of short duration, wine or brandy may generally be dispensed with; but in malignant cases, stimulants, Liebig's extract of beef, etc., should be given as directed in the section on Typhoid-fever, under "Diet and Stimulants." The patient should be frequently sponged over with tepid water, and dried as rapidly as possible, to obviate too long exposure. Other measures are often necessary; *poultices*, frequently renewed, or spongio-piline, squeezed out from hot water, if the glands are swollen; the *inhalation of the steam of hot water*, as described in Part IV, as long as the throat is sore and painful; *injections* of tepid water, if the bowels are costive. During convalescence, warm clothing, including flannel, is necessary, and subsequently, a change of air, if possible to the sea-side.

Secondary Diseases *(Sequelæ)*.—If there are no complications or sequelæ, scarlet-fever may be expected to terminate favourably within a week from the setting in of the disease; but in weakly or scrofulous children the disease is liable to be followed by troublesome or even dangerous maladies, especially if the treatment and nursing have not been skilful and careful.

Affections of the kidney, dropsy, and other secondary

diseases, are infrequent after Homœopathic treatment. The most frequent sequelæ, with the remedies generally useful, are the following:—

Glandular swellings, discharges from the ears, or deafness.—Merc. Iod., Mur. Ac., Calc. Carb., Phos., Sulph., Bell.

Pains in the ear.—Puls., Bell.

Croupy cough.—Hepar Sulph., Iod.

Inflammatory affections of the eyes.—Bell., Acon., Sulph.

Anasarca (dropsy).—Apis, Canth., Ars.

In post-scarlatinal dropsy, when the swelling is considerable and rapid, and involves the subcutaneous tissue rather than the skin, *Apis* is most useful. Its curative action is generally indicated by a large secretion of urine *(Hughes)*.

The last affection is the most common sequel of scarlet-fever, and it has been observed to result more frequently from a mild than from a severe form of the disease. This is probably owing to the disease not having expended all its force, so that some of the poison remains in the system; or it may be due to the neglect of proper caution during the period of recovery; or, again, to the patient having been in a debilitated condition previously to the attack of fever. The *symptoms* of this disease are,—puffiness of the eyelids and face, followed by general swelling of the whole body; frequent desire to pass urine, which is scanty, and of a smoky colour, and if tested by heat and nitric acid, is found to deposit *albumen*.

6.—Typhus-Fever *(Febris Typhus)*.

Definition.—Typhus is an acute specific form of fever, highly contagious and infectious, continuing from fourteen to twenty-one days, attended with a lethargic or confused condition of the intellect, and an eruption on the skin of a measly or mulberry appearance, and is the accompaniment of privation, overcrowding, and defective ventilation.

agnosis of Typhus- from Typhoid-fever is not diffi-
chief differences are, however, arranged below.

RENCES BETWEEN TYPHUS- AND TYPHOID-FEVER.

TYPHUS.	TYPHOID.
on *quickly*.	1.—Commences *slowly* and insidiously, the premonitory stage lasting a week or more.
at *any age*.	2.—Seldom attacks persons after forty, and is most common in *youth*, including childhood.
re among the wealthy pting doctors, students, clergymen.	3.—Is more common among the *rich than the poor*.
ruption is of a MULBERRY nes out in a single crop rth or fifth day, and lasts mination of the disease.	4.—The eruption of the skin consists of ROSE-COLOURED spots, comes in successive crops, which in their turn fade and disappear.
brain is chiefly affected, els are but little so.	5.—The *bowels* are chiefly affected, the evacuations being ochre-coloured and watery, with congestion of the mucous membrane of the intestines, sometimes hæmorrhage, or even ulceration.
is a *dusky blush* on the and shoulders, injected ntracted pupils.	6.—The expression is *bright*, the hectic blush is limited to the cheeks, and the pupils are dilated.
its course in about a	7.—Continues at least *three weeks*, and often five or six, or even more.
pses are of *rare* occurrence.	8.—*Relapses*, marked by a return of all the former symptoms, frequently occur, especially in certain epidemics.
tendency to death is by bid drowsiness), or *conges-* *lungs*.	9.—The tendency to death is by *Asthenia* (exhaustion), *pneumonia*, *hæmorrhage*, or *perforation of the intestine*.
phus arises from *overcrowd-* *defective ventilation*, and contagion.	10.—*Typhoid* arises from *bad drainage*, foul drinking-water,—as from a drain leaking into a well—decomposing animal matter, etc., often with *high temperature*, deficient rain-fall, certain electrical conditions, or an insufficient supply of ozone.

SYMPTOMS.—The precursory stage varies, but is usually short, so that the patient yields to the disease within the first three days, giving up his employment and taking to his bed; in this respect strongly contrasting with the protracted invasive stage of Typhoid. Sensations of uneasiness, soreness, or fatigue, loss of appetite, *frontal headache*, and disturbed sleep, are the early symptoms. The patient is often seized with a rigor, but less marked and severe than in small-pox or internal inflammations, usually succeeded by dry heat of skin, thirst, quick pulse, white, dry, often tremulous tongue, scanty and highly-coloured urine, sometimes vomiting, heavy look or stupor, prostration, and muscular pains; towards evening there is irritability or restlessness, and if sleep occurs, it is disturbed by dreams, or frequent sudden starts, and is in consequence unrefreshing.

The general appearance of a typhus-patient is very marked, and affords to the practised eye a ready means of diagnosis. "In an average attack the patient lies prostrate on his back with a most weary and dull expression of face, his eyes heavy, and with some dusky flush spread uniformly over his cheeks. In the advanced stage of a severe attack he lies with his eyes shut or half-shut, moaning, and too prostrate to answer questions, to protrude his tongue, or to move himself in bed; or the mouth is clenched, the tongue and hands tremble, and the muscles are twitching and half rigid. The dryness of the mouth, the sordes on the teeth and lips, the hot, dry skin, and the deafness, are other symptoms which strike an observer so immediately as to deserve to be included in the physiognomy of the disease."*

During the first week the patient complains much of headache, noises in the ears, and, subsequently, deafness; the

* "A System of Medicine," vol. i.

unctivæ are injected, the pupils contracted, painfully itive to light, and therefore often closed. He becomes able, and his answers short and fretful. After the lapse short period, usually between the fourth and eighth days, mind passes from a state of excitement to one of delirium. s symptom is usually more severe, and appears earlier, n the disease attacks persons in the upper classes of ety, in consequence, no doubt, of the greater activity of r brains. It is at first one of confusion of ideas as to e, place, persons, and even personal identity, with vague bling talk, of which occasionally he seems conscious, and n which he can be roused. Afterwards the delirium may ome active and maniacal, or low and muttering. The ent often fancies that he is two or three persons, and the ject of a series of miseries and violence: confined in a geon, pursued by enemies from whom he vainly flies, with whom he struggles, and he attempts to spring from to reach the door or window to fly from his tormentors. netimes the delirium passes into a heavy stupor, with nulousness of the tongue and hands, and twitching of the scles *(subsultus tendinum)*; but in favourable cases it subs in two or three days, the powers of the mind begin in to dawn, the countenance assumes a more tranquil ect, sleep becomes natural, and at length convalescence is y established.

Diarrhœa is not of infrequent occurrence, but sometimes bowels are confined; the evacuations are natural or dark, l contrast strongly with the yellow-ochre colour of the ols in *enteric-fever;* finally, the evacuations may be inuntary.

THE PULSE.—In typhus the pulse is rarely less than 100, netimes 120, or 130, or even 140 in the minute. In the case, however, in adults, it is indicative of great danger.

As a rule the pulse pursues a gradually increasing rate of frequency up to the ninth or twelfth day, and afterwards undergoes, in favourable cases, a somewhat sudden decline. Cases so marked almost invariably get well. On the other hand, departures from the gradual rise in the pulse, especially if considerable, mark the existence of complications or dangerous symptoms. In fatal cases of typhus the pulse becomes more and more rapid, and also weaker and smaller up to the very hour of death. The first glimpse of dawning convalescence is afforded by watching the pulse; the temperature, as measured by the thermometer, is a valuable but less available sign; and whenever the pulse is fairly on the decline, especially if it gets stronger and fuller, we may confidently conclude that the patient will recover. The *crisis* of typhus is often indicated by no other symptoms than the fall of temperature indicated by the thermometer, and the decline of the pulse after having gradually reached its maximum degree of rapidity. There may be no marked perspiration, no critical diarrhœa, no striking alteration in the urine, or notable phenomena of any kind besides.

DISTINCTIVE CHARACTERS.—The *typhus-rash* appears between the fourth and seventh days, and consists of irregular, slightly elevated spots, of a mulberry hue, which disappear on pressure, and may be singly scattered and minute, or numerous and large; in the latter case two or more spots coalesce. They are usually first seen on the abdomen, and afterwards on the chest and extremities. From the first to the third day after the appearance of the rash, no fresh spots appear; but each spot, although it undergoes certain changes, continues visible till the whole rash disappears, and the disease terminates. In fatal cases, the typhus-spots remain after death.

The *odour* of typhus-patients is very characteristic, and

is described as offensive, pungent, and ammoniacal. Nurses, familiar with the disease, are thus alone able to recognise it, and they estimate the amount of danger by the badness of the smell.

Prominence of Nervous Symptoms.—It is from the constancy and prominence of these symptoms that the name of typhus was first employed, and it is almost certain that it is through the nervous system that the poison of the disease chiefly operates. Hence extreme restlessness, ringing noises in the ears, and low delirium or stupor, are invariably present to a greater or less extent. In fatal cases, about the ninth or tenth day, delirium merges into profound coma, or the condition described as *coma-vigil* may come on. In this latter condition, the patient lies on his back with his eyes wide open, and certainly awake, but indifferent or insensible to everything transpiring around him. His mouth is partially open, his face expressionless, and he is incapable of being roused. At length the breathing becomes nearly imperceptible, the pulse rapid and feeble, or it cannot be felt, and the transition from life to death occurs without any gleam of returning consciousness, and can only be recognised by the eyes losing their little lustre, and the chest no longer performing its slow and feeble movements.

UNFAVOURABLE INDICATIONS.—Early, furious, and persistent delirium, with complete sleeplessness; *coma-vigil; convulsions;* involuntary twitchings of the muscles of the face and arms; abundant and *dark rash*, nearly unaffected by pressure; great duskiness of the countenance, or lividity of the surface; involuntary, uncontrollable diarrhœa; suppression of urine, or albuminuria; a brown, hard, *tremulous tongue;* a temperature gradually rising to 107° Fahr., or higher; a great sudden elevation of temperature in the third week; a small, weak, irregular, or imperceptible pulse, stationary at above 120°; bed-sores, or inflammatory or erysipelatous swellings; a strong presentiment of death on the part of the patient; etc.

Causes.—*Overcrowding, with defective ventilation, and destitution;* thus it is the scourge of the poor inhabitants of our large towns. *Overcrowding* includes the several conditions of overcrowding of rooms by too many occupants; overcrowding of dwelling-houses upon too circumscribed area, preventing the proper ventilation of streets and houses; and want of personal and domestic cleanliness. A spacious dwelling, with free ventilation, robs the disease of half its power, and the danger of its spread to others is reduced to a minimum. *Privation*—famine through failure of crops, commercial distress, strikes, hardships in war, etc.—predispose to typhus by deteriorating the constitution. Before the days of Howard, typhus was never absent from our prisons and hospitals; it was the scourge of the armies of the first Napoleon, and it decimated those of the Allies in the Crimea, the disease varying among the troops exactly in proportion to the degree of privation and overcrowding. In 1818, and again in 1847, the failure of the potato crop in Ireland gave rise to an epidemic of this fever, so that it is estimated that an eighth part of the entire population was attacked. There is undoubted evidence that the poison of typhus may be generated *de novo*, and that the circumstances under which this occurs are those above stated, namely overcrowding, defective ventilation, and destitution. There seems ground for believing that the poison is chiefly transmitted by the exhalations from the lungs and skin; the *materies morbi* (material poison) being inhaled or swallowed, so finding ready admission to the blood, upon which it exerts its morbid influence. The effects of bad ventilation in the development of typhus is well expressed in the following words: "If any person will take the trouble to stand in the sun, and look at his own shadow on a white-plastered wall, he will easily perceive that his whole body is a smoking mass of corruption, with a vapour exhaling from every part of it. This vapour is subtle, acrid, and offensive to the smell; if retained in the body it becomes morbid; but if re-absorbed, highly deleterious. If a number of persons, therefore, are long confined in any unventilated place, they inspire and swallow with their spittle the vapours thus generated, and must soon feel their effects. Bad provisions and gloomy thoughts will add to their misery, and soon breed the *seminium* of a pestilential fever, dangerous not only to themselves, but also to every person who visits them, or even communicates with them at second hand. Hence it is so frequently bred in gaols, hospitals, ships, camps, and besieged towns. A *seminium* once produced is easily spread by contagion."

TREATMENT.—It is a question whether typhus can ever be cut short, or the definite course of the disease altered by the administration of remedies; some contend that it may be broken up in the first stage, especially by the combination of Hydropathic appliances with the use of Homœopathic remedies; others believe that the disease must have its course. However, we have ample experience to prove that in the great majority of cases the violence of the symptoms can be held in check, the patient's comfort greatly promoted, and convalescence hastened, by judicious treatment.

EPITOME OF TREATMENT.—

1. *Febrile symptoms.*—Acon., Bry.
2. *Cerebral symptoms.*—Hyos., Bell., Opi., Rhus Tox.
3. *Sleeplessness.*—Coffæa, Bell.
4. *Stupor.*—Opi., Rhus.
5. *Extreme prostration.*—Mur. Ac., Ars., Phos. Ac.
6. *Pulmonary complications.*—Phos., Bry., Acon. *(congestion)*.
7. *Putrescence.*—Carbo Veg., Ars., Rhus Tox.
8. *Convalescence.*—Phos. Ac., Nit. Ac., China, Sulph.

SPECIAL INDICATIONS.—*Aconitum.*—Thickly-furred tongue, foul taste, thirst; heavy, aching pain in the head; soreness and heaviness in the bowels and other parts of the body; exacerbations towards evening; the urine becomes dark and foul; the patient is restless, depressed in spirits, wakeful or drowsy, and dreams heavily in sleep. *Acon.* will be of great service in the first stage, before the brain is much involved, and when the above symptoms, as indications of severe febrile disturbance, are present: but not afterwards probably, except as an intercurrent remedy, and for inflammation or local congestion.

Gelseminum Semper.—"Specifically indicated in cases in which the patient, from some great excitement or over-exertion, suddenly sinks into a low typhoid state, with great prostration of all the vital forces, and when he experiences strange sensations in the head, with morbid condition of the motor nerves, manifested by local paralysis, or continued jactitation of certain muscles" *(Hale).*

Baptisia.—Should typhoid symptoms appear, and there is difficulty in determining the exact nature of the disease, this remedy should be at once administered, and repeated several times. If improvement does not immediately follow the use of *Baptisia*, other remedies should be given.

Hyoscyamus.—*Severe pains in the head;* dull, distressed, or haggard expression of the face; dry and glazed brown tongue; sordes on the teeth, noises in the ears, deafness, and *aberration of sight*—the patient seeing double or treble; delirium, in which the patient frequently manifests a *desire to escape* from some imaginary enemy or evil. *Hyos.* is probably one of the best remedies in this disease.

Belladonna.—The symptoms indicating this medicine are of a very decided character, and are usually the following:—Great *cerebral congestion,*—bright-red, even bloated, face; *throbbing* of the temples and carotids; glistening and staring of the eyes; partial loss of the use of the tongue, so that the patient can scarcely articulate; much *thirst;* confusion of ideas; picking at the bed-clothes; furious *delirium.*

Opium.—Stertorous breathing; low muttering delirium; stupor; dark-red face; hot and dry, or clammy, skin; thick brownish-coated tongue; complaint of thirst (if the patient can express his sensations).

Muriatic. Ac.—In an advanced stage this acid is sometimes capable of effecting a most beneficial influence; especially when there are,—complete loss of muscular power; extreme dryness and parched appearance of the skin, which is cold; quick, feeble pulse; low delirium; slavering; foul exhalations from the ulcerated throat; etc.

Rhus Tox.—Blackish-brown mucus on the tongue; thirst; bleeding from the nose; discharge of fœtid urine; involuntary, bad-smelling alvine evacuations; small and rapid pulse; stupor.

Arsenicum.—Sunken countenance and eyes; *dry,* cracked *tongue; burning thirst; involuntary diarrhœa.*

Nitric. Ac.—This remedy may be given occasionally throughout the course of the disease: it has sometimes a very salutary influence.

Accessory Measures.—The points of greatest importance may be briefly summed up as under: (1.) The patient should be placed in a large, or at least in a well-ventilated, room, so as to secure a continuous and ample supply of fresh air. Cases occurring in close, crowded rooms, in which this prime hygienic condition cannot be secured, should be removed to a hospital. (2.) Frequent changes of personal- and bed-linen, and changes of posture to avoid congestion and bed-sores; if bed-sores form notwithstanding, the patient should be placed on a *water-bed.* The *wet-pack* (see Part IV) is a valuable measure, especially early in the disease, and when the skin is dry and hot. (3.) Food or beverages should be given in small quantities at regular and frequent intervals, including water, milk-and-water, tea, broth, beef-tea; and, if prostration, feeble and irregular circulation, or complications, indicate their use, wine or brandy. In some cases in which patients obstinately refuse all food, or are unable to swallow, life is often saved by nutritious or stimulating enematæ. (4.) Quiet; in noisy streets stuffing the ears with cotton-wool; cleanliness; sponging the whole surface of the body and carefully drying at least once a day; and intelligent and unremitting watching.

The hints on nursing fever-patients in the following section, and the general accessory measures described in Part IV, should be studied.

PROPHYLACTICS.—As disinfectants,—fresh air, efficient ventilation, and cleanliness are of paramount importance; as additional means for avoiding contagion, but by no means as substitutes,—whitewashing with quick-lime, washing the woodwork with soap and water, repapering infected rooms, cleansing the linen in water to which chloride-of-lime has been added, and the use of this substance or of *carbolic-acid* in the water employed in sponging the patient. Without cleanliness and fresh air, vinegar, camphor, and other so-called preventives, are useless, and only disguise noxious vapours. Persons in attendance on the sick should especially avoid the odour from the breath and the exhalations which arise on turning down the bed-clothes. Nurses should not be overworked, deprived of repose in bed, or of daily out-of-door exercise. If there is any ground to fear an attack of typhus, *Hyos.* and *Baptisia* are probably the best preventives.

7.—Enteric-Fever—Typhoid-Fever *(Febris Typhoides).*

DEFINITION.—*Enteric-*, also called *Typhoid-fever*, from its chief pathological effects being evident in the bowels, is a continued fever, lasting about twenty-three days, often ger, with an eruption on the chest, abdomen, or back, and

of these fevers are different, and suggest sanitary regulations of an opposite nature: Typhoid is less contagious than Typhus; the tendency to a fatal issue varying, the treatment must be regulated accordingly; and, further, if not early recognized, patients may persist in their usual occupations at a time when rest in bed would conserve the strength and moderate the progress of the disease. For the easy recognition of these fevers, consult the table of differences, page 101.

SYMPTOMS.—These may be divided into (1) those of the *accession*, and (2) those of the *three weekly periods*.

Unless the poison is very concentrated, there is a period of *incubation*, varying from seven to fourteen days, after which the disease sets in slowly and insidiously. The patient becomes languid and indisposed to exertion; is chilly and unwilling to leave the fire; the back aches, and the legs tremble; the appetite fails, and there are even nausea and sickness; the tongue is white, the breath offensive, and often the throat is sore; the bowels are generally relaxed; the pulse is quickened, and the sleep disturbed. These symptoms gradually increasing, the patient has probably severe rigors, succeeded by heightened temperature, severe headache, and such muscular debility that he takes to his bed. This is the accession. The course of the fever may now be divided into

1st Week.—The prominent symptoms are,—vascular excitement and nervous oppression, including a bounding pulse, 90 per minute, great heat of skin, thirst, and obscured mental faculties; the patient cannot give a coherent account of himself, complains of little except his head, and is usually delirious at night. The abdomen enlarges, is resonant on percussion, and there is tenderness or even pain on firm pressure, especially in the right *iliac fossa*, near the termination of the small intestine; a peculiar *gurgling* sensation is conveyed to the fingers on pressure, arising from the mixing of the gastric fluids.

2nd Week.—Debility and emaciation become very marked, the muscles wasting as well as the fat; the urine becomes scanty and heavy, being loaded with urea from wasting of the nitrogenized tissues. During the second week also there is frequently *diarrhœa*, which generally increases towards the end of the week, and consists of semi-fluid, pale yellow, frothy motions, of which there may be five, six, or even more in twenty-four hours. The *specific characters* of the evacuations in enteric-fever are the following:—*fluidity; pale-ochre* or *drab-colour; sickly, putrid odour; absence of bile;* and *a floculent debris* of disintegrated glands of the ileum. The floculent debris may be discovered by washing the discharges. In reference to the *colour* of the stools, it is worth notice that often before a patient takes to his bed, or looseness of the bowels sets in, the fæces are of a light-ochre colour, and furnish the most marked early sign of enteric-fever.

3rd Week.—The debility and emaciation become extreme; the patient lies extended on his back, sinking towards the foot of the bed, without making an effort to change or preserve his position. There is a bright and pinkish flush of the cheeks, which strongly contrasts with the surrounding s skin; *sordes* occur on the mucous membrane of the ath and lips; the tongue is dry and brown, or red and glased, and often rough and stiff, like old leather; the urine is frequently retained from inaction of the bladder; the fæces pass without control, the tendons start from irregular, feeble contractions of the muscles; the patient picks vacantly at the bedclothes, or grasps at black spots, like flies on the wing *(muscæ volitantes)*, which appear before his eyes; he becomes deaf, no longer knows his friends, and on recovery will have little or no remembrance of anything that has at this time occurred, and in all probability his intellectual powers will be impaired for some time after convalescence.

In the majority of fatal cases, death occurs about the end of the third week; and it is a notable fact that there seems to be no relation between the general symptoms and the ultimate issue, rendering the disease one of great uncertainty and perplexity.

The Eruption.—At this time, from the seventh to the fourteenth day, the characteristic *eruption* generally begins to show itself, chiefly on the sternum and epigastrium, in the form of rose-coloured dots; which are few in number, round, scarcely elevated, and insensibly fade into the natural hue of the surrounding skin. The quantity of the rash bears no proportion to the severity of the disease. "This successive daily eruption, disappearing on pressure, each spot continuing visible for three or four days only, is peculiar to, and absolutely diagnostic of, typhoid fever *(Aitken)*. The first crop of the eruption is rarely fully conclusive, but successive crops, even of not more than two or three spots each, remove all doubt. Although the rose-coloured rash is never met with in any other disease, yet we have treated cases of true typhoid without being able to detect a solitary spot. Occasionally, also, *sudamina* appear, which are very minute vesicles, looking like drops of sweat, chiefly on the neck, chest, or abdomen.

Enlargement of the spleen, Dr. Jenner remarks, in doubtful cases enables him to diagnose positively this variety of fever, as this enlargement commonly occurs in typhoid-fever.

TEMPERATURE.—The information afforded by the application of the clinical thermometer to the body in the diagnosis of enteric-fever is very important. In all the acute specific fevers the temperature is abnormally raised; in typhoid this elevation is *gradual*, while in most others it is *abrupt*. During the first three or four days we have scarcely any symptoms to indicate the *invasion* of so serious a disease except a *gradual* elevation of the temperature; but if, on the fourth or fifth day, the maximum temperature attained during the twenty-four hours be not 104°, the disease is most probably not typhoid fever. And, further, if on the first or second day the maximum temperature reaches 104°, the disease is some other acute fever, as the temperature only *gradually* attains such a degree in typhoid-fever. At the commencement the diagnosis is difficult, inasmuch as the characteristic rash does not usually appear before the sixth, sometimes not till the twelfth, day of the disease; and, indeed, in children, cannot sometimes be observed at any stage of the disease. Temperature is also an important element in the *prognosis*. Thus we have great *variations* in the temperature in typhoid-fever, being low in the morning, and attaining its maximum degree in the evening. The greater these fluctuations at the end of the second week, the more favourable is the attack, and the shorter will be its duration. If the temperature falls considerably in the morning, even though the evening rise is considerable, the prognosis is favourable. On the other hand, should the temperature during the second week remain continuously high, we may predicate a severe and prolonged attack. Again, probably the first indication of improvement in cases of persistent elevation of the temperature, is a decline in the morning temperature. When such a decline occurs, especially if it be repeated on subsequent days, even though the maximum temperature reached in the evening remain the same, we may be certain that the fever has begun to abate. It is true, a sudden fall in the temperature may be consequent on diarrhœa or hæmorrhage—probably the latter if it occurs very suddenly; but, usually, other symptoms would indicate such an occurrence.

Dangers.—(1) *Hæmorrhage.*—This may occur from the ulcerated patches in the *ileum*, during the separation of the gland-sloughs, and may be either capillary or from the opening of a large vessel. The discharge of blood may be so great as to be immediately fatal by syncope, or it may be remotely fatal, by exhausting the patient so that he has no power to bear up against the fever in its subsequent course. Sometimes without any escape of blood from the orifice of the bowel, the patient becomes suddenly blanched and dies of syncope. In such a case a *post-mortem* examination finds the intestines distended with clotted blood. (2) *Exhaustion from profuse and persistent diarrhœa*, in cases in which the affection of the mucous membrane has been very severe and obstinate. The evacuations weaken the patient rapidly, and hasten the fatal termination. (3) *Perforation.*—The ulceration may extend till the coats of the bowel are perforated and cause fatal peritonitis; this may happen during the second or third week, or, more frequently, during prolonged and imperfect convalescence. The symptoms of this occurrence are,—a sudden pain and tenderness in the abdomen, with swelling, altered expression of the features, more or less nausea and vomiting, and death in one or two days. (4) *Congestion.*—The lungs may become congested, giving rise to bronchitis, pleurisy with effusion, pneumonia, or latent tubercle may be called into fatal activity; in short, there is a tendency, from the poisoned state of the blood, to congestion in the three great visceral cavities of the body—the head, the chest, and the abdomen.

Typhoid-fever presents, in the mode of its accession, in the course, gravity, and termination of the symptoms, so many varieties, complications, and accidents, that it has been considered almost as an *epitome of the whole practice of medicine.*

Mortality.—The reports of the Registrar-General show that in this country alone about 20,000 persons die annually of typhoid-fever, and that probably 150,000 persons are laid prostrate by it. It proved fatal to the Prince Consort on the 14th December, 1861, twenty-one days from the commencement of the attack. Several members of the royal family of Portugal came to an untimely end by it; and also Count Cavour, but the death of the latter was accelerated by venesection.

Cause.—According to Drs. Budd, Aitken, and others, the poison of typhoid-fever does not *originate* in decomposing sewage, but is transmitted by the specific poison contained in the discharges from the bowels of the person infected with the fever. The contagious matter may convey the fever in two principal ways:—(1) By percolating the soil into the wells which furnish drinking-water; (2) By infecting the air through defective sewers or water-closets. In opposition to this hypothesis, Dr. Murchison makes the following objections:—"(1) There are many facts which show that enteric-fever often arises from bad drainage, independent of any transmission from the sick. The danger ensues when the drain becomes choked up, when the sewage stagnates and ferments, and when the transmission of the poison to any distant locality is impeded, if not completely arrested. (2) There are numerous instances of enteric-fever appearing in houses having no communication by drain with any other dwelling. (3) There is no evidence that the stools of enteric-fever are of such a virulent nature as has been stated. The attendants on the sick are rarely attacked. (4) The fact that the prevalence of the disease is influenced by temperature is opposed to the idea that it depends on a specific poison derived from the sick; but is readily accounted for on the supposition that the poison is generated by fermentation or decomposition."

We conclude, therefore, *that refuse animal and vegetable matters, if permitted to accumulate and decompose in seasons of drought, generate a poison, which, if not washed away or diluted by sufficient rain, rises into the air, or becomes diffused in the water; and which, when introduced into the body by these media, may produce enteric-fever (Harley).* Hence we find it most prevalent in autumn, and at the commencement of winter, after a long season of heat and drought. *The* BEST PROPHYLAXIS, *therefore, include an* ABUNDANT SUPPLY OF PURE WATER; *sufficiently-inclined and* WELL-CONSTRUCTED SEWERS, WITH IMPERMEABLE WALLS; A WELL-DRAINED SOIL, *regular* FLUSHING OF THE DRAINS WITH WATER DURING DRY WEATHER, and most especially in SUBJECTING THE INTESTINAL DISCHARGES, on their issue, TO THE ACTION OF POWERFUL CHEMICAL AGENTS, *by which they may be entirely deprived of their specific virus. If these measures are efficiently carried out, typhoid-fever may be expected entirely to disappear.*

TREATMENT.—Unless distance absolutely forbids it, the treatment of this disease should only be confided to a medical man. Before the true character of the fever is detected, the remedies prescribed in the section on "Simple Fever" may be given.

EPITOME OF TREATMENT.—

1. *Invasive Stage.*—Bapt.
2. *Great prostration.*—Ars., Mur. Ac., Rhus Tox.
3. *Excessive Diarrhœa.*—Ipec., Ars. *(involuntary).*
4. *Hæmorrhage from the bowels.*—Tereb., Nit. Ac., Ipec.
5. *Complications.*—Phos., Bry., Bell., Hyos., Opi. See also Secondary diseases.
6. *Debility following.*—Phos. Ac., Ign., Ferr., China, Nux Vom.

SPECIAL INDICATIONS.—*Baptisia.*—As soon as typhoid-fever is suspected, this remedy should be administered,—a drop of the 1st dec. dil., or of the mother tincture, every two or three hours. This remedy is of great value in most cases, modifying, and even cutting short, the attack by destroying the poison in the blood. Its influence in this disease is comparable to that of *Acon.* in simple fever; but *Acon.* exercises little or no curative power in typhoid-fever, as it depends on the presence of a specific blood-poison, which requires the action of an antidote. Should, however, the administration of *Baptisia* have been much delayed, and the specific effects of typhoid-poisoning have been produced, this remedy will do little good, and other remedies must be resorted to.

Arsenicum.—The following symptoms specially indicate this remedy:—frequent, copious *diarrhœa*, which may become *involuntary*, of drab or ochre-coloured evacuations; enlargement and sensitiveness of the abdomen; gurgling sounds, before described; excessive *prostration*; *thirst*; nearly imperceptible, intermittent, pulse. This remedy is one of priceless value, and its administration should be persevered with even in the face of the most disheartening symptoms. Sometimes it may be advantageous to alternate *Arsenicum* with

Carbo Veg., when there are offensive smells from the patient, and very *fœtid* evacuations; and also cold extremities, cold perspirations, and rapidly-sinking powers.

Mercurius.—Greenish or yellowish evacuations, but less serious diarrhœa than described under the previous medicines; thickly-coated tongue; copious perspirations.

Belladonna, etc.—When the brain is much involved, *Bell.*, *Hyos.*, or *Opi.*, as prescribed in the treatment of *Typhus-fever*, will be found of great service.

Terebinthina.—Hæmorrhage from the bowels, and retention of urine.

Phosphoric Acid.—In the milder forms of typhoid, this acid is very useful, especially for nervous prostration; and also after the severity of a bad attack has been moderated by other remedies.

Muriatic. Ac.—Great nervous depression; stupor; sinking down in the bed; putrid sore throat; etc. It probably ranks next to *Ars.* in the gravest symptoms of low fever. For the throat it may also be used locally. *Nitric. Ac.* may also be of service in similar conditions.

Secondary Diseases *(Sequelæ).*—During convalescence, various affections are liable to arise, such as troublesome cough, indigestion, headache, deafness, etc. For these it is only necessary to suggest such remedies as are prescribed for these affections in other parts of this manual. *For chest-symptoms, Phos., Bry.,* or *Iod;* for *indigestion, Nux Vom., Carbo Veg., Ign.,* or *Merc.;* for the *brain, Bell., Hyos., Rhus Tox. Deafness* usually disappears, with the general nervous prostration, under the use of *Phos. Acid* or *China.* The latter remedy also moderates the *excessive hunger* often experienced during convalescence, and is especially useful if there has been much waste of the fluids of the body. Lastly, *Sulphur* aids the recuperative efforts of nature, and may be administered for some time after the more specific remedies are discontinued.

Accessory Measures.—The following points require special attention in nursing fever patients; the reader is however requested to study the more detailed hints on nursing the sick, and the various accessory measures that are described in Part IV of this work. Persons having the charge of extreme cases of illness, should be familiar with the several accessories there pointed out, as the efficient carrying out of those directions is second only to the administration of medicine.

1st.—*The apartment.*—The patient should, if possible, be placed in a large, well-ventilated apartment, provided with a window, door, and fire-place, so contrived as to allow of an uninterrupted admission of fresh, and the escape of tainted air. A blazing fire also assists ventilation; but the patient's head should be protected from its immediate effects. The room should be divested of carpets, bed-hangings, and all unnecessary furniture. A second bed or convenient couch should be provided, so that by removing the patient to it for a few hours every day, the fever-atmosphere around his body may be changed. The light from the window may be subdued, and noise and unnecessary talking forbidden.

2nd.—*Rest.*—The patient should be disturbed as little as possible, and enjoy the most complete rest during the whole course of the disease. The importance of this is proved by *post-mortem* examinations, which often show vigorous attempts on the part of neighbouring structures to limit, by union and adhesion, the results of perforation, obviously indicating, in practice, the necessity of absolute rest throughout the disease *(Aitken)*. Any efforts made when the ulcers in the ileum are healing might affect that progress unfavourably, and even re-excite that morbid action which might end in perforation of the bowel.

3rd.—*Cleanliness.*—The body- and bed-linen should be frequently changed, and all matters discharged from the patient immediately removed. The mouth should be frequently wiped out with a soft wet towel, to remove the *sordes* which gather there in severe forms of fever. The patient's body should be sponged over as completely as possible at suitable intervals with tepid or cold water, as may be most agreeable to the feelings, and quickly dried with a soft towel. *Vinegar and water* may sometimes be substituted for simple tepid water. Vinegar used in this way is generally grateful to the patient, and hastens recovery.

nging the whole surface of the body with cold or tepid er should never be omitted in fever, as it reduces the ssive heat, soothes the uneasy sensations, and is indissable in maintaining that cleanliness which is so desirable the sick-room. Cold water thus applied acts as a tonic, ng vigour and tone to the relaxed capillaries, in which morbid action goes on. Frequent washing with soap and er also tends to prevent the occurrence of *bed-sores*, by ping the skin in a healthy condition. If bed-sores have ned, they should be protected by *Arnica-* or *Calendula-* ter. In bad cases, the patient should lie on a water- or bed.

th. *Hydropathic Applications.*—In addition to the spong- and washing just recommended, we have found the minal wet compress of great utility; and we refer the ler to the detailed directions for its use given in Part IV. abdominal compress tends to diminish extensive diarrhœa, cks the spread of ulceration of the ileum, and obviates foration. Should lung-complications arise, the compress uld be applied to the chest as well as the abdomen.

During the early course of the fever, the *wet-pack*, also cribed in Part IV, is an invaluable application, and tends, we have found, to give a mild character to the disease.

th. *Beverages.*—At the commencement of the fever, e water, toast-and-water, gum-water sweetened with a e sugar (one ounce of gum-arabic, half-an-ounce of loaf ar, one pint of hot water), barley-water, lemonade, or -water, is nearly all that is necessary. Cold water is an nt of supreme importance, and acts favourably by lowering excessive temperature, and proves a valuable adjunct to medicinal treatment prescribed.

th. *Diet and Stimulants.*—In a disease which lasts three ks, sometimes five or six, in which the waste of tissue is t, and when common food cannot be taken, it is a point of high importance to supply the patient with nourishment appropriate to his condition; otherwise he will sink before the disease has completed its course. The following are points requiring attention in the subject of diet.—Typhoid patients are often unable to swallow or relish nourishment in consequence of the dry and shrivelled state of the tongue, when it will be found necessary to soften the mucous lining by putting a little lemon-juice and water into the mouth a few minutes before offering food. All the aliments given should combine both food and drink in a *fluid* or semi-fluid form, until recovery has fully set in. The digestive functions being more or less completely suspended, the nourishment given must be only such as requires the simplest processes for its assimilation. The following are examples of this form of nutriment:—*Milk* (a most important article in the treatment of fever patients), *thin arrowroot with milk; wine whey*, prepared by adding half a pint of good sherry to one pint of boiling milk, and straining after coagulation; *blancmange of isinglass or ground-rice; yolk-of-egg*, beaten up with a little brandy, wine, tea, cocoa, or milk; *beef-tea and animal broths* (a little thickened with well-cooked rice, vermicelli, isinglass, or a few crumbs of bread); and *alcoholic drinks*.*

A little good wine with an equal quantity of water may be given every hour or two. *Effervescent* wines must be avoided.

* "The writer has no intention to side in the controversy concerning the food-character of alcohol. He accepts the evidence that much ingested alcohol is got rid of by the excretory organs, or is retained for some time in the tissues after the manner of many medicines. But with food in its widest sense, viz., that which keeps up the vital functions, the physician will have little hesitation in classing alcohol, who has observed the common case of an habitual tippler maintaining for years a fair standard of bodily health upon a quantity of other nutriment wholly insufficient by itself to maintain such health. And to such a case a fever patient offers some resemblance. He, too, may not be able to take enough of other food to maintain him, but alcoholic drinks will help him not to starve. And thus the writer judges them to have food-value apart from their medicinal action" (*Buchanan*).

Dr. Harley advises six to eight ounces of wine or four ounces of brandy every twenty-four hours when the pulse is of moderate force and under 120. When the pulse ranges between 120 and 130, and is small, double these quantities. If the patient enjoy these stimulants, it may be regarded as a sign of their utility. But the effects of the wine or brandy should be carefully watched by the medical attendant, and only given in proportion to the demands of the system, the bulk and force of the pulse being the main guides. Except in small quantities stimulants are not required by children, nor by persons who can take a sufficient quantity of other kinds of nourishment, nor early in the disease. On the other hand, aged persons, and patients greatly prostrated, or with cold extremities, and livid surface, almost invariably require alcoholic stimulants. Under any circumstances, if stimulants aggravate existing symptoms, their employment should be modified or altogether discontinued.

Again, nourishment should be given with strict *regularity*; in extreme and long-continued cases of prostration, every one or two hours, or even oftener, both day and night. Frequently the functions of digestion and assimilation are so greatly impaired, that the largest quantity of nourishment must be given to sustain the patient till the disease has passed through its stages. Dr. Graves was so strongly impressed with the importance of nourishment in fevers, as to have said that he desired no other epitaph than that *he fed fevers*.

7th. *Watching Patients.*—Fever-patients should be attended and watched day and night. Their urgent and incessant *wants* require] this, and their *safety* demands it. Instances have occurred of patients, in the delirium which so frequently attends this disease, getting out of bed, and even out of the window, during the absence of the nurse, and losing their lives from injuries thus sustained.

8th. *Moderation in convalescence.*—Food should only be allowed in great moderation, and never to the capacity of the appetite, till the tongue is quite clean and moist, and the pulse and skin have become natural. In typhoid fever, and in other conditions in which the bowels have been inflamed, this caution is especially necessary during convalescence. Solid meat given too early may bring back the most severe features of the disease. If stimulants have been given they should be gradually withdrawn as the quantity of nutritious food is increased. Even when convalescence has somewhat advanced, moderation should still be exercised, as the appetite is often excessively craving.

9th. *Precautionary Measures.*—The following precautions are suggested with the view of checking the contagion :—

(1.) All discharges from fever-patients should be received on their issue from the body into vessels containing a concentrated solution of chloride of zinc.

(2.) All tainted bed or body linen should, immediately on its removal, be placed in water, strongly impregnated with the same agent.

(3.) The water-closet should be flooded several times a day with a strong solution of chloride of zinc; and some chloride of lime should be also placed there, to serve as a source of chlorine in the gaseous form.

(4.) So long as fever lasts, the water-closets only should be used as receptacles for the discharges from the sick.

10th. *Change of air.*—The salutary influence of change of climate and scene to persons who have suffered from a serious attack of fever can scarcely be over-estimated; and if the place or climate have been intelligently chosen, the ppiest results may be anticipated.

fter recovery from a serious attack of fever, the whole becomes changed, and there seems to be a renewal of th. Nothing gives such a beneficial direction to this change, nor renders it so perfect, as a temporary removal to a suitable climate and locality. We fully endorse Dr. Aitken's statement,—*No man can be considered as fit for work for three or four months after an attack of severe typhoid-fever.*

8.—Relapsing-Fever *(Febris recidiva)*.

This disease—sometimes called *famine-fever*, and in Germany, *hunger-pest*—is not common in England, but has been epidemic in Dublin, Edinburgh, and Glasgow. It does not occur in tropical climates, in France nor in other parts of the continent, except in some of the Prussian territories, and the Crimea, where it attacked our army during the Russian war. It has occurred also in North America. Its cause is unknown; but it visits chiefly those who are ill-fed, live in crowded, filthy, ill-ventilated houses, and have but few comforts.

SYMPTOMS.—The seizure is sudden: there are rigors, and headache even more severe than that of the invasive stage of Typhus, but the prostration is much slighter. There are, also, pains in the muscles and joints resembling those of rheumatism. After a short time violent reaction sets in—great heat of skin; headache, throbbing in the temples, intolerance of light and sound, and sleeplessness; anxious expression of the countenance; rapid pulse—110 to 140; white-furred tongue, and, perhaps, vomiting, or even jaundice; thirst, etc. The temperature is from 102° to 107°; and at the height of the fever delirium may occur. Sweating may come on without relief. After continuing from five to eight days, the symptoms suddenly abate—usually about the seventh day from the commencement—and the *crisis* is indicated by *profuse perspiration*. Sometimes a miliary eruption occurs; or epistaxis, diarrhœa, menstrual discharge (in women), or hæmorrhage from the bowels; after a few hours there is an abrupt cessation of all bad symptoms; the patient feels much better in a short time, and appears to convalesce rapidly for four or five days; when, about the seventh day from the last attack, or the *fourteenth* from the commencement, a *sudden*

Relapse occurs, a repetition of the first attack. Perspiration again comes on, in from two to five days in favourable cases. The sweat has a very sour and peculiar odour. In other instances, however, uncontrollable vomiting, great thirst, very rapid pulse, jaundice, delirium, and death, may terminate the case *(Aitken)*.

The *Sequelæ* of Relapsing-fever consist commonly of excessive pains in the limbs; sometimes the kidneys are involved; but the dangers are similar, in some respects, to those attending *Scarlatina*. A species of ophthalmia is a frequent consequence.

Treatment.—*Aconitum* may be given during the first stage, for the rigors and following feverishness.

Bryonia.—Dr. Kidd, who treated an epidemic of the disease in Ireland, relied chiefly on *Bry.*, and had great success. It is certainly homœopathic to the nausea and vomiting, sensitiveness of the abdomen, sallowness and anxiety of the countenance, the throbbing and heat of the head, the rheumatoid pains, and the perspiration. It should follow the administration of a few doses of *Acon.*, or be alternated with that remedy from the commencement.

Gelseminum, *Eupatorium Per.*, and *Podophyllum*, are deserving of notice as being likely to influence the disease favourably. The last-named remedy is recommended to be administered in alternation with *Nux Vom.*

Camphor, and also *Nux Vomica*, may be used as *prophylactics*.

For *Accessory treatment* the reader is referred to the measures prescribed in the section on Typhoid-fever; also to Part IV.

9.—Simple Continued Fever and Febricula.

Fever, its nature, forms, etc. The term *Fever* (from *Ferveo*, to be hot) includes various forms of disease in which there are, shivering or chilliness succeeded by preternatural heat, quickened pulse, muscular debility, and general functional disturbance. This morbid condition accompanies many diseases as one of their phenomena, and is then called *symptomatic* fever; as in phthisis, abscesses, etc.; but under certain circumstances we meet with *idiopathic* or *essential* fevers, which are quite independent of any local inflammation, as Typhoid and Typhus, which are the result of a specific poison contaminating the blood. Again, fever may be of an *ephemeral* character, dependent on some cause which is merely sufficient to produce febrile disturbance without further mischief, as *simple continued fever* and *febricula*.

Symptoms.—Simple continued fever is usually ushered in by chills, or alternate chills and flushes, followed by burning heat and dryness of the skin; full, quickened pulse; dryness of the mouth, lips, and tongue, the tongue being red or coated white; thirst; high-coloured, scanty urine; and constipation. To these may be added—pains in the loins, headache, loss of appetite, hurried breathing, delirium, etc.; most of the symptoms usually being more severe at night. *Profuse perspiration*, bleeding of the nose, diarrhœa, or herpetic eruptions, are generally associated with the decline of the fever, and the patient is left weak, but otherwise well.

Duration.—The period of this fever varies from one to three days, or longer. When the symptoms disappear in twelve or twenty-four hours it is said to be an *ephemeral* disorder. The severe forms are often precursors of more serious diseases, as *Typhus*, *Pneumonia*, *Acute Rheumatism*, etc.

Causes.—Great sudden changes of temperature; damp linen or houses; poor, or insufficient diet, or, on the other hand, overfeeding, the action of small or uncertain quantities of specific poisons, as of typhoid or typhus poisons; inebriety; injuries; mental or bodily fatigue or excitement, or any circumstances which shock the nervous system. It may also be associated with various local or functional disturbances, as bronchial or gastric catarrhs, milk-fever, etc.

TREATMENT.—*Aconitum.*—Alternate chills and flushes, hot and dry skin, and other symptoms mentioned above. A dose every two hours, or in urgent cases, every thirty or forty minutes, until the skin becomes moist, and the pulse less frequent. Should the attack be one of *simple* fever merely, this remedy will be rapidly effectual; if it be the precursor of a more severe disease, it is still the best remedy at this stage. A profuse perspiration following its administration may be regarded as an indication of its beneficial action, and it should then be given less frequently, or discontinued.

Belladonna.—This remedy is required, if, after repeated doses of *Aconitum*, there should remain violent headache, redness of the face; confusion of ideas; a wild, fiery appearance of the eyes; throbbing of the blood-vessels in the temples; wakefulness, or even furious nocturnal delirium, and other well-marked cerebral symptoms. Sometimes it is best to alternate it with *Aconitum*. A dose every one to four hours.

Bryonia.—A *heavy, stupifying headache*, aggravated by movement, with a sensation as if the head would burst; cough and oppressed breathing; oppression at the pit of the stomach, yellow-coated tongue, nausea, constipation, brown or yellow urine; *shooting pains in the limbs;* irritability, etc.

Arsenicum.—Severe or prolonged cases of *Febricula*, with much prostration, or occurring in feeble patients, may require the use of this remedy.

If the symptoms do not yield to the remedies prescribed, but increase in severity when they are expected to be declining, case will probably prove to be one of Typhoid-fever, the previous section should be referred to.

ccessory Treatment.—The patient should be protected too much light, heat, noise, company, too many or thick -coverings, and everything likely to cause excitement or ent sleep. In the early stage of the fever, the adoption he *hot foot-bath*, described in Part IV, or the *wet-pack*, described in Part IV, will often at once restore the librium of the system, or, at least, greatly hasten the . Water should be the principal beverage, given in ll draughts, frequently repeated; it encourages perspira-, and promotes the favourable action of the baths just cribed. In acute fever, cold water is like the "Balm of ad."

10.—Yellow-Fever *(Febris flava)*.

his fever is a *specific* disease, and must not be confounded fevers of a malarial type, or others in which yellowness he skin, delirium, etc., also occur. It is described as the agastric pestilence*, is *malignant* in character, *rapidly fatal*, lly happens but once to the same patient, is *contagious*, chiefly endemic in low districts on the sea-coast. It occurred (by importation) in Plymouth, Southampton, on, and other sea-port towns; but has never been known ropagate beyond 48° north latitude, nor without a tem-ture of at least 72° Fahr.

hief Symptoms.—After a period of incubation of un-ain length—during which there may be merely a little ression, loss of appetite, and nausea—violent shivering, or of the face, congested lips, and continued delirium, rvene; the urine is suppressed; and a thick fur lies on tongue, in white heavy flakes, which afterwards peels off, ing the organ like a piece of raw beef; this condition is generally associated with *exudation of blood*. In an advanced stage, *bloody furuncles* occur, or *hæmorrhage from various parts or organs simultaneously*; the urine is albuminous; and there is *vomiting of black fluid*. If the disease be not checked, the life of the patient is terminated by *exhaustion* or *syncope*.

Epitome of Treatment.—

1. *Chill stage*.—Camphor.
2. *The Fever*.—Acon. and Bell.
3. *Second stage*.—Bry., Hyos., Ipec.
4. *Advanced stage*.—Phos., Lach., Ars., Canth. (*urinary derangements*); Arg. Nit. (*black-vomit*); Nit. Ac. (*as a weak gargle*); gum-water, or Calendula lotion, as an application to the raw surfaces.

See also the sections on "Jaundice," and "Typhoid-Fever." Under the latter disease will be found nearly all that it is requisite to say further about curative, preventive, and accessory treatment.

11.—Intermittent Fever (*Febris Intermittens*)—Ague.

Two centuries ago, when the soil around London was neither cultivated nor drained, and when, during portions of every year, the marshes of Lincolnshire, Cambridgeshire, and adjoining counties sent forth their emanations of malaria, ague was a very fatal disease in this country. James I. succumbed to its power in London, in 1625, and Oliver Cromwell died from it at Somerset House, in 1658.

Geographical facts, collected by medical writers from Hippocrates downwards, show that every country is unhealthy in proportion to the quantity of marshy or undrained alluvial soil it contains, the inhabitants of such districts dying often in the ratio of 1 in 20 instead of 1 in 38—the average mortality in healthy districts. The connexion of a given class of disease—represented by remittent and intermittent fever—with marshy districts is now distinctly established and generally recognised (*Aitken*); also, *per contra*, the disappearance of this class of disease has always been in direct relation to the drainage and cultivation of the soil.

Definition.—The disease known as Ague, consists of severe paroxysms of fever, characterized by a cold, a hot, and a sweating stage, between which there is a period of comparative health, in which the patient is able to follow his usual occupation.

Symptoms.—These may set in suddenly, or they may appear gradually, until a regular paroxysm occur. An ague-fit has three stages—the cold, the hot, and the perspiring. The *first stage* comes on with a feeling of debility, weariness, chilliness, and rigors; then follow sensations as of cold water trickling down the spine and a shivering of the whole body; the teeth chatter, the nails turn blue, and the whole frame trembles, often with such violence as to shake the bed on which the patient may be lying. The face becomes pale, the features and skin contracted, and the papillæ of the skin are rendered so prominent as to give it the appearance aptly described as *goose-skin*, such as may at any time be produced by exposure to cold. These symptoms are accompanied by an anxious expression of countenance, the eyes are dull and sunken, the pulse frequent and small, the breathing hurried and oppressed, the tongue white, and the urine scanty and frequently passed. After a period, varying from half an hour to three or four hours, the *second* or *hot stage* comes on with flushings, until the entire body becomes hot, with extreme thirst, full bounding pulse, throbbing headache, and restlessness, the urine being still scanty, but high-coloured. At length, after two, three, and even six or twelve hours, the *third* or *perspiring stage* succeeds, and the patient feels much relieved. Thirst diminishes, the pulse declines in frequency, and the appetite returns; at the same time there is a red deposit of *urates* in the urine. The perspiration first breaks out on the forehead and chest, and gradually extends over the entire surface of the body; sometimes it is only slight, but at other times it is very copious, saturating the patient's linen and bed-clothes. A paroxysm usually lasts about six hours, allowing two hours for each stage. The period between the paroxysms, as already explained, is called the *intermission;* but by an *interval* is meant the whole period or cycle between the beginning of one paroxysm, and the beginning of the next.

TYPES.—There are three chief types of ague: 1st.—*The Quotidian*, has a paroxysm daily, an interval of twenty-four hours, and is most common in the spring. 2nd.—*The Tertian*, has a paroxysm every other day, an interval of forty-eight hours, and is most frequent in the spring and autumn. 3rd.—*The Quartan*, has a paroxysm every third day, an interval of seventy-two hours, and is most common in the autumn. The hours of the day during which the paroxysms occur are by no means uniform. The tertian is perhaps the most frequent, and has the most marked hot stage; but the quartan is the most obstinate. There is still another type in which, though there is an attack every day, those only resemble each other which occur on alternate days.

LAWS.—Although at present ignorant of the physical or chemical nature of this *aërial poison*, we know that malaria obeys the following laws, which, from their great practical use, are worth remembering. 1st.—It spreads in the course of *prevailing winds*. It has always been observed that when the wind blows across malarious tracts of land, the disease spreads in the direction of the current; while the inhabitants of the opposite district escape. 2nd.—Its progress is arrested by *water*, especially by *rivers* and large *running streams*. Thus [illegible] on board ship, or at the side of water opposite to a h, are unaffected by it, although a favourable wind mit the poison to a far greater distance by land. Water ably absorbs malaria; and it is a common opinion in that water so charged produces periodic fevers in those drink it. In like manner, thick *rows of trees* intercept progress of the poison. 3rd.—Malaria does not rise e the *low level*. It seems to be of greater specific gravity atmospheric air, its power diminishing as we rise from surface of the earth. Persons occupying the upper stories house in an infected locality suffer to a far less extent those living on a ground floor. 4th.—It is most dangus at *night*. It has been often observed that sailors who n shore in the day-time, when off a malarious coast, do so out any bad results; but that those who remain on the e during the night are almost invariably seized with r.

FFECTS.—From the recurrence of internal congestions in cold stage, the functions of the liver, bowels, and somes the kidneys, are disordered; the patient becomes w, his limbs waste, the abdomen is distended, and the els are constipated. The spleen is especially liable to be rged, sometimes to a great extent, when it can be felt rnally, attaining a weight of many pounds. An enlarged en is popularly called *ague-cake*. "The heat-generating er of all victims to malaria is impaired; hence they suffer atmospheric changes, of which healthy men take no " (*Maclean*). Another result is extreme liability to ated attacks; for the disease often leaves the body so ebled, that ague may be reproduced by agencies which, er other circumstances, would produce no ill effects. e of the symptoms supposed to be due to malaria are, ever, the effects of over-doses of *quinine or arsenic*, and received the designation of *dumb-ague*.

DUMB-AGUE.—Dr. Bayes, in an excellent pamphlet on "Homœopathy in 1869," clearly shows that what Dr. Golding Bird describes in his work on Urinary Deposits, as *dumb-ague*, with its "sallow aspect, depressed health, and visceral engorgement," is now known to be no ague at all, but is, in reality, slow *quinine-* or *arsenical-poisoning*. The overdosing with *quinine* or *arsenic*, not the ague, is "the poison which remains in the system, and is continuing its work." Indeed, this is proved by Dr. Bird's own experience, for he proposed to cure the so-called "dumb-ague" by eliminating doses of *acetate of potash* and small doses of *mercury*. In short, as Dr. Bayes remarks, the teaching of Dr. Bird may be thus summarised:—*the most successful practice in the treatment of cases originally of ague, where the patient has been slowly saturated with quinine, consists in stimulating the liver by minute doses of mild mercurials, and the kidneys by mild diuretics, to enable them to eliminate and cast out the drug which has caused and is sustaining, an artificial disease in the system.*

CAUSES.—Ague is called an *endemic* disease, because it is peculiar to a particular locality or country. The *exciting cause* is an exhalation of invisible particles from the surface of the ground, known by the term *malaria* or *marsh-miasma*. Malaria is thought to be the product of *vegetable* decomposition in soils, and is inhaled by the lungs during breathing, and thence absorbed into the system. The emanation takes place from marshy lands which have been flooded with water and dried under the influence of the sun's heat, and is most rife in the spring, and when the rains fall upon the decaying leaves of autumn. It is not due, as was formerly supposed, to putrefaction of animal matter. All that seems to be essential to the production of malaria, is the continued action of the sun on moisture stagnant upon or near the surface of the ground. A certain amount of moisture is necessary; for a —— dry season which desiccates a marsh stops the malaria;

while the deposit of the evening dew always favours its production. Excess of moisture, on the other hand, checks its development, so that a very wet season, as well as a very dry one, may render a marsh less unhealthy. But extreme heat does not diminish malaria on the banks of rivers, because portions of these are never dry. The shores of the Black Sea and the Mediterranean are always malarious at the commencement of hot weather, as in the absence of a tide there is none of that frequent salt washing and drainage which purifies other European shores (*Williams*).

The *predisposing causes* are fatigue, exhaustion, insufficient or improper diet, intemperance, exposure to night air, and previous attacks of ague.

Epitome of Treatment.—

1. *Palliatives, during paroxysms.*—Acon., frequently repeated in the cold and hot stages, Ipec., Carbo Veg., or Verat.; also, and chiefly, mitigating the symptoms as they arise, by imparting warmth during the cold stage, removing the patients' coverings and giving cooling drinks during the hot; and supplying him with *warm* and *dry* linen when the perspiring stage has passed by.

2. *Curatives, during the intermission.*—China, Ars., Carbo. Veg., Nat. Mur., Cedron, Nux. Vom., etc.

3. *Consequences of ague.*—Merc. Biniod. (*enlarged spleen*) both internally and as an ointment over the gland; Phos. (*deranged liver*).

4. *Over-dosing by Quinine and Arsenic (Dumb-ague).*—Ipec., Carbo Veg., Cedron.

The *Curative* treatment is of the highest importance, the object being, not directly to arrest the paroxysms, but to bring about such a healthy condition of the system that the disease may gradually decline. It may sometimes be necessary to persevere for several weeks with the appropriate remedy, and not to change it too frequently, or at all, if the paroxysms occur at later periods of the day, and become less severe.

Special Indications.—*China.*—This is a great remedy in recent cases, especially in aguish districts, and when the symptoms are well defined, and take place in the regular order, and with an intermission of comparative health. The symptoms are—*yellowish complexion*; drowsiness after a meal; a sinking or empty sensation, without hunger, or hunger easily satisfied; soreness or swelling of the liver or spleen; watery, slimy, or bilious diarrhœa; extreme sensibility to currents of air; depression and irritability. If preferred, a trituration of *Quinine* may be used in grain doses of the first dec. potency; or four grains of *Quinine* with one drop of *Sulphuric Acid*, may be put into a four-ounce bottle of water, and a dessert-spoonful taken as a dose, every four or six hours, one being administered an hour before a paroxysm is expected to occur. Should *Quinine* have been administered in excessive quantities, *Ars.*, *Cedron*, *Nat. Mur.*, or *Carbo Veg.*, may be substituted.

Arsenicum.—*Chronic ague;* irregular forms of ague, when the stages are not clearly marked, as in simultaneous or alternate shivering and heat, or internal shivering with external heat; *burning heat; insatiable thirst; great debility;* tenderness of the liver and spleen; nausea; *violent pains in the stomach;* great anxiety; tendency to *dropsical affections;* also when *Cinchona* has been used in excess. In *Chronic* ague, *Ars.* is probably the best remedy; in *brow-ague* and *hemicrania*, occurring in marshy districts, it is also very efficacious. A dose every four hours between the paroxysms if they occur daily, or once in six or eight hours if they occur every second or third day.

Ipecacuanha.—Nausea, vomiting, and other *gastric disturbances*, with a thickly-coated, yellowish, moist fur on the

Cedron.—This remedy is considered as a true anti-periodic, and in simple intermittents is said to be infallible. It is also recommended for neuralgia and other disorders when appearing in regularly recurring paroxysms.

Nat. Mur.—This remedy is in high repute in America for chronic intermittents, and is indicated by "bilious vomiting before and during the chill, with great thirst, and sores on the lips or corners of the mouth" (*Pearson*).

Carbo Veg.—This remedy is recommended by Dr. Bayes in the cold stage of ague, when this stage has greatly predominated. We have found it valuable in chronic cases of ague, and have witnessed its power in eliminating from the system the morbid products of the disease; we have proved it also curative of the artificial disease induced by over-doses of *Quinine*,—the *dumb-ague* before referred to.

A much larger list of remedies is often prescribed, but we have treated most unpromising cases with complete success, by means of a small selection.

ACCESSORY MEANS.—One of the first and most essential points is, if possible, removal to a healthy locality; this is often immediately attended by a very marked improvement in the health. If compelled to remain in an aguish district, particular caution is necessary against exposure; patients should not remain out of doors in the evening, or go out too early in the morning, at least not without first taking breakfast; they should also select the loftiest part of the house to sleep in. The light and heat of the sun and the air should be freely admitted during the middle of the day, but the night air carefully excluded. Fatigue should be avoided; also sitting or standing in a current of air.

DIET.—On the days in which the fits occur, the food should be light, and taken in small quantities, observing great care until the paroxysms entirely disappear, not to over-tax the digestive system. Gruel, arrowroot, tapioca, sago, or corn-flour; a little mutton or chicken broth, or tender meat, well masticated, may be taken in the intervals between the fits.

PREVENTIVES.—Persons living in aguish districts should take a dose of *China* morning and night, during the prevalence of the disease. When compelled to be in a malarious atmosphere early in the morning or late in the evening, a good *respirator* should be worn, or, in the case of men, the beard should be cultivated.

12.—Remittent Fever *(Febris remittens)*.

DEFINITION.—Febrile phenomena, with exacerbations and remissions, the remissions being less distinct in proportion to the intensity of the fever, which is *malarious*, and characterized by *great intensity of headache*, the pain darting with a sense of tension across the forehead. It is accompanied by *functional disturbance of the liver*, and frequently *yellowness of the skin*. The *malignant local fevers* of warm climates *are usually of this class (Aitken)*.

SYMPTOMS.—Besides what is stated above, the following details are added.—An attack may come on *suddenly;* or be gradual in its development, and accompanied by the usual precursory chills. The hot stage, or period of *exacerbation*, commences before or about noon and subsides before night, or the reverse; there is much headache, "a painfully acute state of every sense," and great throbbing in the arteries of the neck. There is dry tongue, excessive thirst, tenderness at the epigastrium, and pain in the region of the liver.

Delirium is a frequent accompaniment, being preceded by distressing giddiness; when these symptoms are very marked, or there is lethargy or coma, a severe form of the disease may be expected; there is also sometimes vomiting of colourless, bilious, or bloody matters. The paroxysms may terminate in from six or seven to thirty-six or forty-eight hours. Inability to sleep is most constant. The first exacerbation is the longest; but generally after twelve or sixteen hours the symptoms remit. The duration of the *remission* is as various as that of the hot stage; the second paroxysm is more severe than the first, and is not preceded by chills, etc., but the febrile phenomena are more marked. In bad cases there is jaundice; typhoid symptoms supervene; black vomit may occur, the breath become fœtid, convulsions arise, and death follow. In favourable cases, the disease shews signs of decline after the fifth exacerbation.

TREATMENT.—Dr. Aitken remarks of this fever—"*The first and most immediate object of treatment is to reduce the force and frequency of arterial action during the paroxysm.*" This, to the homœopath, is equal to prescribing *Aconitum*; and though that remedy has no specific relation to the blood-poison itself, it is capable of effecting "the first and most immediate object of treatment."

EPITOME OF TREATMENT.—

1. *Precursory stage.*—Gels., Camph. *(chills)*.
2. *Hot stage.*—Acon. and Bell.
3. *Advanced stage.*—Ipec. *(gastric disturbance)*; Baptisia or Ars. *(typhoid condition)*; Hyos. or Bell. *(delirium)*; Coffæa *(sleeplessness)*; Opi. or Rhus Tox *(coma, or stupor)*; Phos. *(jaundice)*; Ars., Arg. Nit., or Verat. *(excessive vomiting, or black vomit, etc.)*.
4. *During the Remission.*—Quinine.
5. *Prophylactic.*—Gels.

See also "Jaundice," and "Typhoid-Fever." The "Accessory treatment" prescribed in the last-named disease is in most respects suitable to Remittent Fever.

13.—Simple Cholera *(Cholera Simplex)*—English Cholera—Sporadic Cholera.

Definition.—A disease accompanied by *vomiting and purging*, the discharges being of a *bilious* character (distinguishing it from Malignant Cholera, in which the discharges are not bilious), and which, if unchecked, may be followed by *cramps* and a state of *collapse*. It occurs only from occasional causes and in single or scattered cases, hence called *sporadic*.

Summer-diarrhœa, by which is meant the diarrhœa prevalent in autumn and in hot weather generally, is of the same character, and requires similar treatment.

Epitome of Treatment.—Camph. (*Chills*); China (*simple diarrhœic evacuations with griping*); Verat. (*sudden and violent attacks of vomiting and watery diarrhœa, even with cramps and collapse*); Iris Vers. (*bilious motions with colicky pains*); Ars. or Acon. (*collapse*).

For more detailed indications and *Accessory treatment;* the reader is referred to the section on "Diarrhœa."

14.—Malignant Cholera *(Cholera pestifera)*—Asiatic Cholera *(Cholera Asiatica)*—Cholera Morbus—Choleraic Diarrhœa—Cholerine.

In this disease, which resists the efforts of the old system, Homœopathy has won brilliant and undying triumphs. The success of our system in the prevention and cure of Cholera, and other violent diseases, has contributed greatly to its rapid spread in every part of the world. It may be interesting to refer here to the visitation of cholera in 1848–49, when the Government, concerned for the future welfare of the community, determined to adopt the surest means of deciding what was really the most efficient treatment of this disease. A medical committee of the Board of Health, with the President of the Royal College of Physicians at its head, was formed, and an experienced Medical Inspector of the Cholera Hospitals appointed. Printed forms were furnished to each hospital, so that all the circumstances of each case, its symptoms, treatment, and results, might be recorded daily, under the constant supervision of the appointed inspector. The statistics thus obtained were considered and digested by this medical board, and, finally, reported to the Government. It is indeed a humiliating fact to record that this paid board, to whom the Government had confided so important a trust, actually suppressed the statistical report of the Homœopathic Cholera Hospital! This report was afterwards obtained by order of Parliament, and published in a Parliamentary return, dated May 21st, 1855, entitled "Cholera." It testified that, by the Homœopathic treatment of Asiatic Cholera, the death-rate was 16·4 per cent., while according to the aggregate statistics of the other hospitals, it was 59·2 per cent.* "In what language," said the late Dr. Horner, "can I truly designate this conduct of the medical board, but as a conspiracy against the truth and against humanity?"

The history of cholera furnishes a beautiful practical illustration of the worth of that fundamental principle of Homœopathy, namely, that we must ascertain the powers of medicines by testing them upon the healthy body, before they can be properly applied to the removal of disease. Possessed of this knowledge, a medical man can treat a perfectly new disease, or one with which he is totally unacquainted, the symptoms of which correspond with those of

* In an article in the *Lancet* of July 28th, 1866, entitled "Cholera in the Metropolitan Hospitals," the writer states, "It is a melancholy fact to record, but at the time of our last visit no case of undoubted cholera had recovered."

any medicine previously so tested. Thus Hahnemann, from a mere description of the symptoms of cholera, and before he had seen a single case, selected from his Materia Medica those very remedies which have been so triumphantly successful in the hands of Homœopathic practitioners.

DEFINITION.—Malignant cholera, a *miasmatic* disease, *propagated* through the air, and *communicable* from one person to another, is usually ushered in by premonitory diarrhœa, and accompanied by *sudden prostration*, tremors, dizziness, *spasm of the bowels*, faintness, *profuse* serous (rice-water) or bloody *alvine discharges*, *vomiting*, burning heat at the stomach, *coldness and dampness of the whole surface of the body, cold tongue and breath*, *unquenchable thirst*, feeble rapid pulse, extreme restlessness, oppressed breathing, *suppressed urine*, blueness of the body, sunken and appalling countenance, *peculiar odour* from the body, *collapse*, and finally—unless reaction comes on—death.

Under conditions favourable to its development, it often becomes *epidemic*. *(Abridged from Aitken.)*

SYMPTOMS.—As the above definition gives a fair view of the malady, it is unnecessary to describe it further.

CAUSE.—An aerial, or certainly an air-borne *poison*, which, absorbed, infects the blood, and has the power of multiplying itself in the human body to an enormous extent. Pathologists are not yet agreed as to the exact character of the *materies morbi*; but are unanimous in regarding the disease as a most serious one. In India and other Asiatic countries, it is especially sudden and fatal. Instances of death taking place in two, three, four, or more hours, are extremely common. At Teheran, those who were first attacked dropped suddenly down in a state of lethargy, and at the end of two or three hours expired, without any convulsions or vomiting, but from a complete stagnation of the blood. The experience gained during former visitations of Cholera teaches us that it seizes the poor in a far greater proportion than the rich, that the most potent conditions favourable to its spread are poverty, over-crowding, filth, intemperance, and *impure water*, and that as we prevent the accumulation of filth, foul air, and other causes of general disease, and supply the people with wholesome food and pure water, so we render inoperative the powerful agencies by which this dreaded disease chiefly spreads.*

EPITOME OF TREATMENT.—

1. *Premonitory Diarrhœa.*—Camph.
2. *Invasive stage.*—Camph., Acon. (strong tincture in drop-doses).
3. *Fully developed Cholera.*—If Camph. be insufficient—Ars., Verat., Cuprum.
4. *Collapse.*—Ars., Acon.
5. *Typhoid conditions.*—Phos., Ars., Carbo Veg.
6. *Convalescence.*—China, Phos. Ac.

GENERAL INDICATIONS.—*Camphor* should be administered, at frequent intervals, directly the first symptoms of cholera—diarrhœa, chilliness, and spasmodic pains in the abdomen—are noticed. It is often sufficient to cure the disease *immediately* in that stage. Should the disease have much advanced before the administration of *Camph.*, or not yield to it, administer

Aconitum.—Dr. Hempel has found this remedy "eminently useful, during the first invasion of the disease, in restoring the pulse and rousing the vital re-action generally." It should be given in the 1st dec. dil. or mother-tincture. Our own experience with this agent during the epidemic of 1866–7, when we prescribed it in several cases of diarrhœa

* For a fuller discussion of the history, nature, and treatment of Malignant Cholera, including Dr. Rubini's success and the results of his plan as adopted in our own country during the epidemic of 1866–7, see *The Homœopathic World*, vols. I and II.

with great pain in the bowels, coldness of the body, and cadaverous appearance, fully confirms the foregoing statement.*

Arsenicum should be given, every thirty to sixty minutes, when there are cramps, suppressed urine, and *sudden extreme prostration*, the last symptom being more marked than the profuseness of the discharges. But

Veratrum should have the preference if there be *excessive vomiting and diarrhœa*, with cramps.

Cuprum is said to be of service, especially for the cramps and the cyanotic condition.

The remedies most suitable in COLLAPSE and in the TYPHOID CONDITION into which cholera patients often pass, have already been indicated. For detailed symptoms, see the *Materia Medica*, and the section *Typhoid Fever*.

ACCESSORY MEANS.—*Absolute rest* in the recumbent posture, from the very commencement of the initiatory diarrhœa. A *hopeful and cheerful state of mind* should be fostered: a presentiment of death being unfavourable.

PREVENTIVE TREATMENT.—When cholera is epidemic, *Camphor* (the saturated tincture) should be taken once or twice a day, in doses of two or three drops on sugar. The *simple diarrhœa* which often precedes malignant cholera should be promptly met, as it is a serious symptom. *Camph.*, *Ars.*, or *Acon.* may be prescribed according to the indications.

* As an illustration of the value of *Acon.* in cholera, we mention the following facts from our own practice. In 1866 we prescribed, for a patient at a little distance, *Acon.* in a low dilution for severe pain in the abdomen. The medicine produced such striking results in his own case, that, having a large portion to spare, he gave doses of it to his friends when they suffered in a similar manner. Finding the remedy so useful in relieving acute pain, he requested a supply to keep at hand. We furnished it; and at this time cholera broke out in the village, and, although he did not know the name of the remedy, he gave it to as many as he found suffering from cholera, taking the pain in the abdomen as the indication for its use. Death from cholera occurred, but in every instance the patients who had the *Aconite* treatment gr[illegible]vered.

Sanitary and Hygienic Measures.—The following excellent advice has been given, and should be adopted on the earliest indication of cholera :—

The house should be well aired, especially the sleeping apartments, which should be kept dry and clean.

All *effluvia* arising from decayed animal or vegetable substances ought to be got rid of; consequently, *cesspools and dust-holes should be cleaned out, aud water-closets and drains attended to.*

All exposure to cold and wet should be avoided, and *on no account should anyone sit in damp clothes, particularly in damp shoes and stockings. Care should be taken to avoid chills or checking perspiration.*

The clothing worn must be sufficient to keep the body in a comfortable and even temperature.

Habits of personal cleanliness and regular exercise in the open air should be cultivated; also regularity in the periods of repose and refreshment; anxiety of mind and late hours should be avoided.

The diet should be wholesome, and adapted to each individual habit. *Everyone should, however, be more than ordinarily careful to abstain from any article of food (whether animal or vegetable) which may have disordered his digestion upon former occasions, no matter how nutritious and digestible to the generality, and to avoid all manner of excess in eating and drinking.*

Raw vegetables, sour and unripe fruits, cucumbers, salads, pickles, etc., should not be allowed.

The more wholesome varieties of ripe fruits, whether in their natural or cooked state, and vegetables plainly cooked, may be partaken of in moderation, by those with whom they agree.

15.—Diphtheria (*Diphtheria*).

Definition.—Diphtheria is a specific epidemic disease, in which some morbid material has been received into the blood, and in which there is exudation of lymph on the mucous membrane of the mouth, fauces, and upper part of the air-passages, or, occasionally, on an abraded portion of the skin, and attended with general prostration, and sometimes remarkable nervous phenomena.

As just described, it is a blood disease, manifesting local distinctive symptoms. It would be incorrect in theory therefore, and might lead to grave errors in treatment, if the constitutional disturbances were regarded as the effects of the physical changes about the throat, and so concentrating the attention on the tangible mischief, rather than attempting to cope with the whole systemic depression.

Symptoms.—Diphtheria is divisible into two classes, simple and malignant. In the *simple* variety, happily the most common, the symptoms are at first so mild as to excite little complaint beyond slight difficulty of swallowing, or pain in the throat, burning skin, pains in the limbs, etc., and is readily cured by one or more remedies selected according to the subsequent indications. In the *malignant* variety the disease is ushered in with severe fever, rigors, vomiting, or purging, sudden, great prostration and restlessness; the patient has an anxious expression of countenance, and it becomes evident that the system is labouring under some overwhelming disease. The skin is hot, the face flushed, the throat sore, and the mucous membrane bright red; the tonsils are swollen, and grey or white patches of deposit appear on them, small at first, but gradually enlarging, so that one patch merges into another, forming a false membrane in the throat; and swallowing and even breathing become difficult. In some cases, the false membrane has been detached, and after extreme efforts ejected, presenting nearly an exact mould of the throat. The exudation of diphtheria may be distinguished from a slough by its easily crumbling, by the facility with which it can often be detached, and by the surface thus exposed being red, but not ulcerated. The false membrane looks like dirty wash-leather; and between it and the true membrane an offensive bloody discharge exudes, imparting to the patient's breath a most repulsive odour. The glands of the neck are always enlarged, sometimes pain is felt in the ear, and there is generally stiffness of the neck; the inflammation is liable to extend rapidly, in consequence of the continuity of the lining membrane of the throat with the mouth, nose, windpipe, and even the air-tubes of the lungs. If the disease progress, the patient passes into a stupor, and the difficulty of swallowing or breathing increases, till the false membrane is forcibly ejected, or the patient dies from suffocation, the exudation blocking up the air-tubes; or he sinks from exhaustion, similar to that observed in *Typhoid Fever*. The latter is the more frequent cause of death.

Dangerous Symptoms.—A quick, feeble pulse, or a very slow pulse; persistent vomiting; drowsiness and delirium; epistaxis; extension of the disease to the mucous membrane of the nose; dyspnœa; suppressed, or albuminous urine.

Diagnosis.—Diphtheria resembles *Croup* in the exudation of a false membrane on a mucous surface, but differs from it in several points. I. The local inflammation begins in the pharynx instead of the trachea, although it may afterwards spread to the fauces, œsophagus, and respiratory tract. 2. It attacks adults as well as children. 3. It is attended with extreme depression of strength, and in adults is usually fatal by asthenia, but in children sometimes by asphyxia, by obstruction of the larynx.

Some have thought that Diphtheria was only *Scarlatina* without an eruption; but, although there is some analogy between these diseases, further investigation has shown that they are distinct affections. An attack of Scarlatina confers no exemption from subsequent Diphtheria, and *vice versâ*. The after-effects of Diphtheria are of a severe *nervous* character; those of Scarlatina involve mischief in the kidneys or the chest.

Causes and Mode of Propagation.—Impure air, from *imperfect drainage*, living too near manure deposits, slaughter-houses, or where animal substances are in a state of decomposition. It commonly occurs as an *epidemic*, and a solitary case may prove a focus for spreading the disease. The severity of the resulting attack seems to depend as much on the health and vigour of the patient as on the character of the infecting source.

Sequelæ.—After a short period of convalescence—a few days to one or two weeks—sequelæ are apt to arise, usually of disorded innervation, varying from defective nervous power in one or more sets of muscles, to a more or less perfectly defined *paralysis*. Nerves about the throat, the seat of the local manifestation of the disease, are especially liable to suffer, causing chronic difficulty of swallowing, hoarseness, etc. The most alarming sequelæ is loss of nervous power of the heart, with feebleness of action, or, in extreme cases, complete cessation. Recovery, however, from impaired nervous power is not infrequent, though it is generally tedious.

Epitome of Treatment.—

1.—*Mild cases.*—Acon., Bell., or Baptisia, at the commencement; afterwards, if necessary, Merc. Iod., or Nit. Ac.

The treatment recommended in the articles on *Quinsy* and *Croup*, should be consulted, as the remedies there prescribed are often sufficient in Diphtheria.

2.—*Malignant Diphtheria.*—Kali Permang., Mur. Ac., Kali Bich., Ars., Ammon. Carb., etc.

3.—*Sequelæ (after-effects).*—Phos.; Phytolacca *(hoarseness, etc.)*; Coni., Gelsem., Rhus Tox., Sulph.; Dig. *(enfeebled heart)*; Chin. or Quinine *(debility)*.

Special Indications.—*Belladonna.*—Mild cases rapidly recover, and more severe cases often yield under this remedy when perseveringly administered in a low dilution (1st dec.) Dr. Hughes recommends a freer resort to the aid of *Belladonna*, but very properly adds, that if decided improvement have not resulted within forty-eight hours of commencing its use, there is no advantage in persevering with it; or if the symptoms disappear at first under the influence of the remedy, but soon return, it should not be continued.

Muriatic. Ac.—Malignant diphtheria, with foul, greyish ulceration of the throat, fœtid breath, and great general prostration of strength. This remedy should be used in a low dilution, and in frequently-repeated doses; also locally, as a paint to the throat, or as a gargle, when the patient is able to use it in this manner.

Merc. Iod.—This remedy has proved of great value in the disease, and should be administered as soon as any diphtheretic patches are observed in the throat, or swelling of the glands of the neck. Difficult swallowing, pain in and swelling of the salivary glands, and putrid sore throat, indicate this remedy. The first or second dec. trituration is the strength and form on which the greatest reliance may be placed.

Kali Permanganicum.—This appears to be well adapted to malignant diphtheria, with extensive swelling of the throat and cervical glands; pseudo-membranous deposit, partially or completely covering the fauces; obstructed swallowing; a thin, or muco-purulent discharge from the nose, excoriating the parts; thick, obstructed speech, and very offensive breath. "There is no remedy with which I am acquainted that will so rapidly and surely remove the offensive odour of the diphtheretic breath as the *Permanganate*. In this respect, the *Chlorate of Potassa* closely resembles it" *(H. C. Allen, M.D.)*.

The *Permanganate*, or *Condy's Fluid*, should be used locally as a gargle or wash to the affected parts, as well as internally. It may also be used by *inhalation* or by the *spray-producer*.

Baptisia and *Phytolacca*.—Both these American remedies are strongly recommended in diphtheria; the former has a more specific relationship with the blood-poison, and the latter with the local effects of the disease. No cases of diphtheria have occurred in our practice since we have been acquainted with these remedies; and we can, therefore, only recommend them on the authority of others, especially of Dr. Hale.

Arsenicum, in the last stages of the disease, is of immense value, particularly when the prostration of strength is very marked, or is increasing; when there are—œdema, putrid odour of the throat and air passages, and tenacious fœtid discharge from the lining membrane of the nostrils.

Ammon. Carb. is also a valuable remedy in extreme cases, and may be administered alternately with *Ars.* whenever the disease assumes a malignant type.

LOCAL TREATMENT.—In the commencement, a large, thick hot poultice should be applied round the throat; but in advanced severe cases external applications are inadmissible, as they rather tend to increase the œdema and extend the disease. The inside of the throat may be steamed with the vapour of water and acetic acid (a wine-glassful of strong vinegar to a pint of water).

A very abundant and fœtid false membrane is liable to re-infect the system secondarily, and hence such solvents and deodorisers as *Mur. Ac.*, *Kali Permang.*, *Glycerine*, and especially *Acet. Ac.*, are of the greatest value.

Tracheotomy is sometimes performed, but it can hardly be expected to save life, inasmuch as the disease and false membrane extend down the trachea to the bronchi, beyond the reach of this operation.

WARM VAPOUR.—The temperature of the room should be

maintained at 68° Fahr., and the atmosphere made moist by the steam from a kettle with a long spout constantly boiling on the fire. Such an atmosphere is easily secured by forming a tent with blankets over the bed, and then bringing a pipe conveying the steam under it.

WARM-BATHS.—These are most valuable accessories in the treatment of diphtheria. The skin is hot and dry, the urine is often suppressed, the bowels confined, and thus the poison is retained in the system. Warm baths, and the free use of cold water as a beverage, often call into vigorous action the functions of the skin, and the secretions from the bowels and bladder are restored.

ICE.—If vomiting occur, constantly sucking small pieces of ice tends to allay it; it also affords comfort to the patient, and as a diluent it favours the action of the kidneys. The use of ice, therefore, in all cases of diphtheria, croup, and all severe sore throats, should not be forgotten.

DIET, ETC.—The strength of the patient must be well sustained, from the very commencement of the disease, by nourishment, and he must be urged to swallow it in spite of the pain which it occasions. Eggs beaten up in brandy, with hot water and sugar; beef-tea thickened with a little rice or pearl-barley; arrowroot or sago, with port or sherry. Sudden, extreme prostration sometimes requires wine or brandy.

In the case of children who persistently refuse to swallow, recourse must be had at the very outset, in bad cases, to nutritive injections. Dr. Kidd recommends the yolk of an egg beaten up with a tablespoonful of new milk, and two teaspoonfuls of fresh essence of rennet, or an ounce of extract of beef with a scruple of pepsine. Injections should be commenced immediately the true character of the disease is recognised, repeated every two to four hours, and consist of about one ounce at a time.

Convalescence.—Much caution and patience are required during convalescence, as relapses are prone to occur. Nourishing diet, rest, and change of air, are of great utility. Nothing does so much good as a thorough change of air.

Preventive Measures.—The cesspools should be emptied, and if too small or defective, new ones built. The house and local drainage should be thoroughly examined, and imperfections scrupulously rectified; the water-closets carefully trapped and ventilated, and, if necessary, chloride of zinc or of lime constantly kept therein, and thrown down the drains. All dust-holes and accumulations of refuse should be cleared away; while a plentiful supply of water should be kept in the house, and every room regularly well cleaned, whitewashed, and thoroughly ventilated.

16.—Hooping-Cough (*Pertussis*).

Definition.—This is paroxysmal cough of an epidemic and contagious nature, consisting of a series of short, spasmodic, forcible expirations, followed by a deep, prolonged inspiration, attended with a peculiar sonorous sound called the "hoop," "whoop," or "kink," the paroxysms terminating in expectoration or vomiting.

It chiefly affects infancy and childhood, and in delicate or scrofulous constitutions is a distressing malady.

Symptoms.—Hooping-cough is generally preceded by a common cold, cough, and febrile symptoms. After the catarrhal stage has existed from seven to ten days, the cough becomes louder and more prolonged, until it assumes the characteristic convulsive character. Each paroxysm consists of a number of sudden, violent and short *expiratory* efforts or coughs, which expel so large an amount of air from the lungs that the patient appears on the point of suffocation; these forcible efforts are followed by a deep-drawn *inspiration*, in which a rush of air through the partially-closed glottis, gives rise to the distinctive crowing or hooping noise. This *hooping* is the signal of the patient's safety, for when suffocation does take place, it is before the crowing inspiration has been made. During the paroxysms, the face becomes deeply red or black, and swells; the eyes protrude, and are suffused with tears; and the expression and appearance of the sufferer are such as apparently indicate imminent suffocation. The paroxysm terminates by the expectoration or vomiting of a considerable quantity of glairy, ropy mucus, almost immediately after which the child returns to his amusements, and appears quite well. The ropy kind of expectoration which follows the cough enables us to distinguish it from common cough even before the hoop has been heard. The attacks recur three or four times a day, or every three or four hours, or oftener; sometimes blood escapes from the nose, mouth, and even from the ears, during the fits.

PATHOLOGY.—A specific blood-poison, producing a peculiar inflammation of the mucous membrane of the bronchi, and as a consequence of this the absorbent glands at the root of the lungs enlarge and then irritate the branches of the *pneumo-gastric nerve*, which are situated there.

CAUSE.—An unknown *materies morbi* acting in the body, transmitted by the air and by *fomites*.* It spreads by infection, and one attack generally protects the system from its recurrence. As a contagious disease it is most dangerous to the unaffected when at the height of its development.

COMPLICATIONS.—Hooping-cough may be complicated with small-pox, measles, bronchitis, pneumonia, pericarditis, etc. It is therefore desirable that the chest should be examined

* "Hooping-cough was some years ago introduced into St. Helena, where it proved very fatal: the captain of a ship, having some children labouring under the disease on board, allowed their dirty linen to be sent on shore to be washed, and so introduced the disease among the inhabitants" (*Aitken*).

occasionally during the disease by *percussion* and *auscultation*, especially in obstinate cases, so that any complications may be early met by appropriate measures. Convulsions are liable to occur if teething be in progress at the time. If there exist a predisposition to consumption, hooping-cough may hasten its development.

TREATMENT.—The ordinary course of hooping-cough—six weeks to three months, or much longer—may be greatly abridged, and its intensity moderated, by medicines Homœopathic to the condition. As it begins in a common cold, medicines for its early treatment may be chosen from the sections "Cold in the Head," and "Cough;" the prompt use of which may prevent the development of the disease.

EPITOME OF TREATMENT.—

1. *Premonitory febrile symptoms.*—Acon., Bell.
2. *Developed hooping-cough.*—Dros., Coral. Rub.
3. *With gastric symptoms.*—Ipec., Puls., or Ant. Tart.
4. *With convulsions.*—Cup., Bell., Opi., Hydroc. Ac.
5. *With lung complications.*—Acon., Phos., Bry.

SPECIAL INDICATIONS.—*Aconitum.*—Dry, hard, or wheezing cough, with burning pains or tickling in the windpipe, most severe at night, dry heat of the skin, scanty, high-coloured urine, and other febrile symptoms.

Belladonna.—Sudden, violent cough, *worse at night*, with *sore throat*, and determination of blood to the head. In the usual course of hooping-cough, it may advantageously follow *Aconitum*.

Drosera.—Hooping stage, with frequent and excessively severe paroxysms of hoarse, loud cough, sometimes with hæmorrhage from the mouth and nose; there may be no fever, or it may be intense, with perspiration, vomiting of food, water, or slimy mucus. *Drosera* is generally efficient in epidemic hooping-cough, except in scrofulous children, who require professional treatment.

Ipecacuanha.—*Vomiting* of mucus and other *gastric* symptoms; sneezing; watery or bloody discharges from the eyes and nose; violent cough, which threatens suffocation, the face becoming blue and turgid.

Veratrum.—The mucous rattle begins low down in the chest, with tickling irritation, constriction of the larynx, fever, thirst, extreme *weakness*, *cold perspirations*, bluish face, protruding eyes, anxious expression, involuntary escape of urine or fœces during the height of the cough, and vomiting of large quantities of mucus at the end of the paroxysm.

Cuprum.—Violent forms of hooping-cough, causing *convulsions;* the body becomes rigid, the cough suffocating, and the breath nearly suspended during the paroxysms, which occur frequently, and are followed by vomiting, great prostration, and slow restoration.

Opium.—*Stupor*, irregular breathing, constipation; also in cases in which a remedy, well indicated, does not produce the desired results. After a few doses of *Opium* the remedy indicated may be administered.

Phosphorus.—Hooping-cough complicated with *diseases of the chest*, fever, pain, etc.

Cina.—Hooping-cough with worm symptoms, paleness, picking of the nose, itching of the anus, irregular appetite, etc. (See the section on "Worms.") *Cina* is often useful in alternation with *Bell.*, especially if there be symptoms of water on the brain.

Sulphur.—Hooping-cough on the decline; this may be recognised by the phlegm losing its tenacious character and becoming opaque.

Diet.—Light, easy of digestion, and only in moderate quantities; all stimulants should be avoided. Indigestible or too large a quantity of food is almost certain to excite a paroxysm. If fever be present, the use of animal food should be restricted. Toast-and-water, barley-water, gum-water, or linseed-tea, varied to meet the patient's taste, are grateful and soothing.

It is necessary to treat children with great consideration during the complaint, and to overlook many of their dereliotions; as violent emotions of the mind, or fits of anger add to the severity and frequency of the paroxysms. Infants must be constantly watched, taken up as soon as a fit comes on, and placed in a favourable posture.

Frictions with olive oil, or simple liniment, over the chest and along the spine, for ten or fifteen minutes, morning and night, in a comfortably warm room without currents of air, are often of great efficacy.

Accessory Treatment.—During fine, warm weather, the patient should remain in the open air as much as possible; but damp, cold, and exposure to draughts should be strictly avoided. In obstinate cases, and in convalescence, *change of air*, if only for a short distance, proves very beneficial. If possible, mountain- or sea-air, or pure country-air should be chosen, as it acts favourably by removing irritation of the nervous system, and completing the restoration to health.

17.—Mumps *(Parotides)*.

Definition.—An epidemic and contagious affection of the parotid and salivary glands, more prone to attack children than adults, and seldom occurring more than once to the the same person.

Symptoms.—Swelling and soreness in one or both parotid regions, preceded by febrile symptoms. The swelling generally extends from the ears to the glands under the jaw and chin, and the parts are hot and tender. Sometimes one side, and sometimes both sides, are affected; there is often considerable deformity, with difficulty and pain in moving the jaws. On or about the fourth day, in favourable cases, the inflammation and swelling have reached their height, and by about the eighth or tenth day all traces of the complaint have disappeared. Mumps never or rarely lead to suppuration.

METASTASIS.—A curious but important circumstance connected with this affection is, that in many cases, as the swelling of the neck and throat subsides, the *testicles* in the male, and the *mammæ* in the female, become tender and swollen. Occasionally the metastasis is from the neck and throat to the brain, and then it becomes a very serious disease. The transference of the disease from the part first implicated to the testicle, mamma, or brain, is much more likely to supervene when the tumefaction *suddenly* subsides, as on exposure to cold, or from cold applications.

CAUSES.—A specific morbid miasm, generated during peculiar conditions of the atmosphere, which spreads by contagion.* Cold and damp are especially favourable to its appearance. It is also liable to occur during the course of severe fevers, in cholera, and from large doses of *iodine* or *mercury*.

EPITOME OF TREATMENT.—

1. *Premonitory fever*.—Acon. (two or three doses usually sufficient).

2. *Swelling of the glands and difficult mastication*.—Merc. Iod.

3. *Metastasis*.—Bell. *(to the brain)*, Puls. *(to the testicles and mammæ)*.

ACCESSORY MEASURES.—Exposure to cold or damp during the progress of the disease should be avoided; also cold local

* The following fact, from Hooper, illustrates its direct propagation from person to person: "A medical student had *mumps* in London, at a time when his mother was staying with him. They remained in town till the swelling disappeared, and then went—a hundred miles into the country—home. There was no mumps in that neighbourhood; but a fortnight after their arrival one of the children was taken with the disease, and it afterwards successively affected, at regular intervals of a fortnight, each member of a large family."

applications, as they would favour the tendency to metastasis of this disease to more important organs. Warm fomentations are beneficial, the parts being covered in the intervals with one or two thicknesses of flannel roller. In mild cases, a flannel roller is the only local application necessary. Complete *rest*, both physical and mental, and liquid food, favour recovery. All excitement should be avoided.

18.—Influenza (*Catarrhus Epidemicus*).

DEFINITION.—A specific epidemic disease with special and early implication of the mucous membrane of the nose and upper part of the throat, accompanied with lassitude, headache, pains in the limbs, and severe prostration, lasting from four to eight days, and one attack is not preservative against a subsequent one in another epidemic.

It was first called *Influenza* in the seventeenth century, in Italy, because it was attributed to the "Influence" of the stars, and this term has now passed into medical use (*Parkes*). It is supposed to travel from east to west, spreads most rapidly and extensively, and rarely remains more than from four to six weeks in one district. It is most severe in low and insalubrious localities, and at the early part of the visitation. In aged persons, and in others whose lungs have been previously diseased, it is a tedious and sometimes fatal complaint. "In the epidemic of 1847 it has been calculated that in London at least 250,000 persons suffered; in Paris between one-fourth and one-half of the population; and in Geneva not less than one-third" (*Peacock*). The disease is not limited to man, but has been noticed especially in horses and dogs.

DIAGNOSIS.—The symptoms differ from those of common cold chiefly in their sudden appearance and rapid extension among a population, their entire disconnection with either a low or a sudden variation of temperature, the great febrile disturbance which prevails, marked general prostration and nervous depression which accompany and follow the disease, and in their protracted duration.

SYMPTOMS.—There exist chilliness or coldness down the spine, anxiety, feverishness, frontal headache, pains in the limbs and back, severe paroxysms of cough, nausea, loss of appetite, vitiated taste, aching pain and suffusion of the eyes, great sneezing, thin acrid discharge from the nostrils, and extreme prostration of muscular strength. In short, all the symptoms which characterize *gravedo*, *coryza*, and *bronchitis* respectively, are often present in *influenza*.

EPITOME OF TREATMENT.—

1. *Uncomplicated Influenza.*—Ars.
2. *With troublesome cough.*—*K*ali Bich.
3. *Tedious or imperfect recovery.*—Sulph., Phos.

DIET AND REGIMEN.—Farinaceous food, and if there be great prostration, beef-tea, with *repose in bed* or on a couch. In many cases, confinement in bed is quite necessary for the safety of the patient, and always hastens recovery. The room should be warm, well ventilated, and the patient placed so as to avoid draughts or chills. If there be much fever present, with loss of appetite, toast-and-water or barley-water will be suitable. When the cough is very severe, the air of the room should be kept moist by conducting the steam into it from a boiling-kettle by means of a tube, or by putting boiling-water into flat shallow vessels; also *inhalation* of hot vapour is useful (see "Inhalation," Part IV). When the fever abates, a more generous diet should be allowed. If prostration be the predominant symptom, *Liebig's Extract of Beef* should be resorted to. After a severe attack, change of air, with walking- or horse-exercise, is very desirable. During an epidemic of influenza, night-air is invariably injurious.

19.—Erysipelas (*Erysipelas*)—St. Anthony's Fire—Rose.

Definition.—An inflammatory affection of the skin (*simple erysipelas*), sometimes extending into the tissues beneath, with diffuse inflammation of cellular tissue (*phlegmonous erysipelas*); and tending to spread indefinitely.

Idiopathic erysipelas arises from constitutional causes, and generally affects the head and neck; *traumatic* follows a wound or injury, and may occur on any wounded part.

Symptoms.—*Simple erysipelas* is known by a spreading redness of the skin, of an inflammatory character, with considerable puffy swelling, tenderness, burning, and a painful sensation of tingling and tension. The colour of the skin varies from a faint-red to a dark-red or purplish colour, becoming white under pressure, but assuming its former colour on the removal of the pressure. An attack is usually ushered in with shivering, languor, headache, nausea, bilious vomiting, and the ordinary symptoms of inflammatory fever, accompanied or followed by inflammation of the part affected.

Phlegmonous erysipelas is marked by a deeper redness, or it may be redness of a dusky or purple hue, which is scarcely, if at all, removed by pressure; the pain is burning and throbbing; the swelling is greater, and the swollen surface is irregular; and there is often deep-pitting upon pressure. Sometimes the swelling and disfigurement are so great that the features are altogether obliterated, and the parts lose all resemblance to anything appertaining to a human being. Delirium often occurs irrespective of any involvement of the membranes of the brain.

Dangers.—Erysipelas may prove fatal in the following ways:—(1) By *exhaustion*: the constitutional symptoms resemble those of typhoid fever, and the degree of blood-poisoning is great, although the local disease may be limited in extent. (2) By *obstruction to the air-passages:* the inflammation may lead to infiltration of the sub-mucous tissues about the windpipe, the opening into which may be closed, and the patient die suddenly of *apnœa.* The symptoms indicating this condition are—impaired respiration, slight lividity of the lips or finger nails, altered tone of voice, or cough, etc. (3) By *coma*, from effusion within the cranium: this may arise from extension of the inflammation to the membranes of the brain.

Causes.—Debility and loss of resisting power, from disease; the habitual use of stimulants; exposure to cold; impaired digestive organs; wounds; badly-ventilated and over-crowded apartments; certain conditions of the atmosphere; and a morbid state of the blood. The tendency of this disease to attack different parts simultaneously or by *metastasis*—that is, leaving one part and flying to another—furnishes evidence of its origin in a vitiated condition of the blood. The chief *exciting* cause of erysipelas is undoubtedly a recent wound, and the *predisposing* cause is inattention to those hygienic conditions that should surround a patient, combined no doubt with the existence of a personal or family proclivity to the disease.

Prognosis.—The simple or cutaneous variety is attended with much less danger than the phlegmonous. The traumatic form is more dangerous than the idiopathic. It is also more serious when it occurs in an epidemic or endemic form. Mere extent of inflammation is not of so much importance as a high degree of blood-poisoning, combined with a rapid and weak pulse, a dry brown tongue, low muttering delirium, and great prostration. When the disease attacks the head, unless it is controlled by skilful treatment, the membranes of the brain are in danger of being implicated. The disease in any of its forms is most serious at either of the extremes of life. Lastly, the habits and health of the patient, prior to the attack, greatly influence the result. It is especially fatal to drunka[rds] and to patients of a broken-down constitution.

EPITOME OF TREATMENT.—

1. *Febrile stage.*—Acon.
2. *Smooth (non-vesicular) variety.*—Bell.
3. *Vesicular (with little bladders).*—Rhus Tox., Can[th.] Verat. Vir.
4. *With much puffy swelling.*—Apis.
5. *Phlegmonous.*—Ars., Carbo Veg., Nit. Ac.
6. *Gangrene.*—Lach., Ars.
7. *Chronic erysipelas.*—Sulph.

SPECIAL INDICATIONS.—*Aconitum.*—General fever, mu[ch] local inflammation and tenderness. A dose, several tim[es] repeated, at intervals of two or three hours. *Acon.* is mos[t] required before the rash appears, but may be given, if in[di]cated, at any stage of the disease. Hempel recommends t[he] concentrated tincture of the root of *Acon.* as one of the b[est] remedies for either smooth or vesicular erysipelas.

Belladonna.—Cutaneous, bright-red inflammation, swelli[ng] the eruption being *non-vesicular.* If there be *excessive* swelli[ng] *Apis* should be preferred. Violent headache, thirst, consti[pa]tion, and brown-red thick urine, often attend this variety [of] the disease. *Bell.* is especially indicated if the inflammati[on] extend towards the brain, and may sometimes be alternat[ed] with *Acon.* in the early stage of the disease.

Rhus Tox.—*Vesicular* erysipelas, whether on the face or ot[her] part of the body, with swelling, shining redness of the pa[rt] and great restlessness.

Veratrum Vir.—This remedy is also adapted to the ve[si]cular form of the disease, when accompanied by cerebral d[is]turbance.

Apis.—Erysipelas with *acute œdema,* without the inte[nse] cutaneous inflammation indicating *Bell.*, or the disposition [to] form vesicles like *Rhus (Hughes).*

Cantharis.—Erysipelas from the improper use of *Arnica*, and *vesicular* erysipelas.

Arsenicum.—This remedy is indicated when the erysipelatous inflammation assumes a gangrenous character, and also when there is great general prostration.

LOCAL MEASURES.—In the local management of erysipelas, the natural functions of the skin are to be promoted, and currents of air, or exposure of the skin to great variations of temperature, guarded against. In mild forms of the disease, no external applications are required; wet compresses, ointments, etc., are not only useless, but favour the spread of the inflammation. But when there is great heat or irritability of the skin, much relief will be experienced by dusting it over with dry flour, finely-powdered starch, or violet-powder. Flour is also useful to absorb any fluid that exudes from the skin. When, however, inflammatory swellings are very tense and painful, warm fomentations may be first applied, and afterwards the parts sprinkled over with flour or fine starch, or painted with collodion, if the inflammation is of limited extent, or any other suitable substance, to keep out the air. If there is much œdema, moderate pressure should be maintained by the application of well-adjusted bandages. If matter forms, incisions are generally necessary to afford openings for its discharge; poultices are then to be applied, and afterwards bandages, to prevent the lodgement of matter.

Dr. Wilkinson recommends lotions of *Veratrum Viride;* he remarks, "The triumph of *Veratrum Viride*, locally applied to pure erysipelas, is as complete as the art of medicine can desire. Diversity of cases of course require corresponding diversity of treatment; yet, from no slight experience, I can declare that *Veratrum Viride* is a cardinal remedy for erysipelas."

DIET.—Pure water, gum-water, or barley-water, with lemon-juice, to allay the thirst. If the attack is severe and protracted, Liebig's beef-tea, and even wine or brandy may be required. Subsequently, a change of air, regular habits, and nourishing diet, essential in the after-treatment of all acute diseases, are necessary after a severe attack of erysipelas.

20.—Puerperal-Fever *(Febris puerperarum)* and Puerperal Ephemera *(Ephemera puerperarum)*.

DEFINITIONS.—*Puerperal-fever* is a continued fever, communicable by contagion, occurring in connection with childbirth, and often *associated with extensive local lesions*, especially of the uterine system.

Puerperal ephemera (sometimes called *weed*) is a fever, consisting of one or more paroxysms, occurring a few days after delivery, generally attended by diminution of the milk and lochia, and *unaccompanied by local lesions*.

EPITOME OF TREATMENT.—

1. *Invasive stage.*—Acon.
2. *Cerebral disturbance.*—Bell.
3. *Complications.*—Bry., Acon., Bell., Merc., Hyos., Stram., Ars., etc.

For *Special Indications* and *Accessory Treatment*, see the author's "Lady's Homœopathic Manual," where these diseases are more fully considered.

CHAPTER II.

General Diseases *(continued)*:—B. Constitutional Diseases.

21.—Acute Rheumatism *(Rheumatismus acutis)*— Rheumatic Fever.

Definition.—A specific febrile disorder, accompanied by acute inflammation of the white fibrous tissues,—ligaments, tendons, sheaths of tendons, aponeuroses, fasciæ, etc., surrounding the joints, of which several are affected simultaneously or in succession. The local symptoms are very erratic; the skin of the affected part is covered with a copious sour, sticking perspiration, containing lactic acid; and the blood has a large excess of fibrine, probably to the extent of thrice the normal quantity.

Sub-acute Rheumatism is the same affection in a modified form, often following upon the acute disorder.

Symptoms.—Acute rheumatism is usually ushered in with febrile disturbances, followed by the local attack of inflammation of the fibrous structures about one or more of the larger joints—the shoulder, elbow, knee, ankle, the fibro-serous covering of the valves of the heart, the pericardial sac, etc. Exposed joints appear to be more prone to attacks than those that are covered, the larger more frequently than the smaller, and the small joints of the hands more frequently than those of the feet. Sprained or otherwise injured joints are particularly liable to suffer. The general febrile condition often precedes the local inflammation one or two days; sometimes the general and local symptoms occur simultaneously, while in others the inflammation of the joints precedes the febrile condition. The affected joints are swollen, tense, surrounded by a rose-coloured blush, and acutely painful; pain, however, is a more constant symptom than swelling, and swelling than redness. The pain of rheumatism has many degrees of intensity, is generally intermittent, abates somewhat in the day, but is aggravated at night, and in all cases is increased by pressure, so that even the touch of the medical attendant or nurse, or the weight of the bed-clothes can scarcely be borne. Often the patient remains fixed, as it were, in one posture, from which he dare not move, and declares that he has lost the use of a limb. The skin is hot, but covered with a sour sweat, having an offensive odour, and so highly acid as to redden litmus paper. The perspirations, although unattended by immediate relief, are nature's mode of elimination, for the pains are always aggravated, and the constitutional symptoms intensified, if they become suppressed. It is only when the perspirations lose their characteristic *sour* character that they become useless. The *urine* in acute rheumatism is scanty, of high specific gravity, and deposits on cooling, deep-coloured sediments of urates. The pulse is round and full; the tongue loaded with a yellowish-white mucus, but the head is unaffected, or but slightly so. The usual absence of headache or delirium is a distinguishing point between acute rheumatism and the continued fevers.

"Such are the general and local expressions of a diseased state of the system in acute rheumatism; and at the height of the disorder it is difficult to conceive a more complete picture of helplessness and suffering than that to which the patient is reduced. A strong and powerful man, generally unused to disease, lies on his back motionless, unable to raise his hand to wipe the drops which flow fast from his brow in the paroxysms of pain, or the mucus which irritates his nostril. Indeed, he is so helpless that he is not only obliged to be fed, but to be assisted at every operation of nature. The sweat in which he lies drenched seems to bring him no relief; his position admits of no change; if he sleeps, it is short, and he wakes up with an exacerbation of suffering which renders him fretful, impatient, and discontented with all around him" (*Aitken*).

The *erratic* character of rheumatism is usually well expressed; it often suddenly quits one joint to appear in another, and then in another, afterwards, perhaps, travelling back to its original seat, the development of inflammation in one joint being often accompanied by its rapid subsidence in another, this alternation occurring many times during an attack. But the most serious metastasis is from the joint-structures to other fibrous tissues, as the pericardium or the valves of the heart. This complication may be expected in very severe attacks, in young persons, in women oftener than in men, in patients who have been weakened by disease or other causes, and in persons troubled with irritability or palpitation of the heart.

Heart-Complications.—When cardiac inflammation arises, the patient's countenance becomes dreadfully anxious, the breathing distressed, and pain is complained of in the heart's region; also there is tenderness between and under the ribs, and there may be palpitation or irregular action of the heart. The physical *signs* of *pericarditis* (inflammation of the membrane or bag that surrounds the heart) may be detected by the stethoscope, and a distinct friction or *to-and-fro* sound heard, like the rubbing of paper, owing to the roughening of the serous surfaces by effusion of fibrine. This sound may soon be lost, either from the opposite surfaces becoming glued together, or separated by serous effusion. If the amount of effusion be large, both the circulation and the respiration become seriously embarrassed, the heart beats tumultuously, the sounds become muffled, and there is increased extent of dulness in the heart's region.

Endocarditis (inflammation of the inside lining of the heart, especially of the valves) may arise, with pericarditis or separately. The *symptoms* are similar to those of pericarditis, but the physical *sign* is a *bruit* (a modification or an unnatural character of one or both of the natural sounds of the heart).

In consequence of the extreme danger of these complications all cases of severe rheumatic fever should be watched daily by a medical man, so that the signs and symptoms of heart-complications, which often come on very insidiously, may be early recognised, and appropriate treatment at once adopted.

RHEUMATISM AND GOUT.—For a tabular statement of the differences between these diseases, see the section on "Gout."

CAUSES.—The *predisposing* cause is some morbid product in the blood, a product probably of unhealthy assimilation. "The circulating blood carries with it a poisonous material, which by virtue of some mutual or elective affinity falls upon the fibrous tissues in particular, visiting them and quitting them with a variableness that resembles caprice, but is ruled, no doubt, by definite laws, to us, as yet, unknown" (*Watson*). These *materies morbi* with which the blood is loaded, constitute that predisposing cause without which it is probable the disease would never occur. Hereditary predisposition exists undoubtedly in many persons. The suppression of an eruption or rash, as measles, or the sudden stoppage of dysentery, may also act as a predisposing cause.

The *exciting* causes are, exposure to cold and wet, especially *evaporation* from wet or damp clothes, causing chill. This is no doubt an explanation why the disease is most common among the poorer classes of society, who cannot protect themselves so effectually as their wealthier brethren. The cold probably excites an attack of acute rheumatism by arresting the secretory functions of the skin, by means of which, in health, morbid substances in the blood are often removed; now, however, the functions of the skin being deranged, unhealthy principles accumulate in the blood, and rheumatism results. Mere cold, however, is not so much a cause of rheumatism as extreme atmospheric vicissitudes. Hence it is found that it does not prevail most, abstractedly, in the coldest regions of the globe, but rather in those climates and during those seasons remarkable for damp and changeable weather.

EPITOME OF TREATMENT.—

1. *Rheumatic Fever.*—Acon., Bry., Bell.

2. *Complications and secondary disorders.*—Cimic., Cactus Grand., Spig., or Ars. *(for the heart)*; Colch., Coloc., Ran. Bulb., Rhodod., Rhus Tox., or *Kali* Iod. *(for the joints)*.

3. *Sub-acute.*—Cimic., Rhus Tox.

4. *Wandering Rheumatism.*—Puls., Cimic. Rac.

5. *Rheumatic Gout.*—Colch., Puls., Coloc. See also under "Chronic Rheumatism."

TREATMENT.—*Aconitum.*—Acute rheumatism, especially at the commencement, *when the fever is high*, and there are violent shooting or tearing pains, worse at night, and aggravated by touch. Also swelling and redness of the affected parts, impaired appetite, high-coloured urine, and other febrile symptoms. *Acon.* may be administered either alone or in alternation with *Bry.*, at intervals of one to three hours; or the latter may be administered in the day time, and the former at night. In numerous instances, *Acon.* is sufficient in the early stage of Acute Rheumatism to cure it without the aid of any other remedy. It should be given in a low dilution.

Bryonia.—This remedy is most frequently required after the use of *Aconitum*, and is chiefly indicated when the pains are lancinating or stitching, and seem to affect the muscles rather than the bones; are worse on *the least movement*, but are relieved by rest; there also exist febrile heat, gastric derangement, profuse perspiration or coldness and shivering, and irritability of temper. *Cardiac, lung,* or *pleuritic complications* are but extensions of the rheumatic disease, and are not, therefore, necessarily indications for any change from *Bry.* or *Acon.* It is sometimes necessary to change the remedy to *Rhus*, if the tendons become implicated.

Sulphur.—This remedy is especially indicated if the constitutional predisposition is strongly marked, and should be given for some time after the acute symptoms have subsided, to complete the cure and prevent obstinate sequelæ; also as an intercurrent remedy. It is especially useful in rheumatism following repelled eruptions, and when the pains are drawing and tearing, *worse when cold*, and *better when warm*.

DIET.—During the fever the diet should be mainly restricted to water, milk-and-water, barley-water, gruel, and arrow-root, at least at first; afterwards, beef-tea, mutton-broth, etc. In rheumatic-fever there is a strong argument for restricting the supply of nutriment to a liquid form. If meat be given before the power of fully converting it into living flesh is restored, a semi-conversion into lactic acid takes place, and then a febrile disturbance is produced, which is followed by a return of the rheumatic pains. Or perhaps rheumatic fever is due to an excess of lactic acid in the blood; and if so, the relapse which ensues on the generation of it is readily explicable. Vegetable matter does not expose patients to the same danger, and thus by dint of rice-puddings, porridge, gruel, bread, mashed potatoes, and the like, we may satisfy the hunger of our patients without provoking a relapse of rheumatic fever, which solid meat is likely to do *(Chambers)*.

HYDROPATHIC TREATMENT in the early stages of the disease is highly beneficial. Warm baths, hot-air baths, or hot compresses, are both useful and comforting. *Spongiopiline*, made into gloves or caps for the hands, feet, elbows, or knees, or shaped to cover any large surface, is an excellent substance for conveying moisture to the parts. The spongy surface should be wetted, and every few hours re-moistened. *Wet-packings*, repeated as often as the fever returns, and enveloping the joints which are chiefly implicated, or even the whole body, with several folds of wet linen, are most useful adjuncts. Except, however, when the skin is *hot and dry*, *cold* applications are contra-indicated, as from the migratory character of the disorder, great risk would be incurred of repelling the poison into the circulating fluid, to settle possibly upon the heart or other internal part. But no danger of this character belongs to warm fomentations, or to hot compresses, which often afford great relief to the patient.

Blankets in Rheumatism.—An invaluable adjunct to the measures already suggested is that of enveloping the patient in blankets and flannel. "Bedding in blankets reduces by a good three-fourths the risk of inflammation of the heart run by patients in rheumatic fever, diminishes the intensity of the inflammation when it does occur, and diminishes still further the danger of death by that or any other lesion; and at the same time it does not protract the convalescence" (*Chambers*).

22.—Muscular Rheumatism (*Rheumatismus musculorum*).

Definition.—"Pain in the muscular structures, increased by motion."

The local varieties of this affection are, *Lumbago* and *Stiff-neck*.

a.—Lumbago (*Lumbago*).

Definition.—Rheumatism of the sheaths of the fleshy mass of the lumbar muscles on one or both sides of the loins, extending often to the ligaments of the sacrum; the pain is aggravated by movement of the back, and by pressure on the affected muscles.

Treatment.—*Rhus Tox.*—Chronic lumbago; lumbago from getting wet: pains increase during repose, at night, and on *first* moving the affected part.

Arnica.—Lumbago implicating muscles that have formerly been injured, as by over-lifting, a sprain, or a blow.

Aconitum.—Recent rheumatism of the lumbar muscles, unassociated with any injury to the affected parts.

ACCESSORY MEANS.—*Liniments*, medicated with the same remedy as administered internally, rubbed into the affected parts, are very useful. The frictions should be performed in a warm room, and currents of air guarded against. A *wet compress*, simple, or medicated with the same remedy as administered internally, greatly assists the cure. In this and other varieties of muscular rheumatism, rest and warmth are of the greatest importance. In lumbago, nothing is so instantaneously beneficial as strapping the back from the level of the "seat" upwards, in layers that overlap each other, with strips of adhesive-plaster, or warm plaster (*Tufnell*).

b.—STIFF-NECK (*Cervix rigida*)—CRICK-IN-THE-NECK.

DEFINITION.—A rheumatic affection of the muscles of the side of the neck, chiefly the sterno-cleido-mastoideus, which become rigid, hard, and swollen, and the least attempt to turn the neck is attended with acute pain. Sometimes the rheumatism extends to the articulations of the clavicle and intercostal muscles.

EPITOME OF TREATMENT.—

1. *From exposure to draughts.*—Acon.
2. *From damp weather.*—Dulc.
3. *With tearing lancinating pains.*—Bell.

RHEUMATISM AND MUSCULAR WEAKNESS.—The diagnosis of muscular rheumatism is apt to be mistaken for painful muscular affections following prolonged or excessive exertion, or soreness or stiffness, which occur during convalescence from any long illness, or accompany general debility from any other cause. These affections are generally better in the morning after the repose of the night, but increase with fatigue; and the pain in the affected part is mitigated by relaxing or supporting it. The diagnosis is important, especially to medical men, because if we fail to prescribe appropriate medicines, nourishing diet, and proper rest and support to the weak muscles until they regain their tone, we shall fail to benefit the patient, who possibly in his contempt for medicine, as Dr. Tanner remarks, will hasten to try the good diet and pure air of some hydropathic establishment, and then circulate reports of his extraordinary cure, "after having been given over by the faculty."

23.—Chronic Rheumatism (*Rheumatismus longus*).

Definition.—Chronic pain, stiffness and swelling of various joints.

This is sometimes a sequel of the acute form of rheumatism; at other times it is a separate constitutional affection, coming on quite independently of any previous attack. It is generally very obstinate, prone to recur, and is often worse at night. In time, the affected limbs lose their power of motion, and lameness results, the knee-joint being often affected; sometimes there is emaciation of the muscles; sometimes permanent contraction of a limb, or bony stiffness of the joint. There is but little febrile disorder, no perspirations, and less swelling than in acute rheumatism.

Varieties.—Rheumatism is variously described according to the parts implicated, and the conditions with which it is associated. When the sheaths of the fleshy mass of muscles on one or both sides of the loins are affected, and the pain is increased by movement of the back, or by pressure, it is called Lumbago. When the neurilemma of the sciatic nerve, in its course along the thigh to the knee, or even to the foot, Sciatica. When the sheaths of the muscles of the neck,

CRICK IN THE NECK. When the fibrous fascia of the intercostal muscles, PLEURODYNIA; etc.

TREATMENT.—In treating chronic rheumatism, the reader must bear in mind that the dyspeptic-symptoms often associated with the disease are primary considerations; and that little hope of a cure can be expected till they are remedied. Suitable medicines will be found in the following list and in the section on "Dyspepsia."

SPECIAL INDICATIONS.—*Rhus Tox.*—When the sheaths of tendons, muscles, etc., are chiefly affected; the pains worse during rest, and at night in the warmth of the bed; also pains much increased on first moving, but wear off with continued exercise. Creeping sensations also may be present. In rheumatic lameness generally, with the above symptoms, it is often curative.*

Bryonia.—Chiefly when the lower limbs are affected; severe pains down the calf of the leg; shining red swellings, with heat and dryness of the parts. The pains are aggravated by motion. It should not be lost sight of in the indigestion, constipation, etc., associated with the disease.

Aconitum.—This remedy is often of service, is sometimes even curative, in chronic rheumatism. It is more especially adapted to rheumatism of the shoulder, and of the large joints generally, when there is no rigidity. Also in rheumatism of the heart, with congestion and sense of anguish. It should always be administered during febrile disturbance.

Rhododendron.—This is a valuable medicine in rheumatism. Three of its most marked indications are—the pains are worse during rest, in the warmth of bed, and with every unfavourable change of the weather. It has cured cases in which there were swelling and redness of both the large and small joints, tension, and rigidity.

* Several interesting cases illustrating the value of *Rhus Tox* in chronic rheumatism, as well as cures by other remedies, may be found in the "Cases from Practice" in *The Homœopathic World*, Vol. III.

Ledum Palustre.—Predominant chilliness, associated with rheumatism of the small joints.

Dulcamara.—Rheumatism from exposure to damp, accompanied by œdematous swellings, and somewhat relieved by rest. Stiff-neck occurring under the same conditions.

Pulsatilla.—When the knee, ankle, or instep is affected; and when there are *fugitive* rheumatic pains in various parts of the body; especially in females with scanty menstruation.

Cimicifuga Rac.—Local manifestations of rheumatism, such as lumbago, pain in the side; also in affections of the heart consequent on rheumatic-fever. Wandering-rheumatism is also within the curative sphere of *Cimic.*

Phytolacca.—This remedy bids fair to become very useful in this disease, and has cured cases of many years standing, with stiffness of the joints, and even loss of the use of the affected limb. If the periostial covering is implicated, *Phyto.* is the more indicated. Dr. Hale considers it an analogue of *Kali Iod.*

Arnica.—Stiffness in the large joints; tearing pains in the small joints, with pricking; sensations in the parts as if they were bruised. Also when rheumatism is associated with a previous wound.

Causticum has been useful in "rheumatism of the joints with swelling and stiffness, contraction of tendons, shooting and tearing pains, especially in scrofulous patients."

Mercurius.—Puffy swelling of the affected parts; the pains feel as if seated in the bones or joints, and are increased by warmth, and at night; there are also chills, and *profuse perspiration*, which do not give relief.

Sulphur.—Either before the above remedies, or after them, to complete the cure; also as an intercurrent remedy. It is especially useful in rheumatism from hereditary taint, and when it follows repelled eruptions; also when the pains are drawing and tearing, *worse when cold*, and *better when warm.*

Kali Iodidum,* *Kali Bichromicum*, *Bell.*, *Coloc.*, *Ranun. Bulb.*, *Mangan.*, and *Colch.*, are also serviceable remedies. The higher dilutions are generally found most useful.

ACCESSORY MEANS.—Patients who are much afflicted with this complaint, and who are in a position to do so, should reside in a warm, *dry* climate. At any rate such patients should wear flannel and other warm clothing, and protect themselves against atmospheric changes. Shoes and boots should have soles sufficiently thick to protect the feet from cold and damp. Wet compresses, covered with dry flannel, over the joints specially attacked, are always useful. Sometimes warm baths, especially of salt water, or vapour, or hot-air, will be found very serviceable. To these means may be added friction with *Liniments*, especially when medicated with *Arnica*, *Rhus Tox.*, or whatever remedy is taken internally. One more point necessary to refer to is the *diet*, which should be easy of digestion, as attacks are often occasioned by disorder of the digestive organs.

24.—Acute Gout *(Podagra acuta)*.

DEFINITION.—A specific febrile disease, usually occurring in paroxysms at longer or shorter intervals, characterised by non-suppurative inflammation, with considerable redness of certain joints—chiefly of the hands and feet, and, especially in the first attack, of the great toe—and accompanied with excess of uric acid in the blood. The disease is largely traceable to hereditary influence, and a "fit of the gout" is always associated with derangement of the digestive and other organs.

SYMPTOMS.—An acute attack of gout is often preceded by an excessive debauch, or by over-fatigue, impairing the di-

* For two remarkable cases cured by this remedy see *The Homœopathic World*, Vol. III.

gestive powers, its onset commonly commencing an hour or two after midnight, when indigestion from a supper or late dinner arises at its acme. Ordinarily a patient retires to rest in his accustomed health, but awakes early in the morning with severe pain, chiefly in the metatarso-phalangeal joint of the great toe, which on examination is found red, hot, swollen, and so exquisitely tender that the mere weight of the bed-clothes is intolerable, and the vibration of a heavy footfall in his room causes great discomfort. The veins proceeding from the toe become turgid with blood, and surrounded with more or less œdema. On the first accession of the pain there is generally cold shivering, which gradually subsides as the pain increases, and is followed by symptomatic fever. The patient is perpetually shifting his foot from place to place, and from posture to posture, change of place giving no relief. At length, if suitable precautions are taken, and the foot kept in a horizontal posture, the pains subside in the early part of the day; but at evening an exacerbation takes place, which persists during most of the night, and subsides again towards morning, when he falls asleep in a gentle perspiration. Sometimes the pains remit so suddenly that the patient attributes the relief to his having at last found an easy posture. The same series of symptoms recur, in a less severe form, for some days and nights, varying considerably in different cases, and greatly influenced by the treatment adopted; and then the attack passes off, not to return for one, two, or after a first attack, perhaps for three years. After the lapse of years, however, the intervals between the attacks are liable to diminish until the patient can scarcely ever calculate upon being free. The joints of the fingers and toes become enlarged and disorganised by deposit within and without the synovial cavity of a white saline matter, commonly called "chalk stones," but really *urate of soda.*

It is not uncommon, even in a first attack of gout, for both great toes to be implicated, generally alternately, the inflammation rapidly subsiding in one joint to appear in the other, but sometimes simultaneously. In many instances, after first attacks, other joints, the instep, ankle, the heel, or the knee are affected at the same time; in rarer cases, some joints of the upper extremities.

SYMPTOMS PRECEDING AN ATTACK.—Flatulence, heartburn, acidity, relaxed or confined bowels, and other disorders of digestion are usually present. In some patients the function of breathing is implicated, or the liver deranged; in others the nervous system is involved, with palpitation; or there may be alteration of the urinary secretion, or a crampy condition of the muscles. Such symptoms are no doubt consequent on the altered state of the blood, which always exists prior to the development of a regular fit of gout. Should any organ or function be specially implicated, it is then termed *irregular gout*.

CAUSES.—Gout is generally hereditary, but it may be acquired. The experience of physicians largely engaged in treating the disease, proves that more than half the gouty patients can trace the disease to hereditary influence; and if the wealthy portion of the community were only included, the proportion would be much greater. Large-built men, of a full and luxurious mode of life, particularly if addicted to indulgence in *wine* and *malt liquor*, and too much animal food, combined with too little exercise, are very liable to the disease, whether a predisposition has been transmitted or not. That wine and malt liquor have a greater tendency to the production of gout than distilled spirits is proved by its prevalence in those countries or cities in which these beverages are largely consumed, and its absence where distilled spirits are almost exclusively made use of. Thus gout is more frequent in London, where porter and beer are largely partaken of, than in Edinburgh, where the favorite beverage is whisky. Gout is very common amongst brewers' men; also amongst ballast men employed on the Thames, who often drink from *two to three gallons of porter daily.** Gout prevails largely in Germany, and in most countries where beer is the ordinary beverage of the people. *Port-wine* has a marked reputation, and probably justly, for causing gout; and sherry is by no means so harmless a beverage as many suppose. It is chiefly a disease of the *male* sex, although occasionally women of a robust and plethoric habit suffer with it, after the cessation of the catamenial function. That luxurious living and an inactive life are at least exciting causes of gout seems evident from the exemption of working people in rural districts from the disease. Even when the disease does occur in poor people it is chiefly in persons who have previously lived fully and inactively, such as the servants of wealthy families—butlers, coachmen, etc.,—men who often live more luxuriously and idly than their masters.

The connexion existing between gout and convivial excesses is proved by the much less frequent occurrence of the disease consequent on improved habits as to diet. The heroic appetite of our chivalrous ancestors, the bold barons of feudal times, who used to treat their guests to an ox roasted whole, and the suppers of Lucullus, are past and gone. We are less partial to animal food, our meals are shorter, our potations

* "Observant men are now inclined to discard the doctrine which teaches the noble origin of gout, and its necessary association with high mental development. The disease is now certainly common and plebian, as well as aristocratic. It may have been, in the days of Sydenham, that the gouty patients of a physician were to be found amongst '*magni reges, dynastæ exercituum, classiumque duces, philosophi, aliique his similes.*' Now-a-days it is no less certain that the physician, in London at least, must pay his visits and prescribe for gout amongst 'the London labour,' as well as among 'the London poor.' And his list will number 'coal-heavers, bakers, brewers, draymen, house-painters, butchers, innkeepers, publicans, butlers, coachmen, and porters in wealthy families especially'" (*Aitken*).

less deep, and consequent on these changes gout has gradually gone out.

Unless the gouty diathesis be very strong, the actual manifestation of the disease may generally be averted. Let the son of a rich gouty nobleman take the place of a farm servant, and earn his temperate meal by daily toil, and very likely he will wholly escape a visitation of the malady. Probably the operation of this cause explains how it is that gout leaps over one generation, while the predisposition descends through those who have never actually had the disease. In fine, gout, in familiar language, is often said to be the result of a surplus of receipts.

The influence of *lead* in the production of gout Dr. Garrod believes to be considerable; he has observed that a large per centage of the gouty patients that come under his care in hospital practice consisted of painters, plumbers, or other workers in lead, forcing him to the conclusion that the influence of this form of metallic impregnation in inducing gout is considerable.

Among the *exciting causes* of gout may be mentioned *indigestion*, especially that form of it which favours the production of an excessive amount of acidity in the system, causing a less alkaline state of the blood, and so tending to the insolubility and deposition of the urate of soda in the tissues. During an attack of gout, uric acid is said to be absent from the urine, the kidneys not excreting it; hence it collects in the blood, and in the serum may be detected by the microscope in minute crystals upon threads immersed in it, after the addition of a little hydrochloric acid.

The influence of *season and climate* has much to do in exciting a paroxysm of gout. First attacks are much more common in spring; as the disease becomes more confirmed, an autumnal seizure is added; after the lapse of a long time, a fit may occur at any season, and at most irregular intervals.

DIFFERENCES BETWEEN GOUT AND RHEUMATISM.

GOUT.	RHEUMATISM.
1. In the earlier attacks, the *small joints* are affected, the metatarsal joint of the great toe being chiefly implicated.	1. The *large joints* are chiefly implicated, several being affected at the same time.
2. Rarely occurs *before* puberty, and generally not till from 35 to 50 years of age.	2. Generally *occurs in the young*, from 20 to 30 years of age, and often earlier.
3. Is more frequent in *men* than women, and in the latter rarely till after the cessation of the menstrual function.	3. Affects *men and women* equally.
4. Is often the punishment of an *idle*, luxurious, and intemperate life.*	4. Is the lot of the *poor*, the hard-working, the exposed, and the ill-clad.
5. Is strongly *hereditary*.	5. Is but *slightly* hereditary.
6. Is associated with *chalk-stones* (urate of soda) in the external ear, on the tops of the fingers, or other situations.	6. Is *never* associated with chalk-stones.
7. A fit of gout often affords great temporary relief, so much so that patients are often sent to Bath to obtain one.	7. An attack of Rheumatism has not one redeeming feature in it, and patients are sent to Buxton to get cured if it be possible.
8. Is confined to the temperate regions of the world.	8. Rheumatism appears to prevail in all climates, and has been called an ubiquitous disease.

EPITOME OF TREATMENT.—

1. *During an attack of Gout.*—Colch., Acon., Bry.

2. *External applications.*—Acetic Ac. *Formula.*—Acet. Ac. Sp. g. 1.044, ʒj., Spt. Vini. ʒvj., Aq. Dest. ℥vj. mix. Dr.

* This, it has been observed, may be illustrated on a large scale by a regiment of soldiers, in which we can scarcely find a case of gout among the privates, whereas, after attaining the rank of quartermaster, diminished exercise and a stimulating diet is found to affect many.

Hastings recommends the inflamed part to be bathed with the lotion, and cloths saturated with it kept constantly applied, and covered with dry flannel. He has adopted this lotion, administering Acon. internally at the same time, with excellent results. For particulars, see *The Homœopathic World*, vol. iv., pp. 74–5.

Lotions of *Acon.* applied locally to the inflamed surface, or of any other drug used internally, are often employed with great success.

3. *Between the paroxysms.*—Puls., Nux. V., Merc. Iod., Bry., Rhodod., Rhus Tox., Arn., Sulph.

LEADING INDICATIONS.—

Colchicum.—This remedy bears a Homœopathic relationship to gout, and is best administered in comparatively large, and frequently-repeated doses, as follows:—Twenty drops of the strong tincture to be added to a tumblerful of water, and a dessert-spoonful given every twenty, thirty, or sixty minutes, according to the intensity of the pain, and until it subsides. *Colchicum* is a drug used both in the new and in the old school of medicine, with this difference, that all the good effects of the remedy are secured by the small doses of the former, without any of the injury the large doses of the latter entail. The following extracts from a leading physician of each school will be read with interest:

"There is one drug (says Dr. Garrod) which has an undoubted influence in controlling gouty inflammation, and its action in articular gout appears as marked as that of *Cinchona Bark* in the cure of ague: this remedy is *Colchicum*. It signifies not what part of the colchicum plant is taken, whether the corn, the seeds, or the flowers, for the same principle pervades the whole plant; neither does it signify what preparations are made use of, whether the wine, the tincture, or the extract, provided equivalent doses be administered, for the effects of all are the same.

"*Colchicum*, as before stated, has a direct controlling power over the joint disease, and I cannot call to mind a single instance in which its in- ...ce was not well marked."

"In adopting *Colch.* as the remedy for the gouty paroxysms, Homœopathy may do something towards removing those inconveniences which beset its administration in the old school. Probably, all the bad effects which result from over-doses may be averted by a reduction of the dose. Should the pain recur in the same, or attack other joints, *Colchicum* should be resumed.

"In the interim, any medicine which seems Homœopathic to the general condition may be given, having especial regard to the digestive organs. *Puls.*, *Nux Vom.*, and *Merc.* are the remedies most frequently indicated: and sometimes the state of the circulation requires *Acon.*

"When the patient has passed through an acute attack, the morbid diathesis has to be corrected; and there seems no doubt but that in gout the fault lies in the primary digestion.

"This part of the treatment is of paramount importance, and here Homœopathy comes to help us with its array of anti-dyspeptic medicines. I cannot enumerate these, or define the place of each: every case must be treated as an individual, and a remedy selected according to the character of the digestive derangement present. In confirmed gout, Dr. Acworth states that he has seen much benefit from the administration of *Sulphur*: and the frequent determination of the poison to the skin in the form of psoriasis or eczema adds force to his recommendation" *(Hughes)*.

Accessory Measures.—During an attack of gout, the affected limb should be raised, so as to favour the free return of blood to the heart; the application of flannels wrung out of hot water, hot bread-and-water poultices, or *spongio-piline*, after immersion in hot water, often do good; or the *acetic acid lotion*, before recommended, may be used. In acute attacks, the patient should be restricted to farinaceous diet—arrowroot, tapioca, sago, bread, etc., and milk; water, or toast-and-water, *ad libitum*. As the febrile symptoms decline, a more generous diet may be gradually allowed; at the same time, the patient should resume daily moderate out-of-door exercise as early as he is able.

Preventive Treatment.—To prevent subsequent attacks of gout, or to diminish their frequency or severity, the following suggestions should be acted upon, and will often prove efficient.

1st. *A well-chosen diet.* This should include both animal and vegetable food, of such quality and quantities as the stomach can easily digest, and as will, at the same time, furnish materials sufficient to nourish the patient, and out of which pure blood can be formed. White fish, soles, whiting, and codfish; mutton, tender beef, fowl, and game may be partaken of with advantage. Salmon, veal, pork, cheese, and highly-seasoned dishes, are unsuitable. The consumption of animal food should be moderate, and the tendency to acidity of the stomach guarded against by avoiding pastry, greasy or twice-cooked meat, raw vegetables, "made dishes," highly-spiced food, and anything likely to lead the patient to eat more than is strictly moderate. The wines most likely to injure are port, sherry, and madeira. If wine be taken at all, probably good claret, free from sugar, and without acidity, is best. If gout attacks a patient early, entire abstinence from all alcoholic beverages is one of the most likely measures for checking the future progress of the malady. Aged persons, however, and others whose health has been much enfeebled, may be allowed a small quantity of stimulants, such as the particular circumstances of each case seem to justify. For, "although a plan can be sketched out which may apply to the majority of cases of gout, still each case not only exhibits its own peculiarities, and becomes a separate study, but likewise demands, in certain respects, a separate treatment" *(Garrod)*.

2nd. *Healthy action of the skin.*—This should be promoted by bathing, warm clothing, Baden towels, bath brushes, etc., for much excrementitious matter is got rid of in this manner. Friction over the whole surface of the body is extremely useful when exercise cannot be taken. The patient should be well rubbed with a flesh-brush, or with the hands, twice a day.

3rd. *Good habits.*—A life of indolence should be exchanged for one of activity and usefulness. Exercise should be *regu-*ly taken, but not of a severe or exhausting nature. Walking exercise, so as to secure an abundance of fresh air, must ever be considered the best, but it may be conjoined, if agreeable, with riding on horseback. Without sufficient walking or horseback exercise, probably every other measure will be unavailing. Early and regular hours should be adopted; and too severe or prolonged mental application avoided. In some cases, removal during the winter and spring to a warm and dry climate may ward off subsequent attacks.*

25.—Chronic Gout (*Podagra longa*).

DEFINITION.—A persistent constitutional affection, characterised by stiffness and swelling of various joints, with deposits of urate of soda.

The deposits in the joints constitute the distinguishing feature; chronic stiffness and swelling of various joints, with pain, are considered as cases of chronic rheumatism.

Chalk-stone Deposits. The original condition of these deposits is that of a liquid, rendered more or less milky or opalescent from the presence of acicular crystals; as the fluid part is absorbed, the consistence becomes creamy, and at last a solid concretion is produced. When the effusion is confined to the cartilages, unless very excessive, the injury to the mobility of the joint is comparatively slight; but when the ligaments are infiltrated, they are made rigid, and the play of the parts is consequently seriously interfered with. If a bursa has been infiltrated, the resulting chalk-stone is free and of uniform composition, but the distortion is considerable. The visible occurrence of chalk-stones is not constant, but when external deposits do occur in any patient,

* For the fuller description of this disease, the reader is referred to *Sir Thomas Watson's Lectures*, *Dr. Aitken's Science and Practice of Medicine*, and Dr. Garrod's article in *Reynolds' System of Medicine*, to which the author is much indebted.

no possible doubt can exist as to the nature of the case, for, as the deposition of urate of soda in the tissues occurs only in gout, its presence constitutes a pathognomonic sign *(Garrod)*.

EPITOME OF TREATMENT.—

Sub-acute Gout.—Colch.

For the gastric symptoms.—Ant. Crud., Puls., Merc., Nux V.

Colchicum.—The virtues of this drug are not restricted to the acute form of the disease, for it exerts a powerful influence in diminishing the sub-acute inflammations in old-standing cases of gout.

Pulsatilla.—*Wandering pains*, especially when those dyspeptic symptoms and characteristics exist for which this remedy is suited.

Antimonium Crud.—Gastric derangements, white-coated tongue, nausea, and increase of the pains after eating; gouty nodes.

Nux Vomica.—Sub-acute attacks brought on or aggravated by indulgence in wine, heavy suppers, or late dinners. Constipation, piles, spasms, etc., are additional indications.

TREATMENT OF GOUTY DEPOSITS.—The following simple method Dr. Broadbent has found effectual:—Wrap the hands in linen or flannel dripping with water, warm or cold, and enclose them in a waterproof bag all night. This very speedily removes inflammatory stiffness, and little by little the concretions of urate of soda soften, frequently disappearing entirely. Dr. Broadbent has, in other cases, applied alkaline solutions, and water acidulated with nitric acid, to one hand, while water alone has been applied to the other, and has come to the conclusion that water is the agent in the process of removal. Urate of soda is soluble in a sufficient quantity of water. When once deposited round the joints it is extra-vascular, and not readily acted on through the blood, but water being absorbed by the skin effects its solution, and when dissolved it is carried away.

26.—Syphilis (*Syphilis*).

Definition.—A specific disease arising from venereal causes, produced by a peculiar poison, which is contagious, and which cannot be otherwise produced.

Primary Syphilis is the name given to the disease while limited to the part inoculated and the lymphatic glands connected with it.

Secondary Syphilis describes the disease when it affects parts not directly inoculated.

Tertiary Syphilis is a term sometimes used to express symptoms which arise later in the disease, after an interval of apparent freedom.

The primary stage of this disease is more prolonged than that of any of the other specific fevers; and, "as is the case in the other Zymotic diseases, the poison of syphilis is one which possesses the power of breeding in the patient's body, and the smallest possible quantity of virus suffices in due time to inoculate all the solids and fluids of the system. The time required, however, is much longer, and the *stages* are much more protracted. Instead of counting by days, we have to count by weeks and even months. It follows that because the disease extends over years, its subject is often not incapacitated by it for social life; many, whilst still infected, become parents, and transmit their own taints to their offspring" (*Hutchinson*).

Symptoms.—In *Primary Syphilis* an ulcer forms on the infected part, having a hard base, and discharges. The lymphatic glands in the locality of the ulcer become hard, without much inflammation or tendency to suppurate. A febrile condition, which is never severe, accompanies these changes, while there is generally an enlargement of the lymphatic glands in all parts. *Secondary* symptoms include ulcers in the tonsils; eruptions on the skin of a warty character; inflammation of some of the membranes of the eye; pains in the bones and joints; febrile disturbance; alopecia; etc. In the *Tertiary* form there are ulcerations of the mouth and throat, tending to spread; ulcerations on the skin; diseases of the periosteum, cellular tissue, muscles, tendons, etc.

EPITOME OF TREATMENT.—

1. *Primary Syphilis.*—Merc., Acon. *(febrile symptoms).*

2. *Secondary.*—Merc., Nit. Ac., Merc. Bin., Kali Bich., Kali Iod., Plat., Aur., Bell., Ars.

3. *Tertiary.*—See the remedies for the "Secondary" form.

The disease requires prompt professional treatment at the outset, when it may, by Homœopathic remedies, generally be quickly brought under; and in the later stages it is equally important to resort to professional skill.

27.—Cancer *(Carcinoma)*—Malignant Disease—*(Morbus malignus).*

DEFINITION.—A deposit or growth that tends to spread indefinitely into the surrounding structures, and in the course of the lymphatics of the part affected, and to reproduce itself in remote parts of the body.

Cancer is in the strictest sense a constitutional disease. By this we intend to express the idea that a special constitutional condition precedes the formation of a local cancerous growth. In by far the largest proportion of patients so afflicted it will be found that grand-parents, parents, uncles or aunts, have died of the same disease. This applies equally to private and hospital patients.

There are several varieties of cancer, but the two principal are, the *scirrhus* or hard cancer, and the *encephaloma* or soft cancer. Malignant or cancerous tumours differ from non-malignant in several important respects, chiefly in the following:—

Distinctions between Malignant and Non-malignant Tumours.

MALIGNANT TUMOURS.	NON-MALIGNANT TUMOURS.
1. Are of *constitutional* origin.	1. Originate in some *local error* of growth.
2. Are not surrounded by any cyst, but *invade the surrounding tissues* and convert them into a structure like their own.	2. Are limited by a cyst, and although they may *compress* they cannot *invade* the neighbouring tissues.
3. *Increase constantly* and often rapidly.	3. Have an *uncertain period of increase*, after which they may remain stationary.
4. Are attended with severe *pain*, which gradually increases in severity.	4. Are usually unattended with pain.
5. Extend to *remote parts* of the body, and re-appear there chiefly in the course of the absorbents and veins.	5. Are local and have *no disposition to spread* to distant parts of the body.
6. Are associated with an *impaired* state of the *general health* called the cancerous cachexia.	6. May impair or obstruct the functions of parts upon which they press, but such *inconveniences cease* when the tumours are removed.
7. *Return*, in the same or other parts, if extirpated, and prove fatal in the end.	7. If effectually removed do *not return* either in the same or in any other part.

Treatment.—The cure of cancer involves the destruction or elimination of the morbid tendency. Whether or not there is any remedy known which is capable of this, is a disputed point. Many vaunted remedies have disappointed those who trusted in them; while others have failed in some cases though they were useful in others. We can assert, however, from our own experience in numerous cases, that the sufferings attendant on this malady may be greatly alleviated, and life prolonged, by the use of our remedies, even when it is impossible to effect a cure.

Arsenicum.—In many cases in our own practice we have witnessed the priceless value of this remedy, in different degrees of strength, perseveringly administered, by its causing arrest of the growth, and the gradual dispersion of cancerous enlargements; these cases having been marked by the severe pain and the general cæchexia of true cancer. The utility of this potent drug is also often strikingly expressed by the restoration and maintenance of the general health in the patient.

Hydrastis Canadensis is a remedy which has been much extolled, and is undoubtedly useful when the seat of the disease is in the *glands*, or the *uterus*. We use it both internally and externally.

Conium seems to be chiefly beneficial in cancer of the *breast*.

Carbo Animalis has effected much improvement in the discharges of cancer, and has also revived the dormant energies of the system.

Thuja may be chiefly depended on in the simpler varieties of disease, as in epithelial cancer.

Acetic. Ac.—In a pamphlet recently published by Dr. Hastings, this remedy is said to have cured the disease in several cases which are narrated. The author states that the acid is capable of dissolving the cancer-cells. He does not profess it to be a panacea, but maintains that it is equal to any other known remedy.

Aconitum Radix.—The writer, in a recent case of cancer of very virulent character, found the tincture of *Acon.* of more service than any other remedy. Its power in relieving the agonising sufferings of the patient was striking; even when *Opium*, *Morphia*, etc., could not be borne, *Acon.* lulled the pain, calmed the nervous excitement, and procured that much-needed blessing—sleep.

Aurum is the best remedy when the disease affects the *bones*.

Phos., *Bell.*, *Sulph.*, *Kreas.*, *Sepia*, *Secale*, *Iod.*, *Carbolic Ac.*,

Plat., and *Calcarea** have each reputed virtues, but we have had little experience with them in the disease.

OPERATIVE MEASURES.—Connected with cancer, the consideration of extirpation by the knife, or by caustics, is important, and an opinion as to its desirableness can only be arived at by the nature and circumstances of individual cases. Life is undoubtedly sometimes prolonged by removal of a cancerous tumour, and although it return afterwards, the operation is now quite painless, and the addition thus made to life, may be one of comfort and usefulness. There is also the chance that the tumour may not be cancer, but a non-malignant growth which excision might cure. On the other hand, it must be remembered that extirpation of the tumour cannot remove the true cancerous cachexia, that a patient may sink under the operation, and that patients have so sunk for tumours that afterwards proved to be non-malignant.

ACCESSORY MEASURES.—In ulcerated cancerous tumours, the fœtor may be greatly diminished, and the patient's and attendant's comfort promoted, by solutions of *Carbolic acid*, *Condy's disinfecting fluid* and the internal and external use of *Carbo Vegetabilis*.

28.—Lupus *(Lupus)*.

DEFINITION.—A spreading tuberculous inflammation of the skin, usually of the nose or face, tending to destructive ulceration, chiefly affecting women of a strumous or delicate constitution.

The above definition applies to *Lupus non-exedens;* there is also a variety described as *Lupus exedens*, marked by the rapidity, depth, and extent of the ulceration, and by occasionally appearing on other parts than the face.

* The treatment of cancerous tumours by Lime *(Calcarea)* is discussed in a paper in the *Homœopathic World*, Vol. II. Persons interested in the subject should peruse the article.

SYMPTOMS.—Lupus "begins either as a shining, soft, circumscribed swelling of the skin, usually on one ala of the nose, which ulcerates; or else as a mere crack or small excoriation, covered with a thin scab, under which it slowly spreads. When the scab is removed, the discharge, which is scanty and viscid, soon dries and forms another large one. The ulcer is constantly spreading in one direction, and healing in another; it may last for years, and wander over the whole face, completely destroying perhaps the alæ of the nose, or the eyelids, but in other parts not penetrating the entire thickness of the true skin. The cicatrix is excessively irregular and shining, of a dense whiteness, causing perhaps eversion of the eyelids and distortion of the features; in some parts it feels soft, and pulpy. The cause and pathology of this affection are unknown."

TREATMENT.—*Arsenicum.*—This is the chief remedy, indeed the only one we have found of any use in the disease. By its persevering use both internally (in various dilutions) and externally, we have witnessed most unpromising cases completely cured.

29.—Scrofula *(Struma)*.

DEFINITION.—A constitutional disease, resulting either in the deposit of tubercle, or in specific forms of inflammation or ulceration. It may be associated with tuberculosis or it may occur without.

a. SCROFULA WITH TUBERCLE *(Tuberculosis)*.—It is at present uncertain whether scrofula and tuberculosis are different diseases or not; but it is highly probable that the disease of the blood which leads to the growth of tubercle, and that which gives the specific character to scrofulous affections, are identical.

Tubercles, so called because they are *small protuberances*, are about as large as millet-seeds, and are of two varieties—the *grey* and the *yellow*: the former is semi-transparent and somewhat firm; the latter of a dull yellow colour, and of a cheesy consistence. The yellow has in it far greater elements of danger: softening takes place earlier, and it has a greater tendency to aggregate in masses. Frequently the two varieties are mixed, but as cases advance towards a fatal termination, the yellow appears to gain the ascendancy. Many pathologists are of opinion that the grey is a previous form of the yellow, and that it passes into it after the lapse of an uncertain time.

Tubercles are usually produced slowly and painlessly, during some period of defective health, and after remaining latent for an indefinite time, they waste, if the general health improves; or soften and cause abscesses and other destructive changes, if the health deteriorates. Unlike cancer, tubercle has no elements of reproduction.

The practical conclusions of Læennec, Clark, Bennett, Pollock, and other scientific observers are, that if the further growth of tubercle can be arrested, those already existing may diminish in size, become absorbed, and the part cicatrize; or they may remain dormant, without exciting any symptoms, after undergoing a process called *cretification*, in which the animal portion is absorbed, the earthy only remaining. Frequently, however, from indigestion, defective hygienic conditions, or other cause, tubercles undergo a succession of changes; they become soft, first in the centre, that part being the oldest and most removed from living influences; then, like foreign bodies, they excite inflammation, suppuration, and ulceration in the neighbouring tissue. The groups often continue to enlarge till several groups communicate and form an abscess, or, in medical language, a *vomica;* this bursts, and if the lungs be the organs involved, its contents are discharged into an adjacent bronchial tube, and the matter is conveyed into the windpipe, and thence to the mouth, to be evacuated. Unless the disease be arrested by remedial measures, other abscesses form and unite, till the lung-substance is so diminished in volume, and its continuity so completely destroyed, as to be incompatible with life, and the patient dies from exhaustion. In other cases, as the result of proper treatment, the tubercular matter, with the inflammatory products it excited, are removed by expectoration or absorption, the tissues around the cavity contract and obliterate it, and so the disease is cured.

The parts most commonly affected by tubercle are—the *lungs*, the *brain and its membranes*, the *intestines*, the *liver*, the *pericardium*, and the *peritoneum*.

b. Scrofula without Tubercle is usually manifested by various local lesions, the most common of which is induration and enlargement of the sub-cutaneous glands—on the neck below the jaws, on the nape of the neck, then in the *axillæ* (armpits), groins, and afterwards in any part of the body. These swellings are at first soft, painless, movable; afterwards, they may enlarge, become painful, inflame, and eventually suppurate, forming scrofulous ulcers. They occur very frequently during childhood, and are excited into activity by cold, measles, scarlatina, hooping-cough, etc., and either remain for a long time inoperative, or proceed to inflammation and suppuration. Not that all enlargements of the lymphatic vessels and glands are due to scrofula; they may arise from temporary causes, and their character as such is readily determined by the history and symptoms of the case.

Other evidences of scrofulous taint are seen in the eyes—as scrofulous ophthalmia; in various cutaneous diseases; otorrhœa; a large and tumid abdomen; swellings and caries of bones, white-swellings, and the hip-joint disease; ozœna;

diseases of the testicle and mammary gland; and convulsions and acute hydrocephalus during infancy.

The following common scrofulous diseases—*Tubercular Meningitis*, *Scrofulous Ophthalmia*, *Scrofulous disease of the glands*, *Phthisis Pulmonalis*, and *Tabes Mesenterica*, are considered in subsequent sections.

CAUSES.—The most important cause is, *hereditary predisposition*: by this is meant the transmission, from parents to children, of a liability to the disease. The subject is fully dwelt upon in the author's work on "Consumption: its Causes, and Preventive and General Treatment," to which the reader is referred.

The *want of pure air* consequent on the imperfect ventilation of sitting- and sleeping-rooms is a frequent and potent cause of tubercular disease, as indeed might be inferred from the physiological evidence of the extreme importance of a due aëration of the blood. Persons breathing, for a considerable period, air which has been rendered impure by respiration, soon become pale, partially lose their appetite, and gradually decline in strength and spirits. Defective aëration leads to imperfect nutrition of the blood; the general tone of the system sinks, and it can offer but a feeble resistance to morbific agencies. Of special diseases, consumption is now known to be frequently induced by the constant breathing of air vitiated by the organic vapours and particles arising from the person. Evidences of this are very numerous. In a school at Norwood, containing 600 boys, scrofula was extremely prevalent, and great mortality occurred, which was supposed to be due to deficient or unwholesome food. The diet was, however, investigated, and found to be good, but the ventilation of the rooms and dormitories was very imperfect. This was corrected, and the disease rapidly disappeared. Even the cow, imprisoned in the town shed, the penned sheep, the confined monkey, the hutched rabbit, the caged lion, tiger, or elephant, almost invariably suffer from tubercular disease, the cause being defective ventilation and want of healthy exercise in a free atmosphere.

In the *working-rooms*, and especially in the *sleeping-apartments*, a large majority of the industrious classes of this country are deprived of an adequate supply of fresh air to support physiological changes in their integrity. Even where proper changes are secured in the day-rooms, ventilation is often neglected in the night, and eight or nine hours are spent in a space so limited, that the impure products of respiration, and the exhalations from the relaxed skin, induce much of the scrofula and consumption prevalent among the working population. The breathing of impure air in work-rooms, dwelling-houses, schools, and in places of public worship or amusement, directly lowers the vital powers, enfeebles the nervous system, diminishes the appetite, deranges the secretions, and favours the retention of worn-out particles in the blood, which may act both as a predisposing and exciting cause of consumption.

Unhealthy occupations occupy a place among the predisposing causes of scrofulous diseases. But occupations are only injurious to health accidentally, and the chief circumstances which render them so are mostly preventible, and are briefly the following:—deficiency of sunlight and pure air, the inhalation of mechanical or poisonous substances, too great prolongation of the hours of work, a bad posture of the body during labour, and the intemperance, and consequent poverty, of those engaged in them. Out-door occupations are much less likely to produce scrofulous or tuberculous diseases than those practised in-doors.

A deficient supply, or an improper quality of food, may serve as an exciting cause of struma and tubercle, although probably to a less extent than causes already pointed out. Even the hand-feeding of infants, as too generally practised, may have a considerable share in the production of the cachexia.

Two other potent causes of scrofula have been pointed out by Dr. Piddock; they are, *tobacco-smoking* on the part of the father, and the existence of *leucorrhœal discharge* on that of the mother. To both of these we would draw special attention.

Indulgence in tobacco-smoking, more especially when the habit becomes frequent and inveterate, or where it has been acquired early in life, is, it is believed, a fruitful cause of struma. The pale, sallow complexion, the frequently disordered digestive functions, and the debilitated or consumptive frames of many young fathers in the present day, attest the pernicious tendency of the habit in question.

Leucorrhœal, hæmorrhagic, or other uterine and vaginal discharges, often generate scrofula in the fœtus during utero-gestation, which declares itself during infancy in convulsions, hydrocephalus, mesenteric disease, or at or after puberty, by tubercular consumption. No observant medical man can doubt the influence of these causes as tending largely to the production of disease.

The scrofulous habit, therefore, even if not congenital, may probably be produced by any cause capable, directly or indirectly, of lowering the vital energies, such as poverty and wretchedness; meagre or insufficient food; neglect of healthy exercise; insufficient clothing; want of cleanliness; frequent exposure to cold and damp; and, especially, want of pure air and sunlight.

Treatment.—The perfection of the treatment of scrofula and tubercle, as, indeed, of disease in general, lies in its adaptation to individual cases. The stock whence the patient has sprung, the circumstances of his birth and early life, his education and general habits, the influences of soil and climate, the diseases he may have passed through, the tendency to disease of the body generally, and of organs and tissues in particular,—these are but illustrations of the points that have to be brought, as it were, into the focus of thought before a course of treatment can be prudently decided upon. We need, therefore, scarcely add, that the knowledge and experience of a physician are pre-eminently necessary.

The treatment is generally tedious, often requiring to be continued for months, and in some cases for years. A dose of one of the following medicines may be given once or twice daily as a modifier of the cachexia. As it is often desirable to persevere with one remedy for a long period, it is necessary occasionally to suspend its use for a few days, then to administer a dose or two of an intercurrent medicine, such as *Sulphur;* and again, after waiting a few days, to resume the former remedy. The most useful remedies are—*Calc.*, *Sulph.*, *Iod.*, *Ferr.*, *Phos.*, *Ars.*, and *Merc.*

Calcarea.—This remedy is well adapted to those constitutions in which the digestion and assimilation of food does not lead to the formation of good blood and healthy tissues; there is an impoverished appearance, notwithstanding that a sufficient supply of good food is taken. Other indications for this remedy are,—a want of firmness of the bones, slow or difficult dentition, scrofulous swellings, extreme sensitiveness to cold and damp, and, in females, too frequent and profuse period. It is specially adapted to children and females.

Phosphorus.—When the lungs are frequently and easily affected, as from a slight cold, with a short, dry cough, pain or soreness of the chest, shortness of breath, tendency to diarrhœa or perspiration, and general feebleness of constitution.

Arsenicum.—This is one of the most important remedial agents in scrofula, when debility is very marked, and the patient has frequent and exhausting discharge from the bowels, sallow complexion, and *emaciation.*

Iodium.—Is adapted to that condition of the system in which swelling or atrophy of the glands, and general emaciation, are prominent symptoms. A chronic diarrhœa, premonitory of consumption of the bowels, is well met by *Iodium*.

Merc. Iod. and *Silicea* are suitable adjuncts in many cases.

Fer. Iod.—This remedy is of great value in the anæmic, impoverished, and cachectic conditions so common in scrofula and tuberculosis, arising from imperfect assimilation of food.

Aurum.—Often of great service in cases improperly treated with large doses of *Mercury*. It is chiefly indicated in *affection of the bones*. *Ferrum* and *China* are deserving of attention in like cases.

Belladonna.—Useful when sensitive organs are affected, such as the eye, the ear, and the throat: there exist heat, redness, and pain in the eye, with great intolerance of light; neuralgic pains; soreness of the throat, rendering swallowing difficult; painful swelling of the parotid and other glands; etc.

Silicea.—Scrofulous ulcers with callous edges, fistulous ulcers, scaldhead, discharge from the ears, and in scrofulous affections of the bones. It may advantageously follow *Calcarea*, especially in disease of the bones.

Mercurius.—Glandular inflammations characterised by a diffused redness, much swelling, and pains worse at night in bed; it is particularly indicated when the glands of the neck are swollen and painful, and there are excessive discharges of saliva, disagreeable taste, frequent and unhealthy-looking stools, and strumous affections of the eyes.

Sepia.—Often required in scrofulous females, who are troubled with menstrual irregularities, corrosive leucorrhœa, indurations of the uterus, etc.

Iodine.—This is an excellent remedy in enlargement of the glands, scrofulous inflammation of the knee, rough, dry skin, enlarged mesenteric glands, enlarged and tender abdomen, and emaciated appearance, with hectic fever.

Sulphur.—An unhealthy condition of the skin; scrofulous ophthalmia of children; humid eruptions behind the ears; purulent discharge from the ears; swelling of the axillary glands, tonsils, nose, or upper lip; swelling of the knee, hip, or other joints; defective nutrition; colicky pains, mucous discharges, etc. Very important also as an intercurrent remedy.

Phyto., *Kali Iod.*, *Baryta Carb.*, *Hep. S.*, *Staph.*, and many other remedies are frequently required.

Remedies for the Indigestion. In order to correct the derangements of the digestive tract—which have an important bearing on the development of the tubercular predisposition—choice may be made from the following short list of remedies:—

Nux Vomica.—This is a prime remedy for indigestion with the following symptoms—flatulence, heart-burn, acid eructations, and constipation or irregular action of the bowels. It is specially indicated in patients of dark complexion, sallow skin, of sedentary habits, or who suffer from much mental fatigue or anxiety.

Pulsatilla.—Adapted to that form of indigestion in which fat, an important constituent of a mixed diet, is distasteful, and is not taken without more or less derangement of the mucous membranes. Except that *Puls.* is generally more suitable to light-complexioned persons, and where there is a tendency to *diarrhœa* rather than to *constipation* from gastric disturbance, the indications are much the same as for *Nux V.*

Calcarea Carb.—In addition to the indications before pointed out, this remedy is very efficient in obstinate acid eructations not cured by *Nux V.* or *Puls.*, and when a debilitating relaxation of the bowels is present.

Mercurius.—Faulty action of the liver shown in yellowish

appearance of the skin and whites of the eyes, mental depression, loss of appetite, etc.

Kali Bich., *Bry.*, *Ant. Crud.*, or *Carbo Veg.*, may likewise be of service in some cases. See the section "Dyspepsia."

ACCESSORY MEANS.—These are of the *greatest* importance, for medicines will be of little use unless hygienic rules are strictly adhered to.

Food.—The food of scrofulous patients should always be of the most nutritious character, light, and digestible. Beef, mutton, venison, and fowls, are the best kind of animal food; to these should be added preparations of eggs and milk, a due quantity of bread, mealy potatoes, rice, and other farinaceous principles, as more suited to this class of patients than very watery and succulent vegetables.

Cod-liver Oil, as a supplemental article of diet, is an agent possessing such remarkable properties of arresting general or local emaciation, so well known as not to require further recommendation here. It may be taken in almost any scrofulous disease, and in any case in which the patient is losing flesh; it may be given in teaspoonful doses, two or three times a day, commencing even with half-a-teaspoonful if it is found at first to disagree with the patient.

Exercise.—Moderate exercise in the open air is most essential; and in carrying out this suggestion the patient should endeavour to take exercise with the mind agreeably occupied, rather than following it as an irksome task. A bracing mountain- or sea-air, if it can be borne, is the best. The patient's room should also be uninterruptedly supplied with pure air. *Bathing*, both in fresh and salt water, is invaluable, as a means of promoting a healthy action of the skin, and of imparting tone to the whole system. The *clothing* should be adapted to the season, and should be warm without being uncomfortable. The extremities especially should be kept warm. As a general rule, flannel (see pp. 47–8) should be worn, but only during the day; in winter it affords direct warmth, and in summer it tends to neutralize the effects of sudden changes of temperature. The linen should be frequently changed, always observing that it is put on perfectly *dry*.

PREVENTION.—The prevention of strumous diseases consists not alone in the hygienic or medical treatment of the patients, but primarily in the correction of the habits and improving the health of the parents, more particularly in respect to the points referred to under "Causes."

30.—Tubercular Meningitis (*Meningitis tuberculosa*)—Acute Hydrocephalus.

This is a disease which is frequently fatal to scrofulous children, though all ages are liable to it. Its essential morbid character consists in the growth of tubercle on the arachnoid membrane of the brain.

SYMPTOMS.—When occurring in children, the usual manifestations of the disease are—febrile disturbance, quick irregular pulse; vomiting; constipation, the motions having the appearance of clay; red tongue; and continuous high temperature. The child is irritable; has disturbed sleep; grinds its teeth; manifests pain in the head intolerance of light and noise; inability to stand from *vertigo*; and becomes generally feeble. He also desires to be quiet; has occasional delirium; looks old and distressed; suddenly cries out; and is very drowsy. Twitching and squinting may also occur. In unfavourable cases, coldness of the extremities, clammy perspiration, an exceedingly rapid and feeble pulse, and death supervene.

TREATMENT.—*Aconitum* at first for the febrile symptoms.

Belladonna is of most importance for the brain-symptoms as above described, except when there is much drowsiness and stupor, when *Hyos.* should be selected in preference.

Bryonia.—If effusion *(water on the brain)* be probable, this remedy should be given.

Helleborus if there be much effusion.

Sulphur, as an occasional remedy, should be administered between the doses of other medicines.

Dig., *Verat. Vir.*, *Ars.*, or *Apocynum* may also be required.

Accessory Treatment.—This should include applications of cold water to the head, liquid diet, sponging the body with cold or tepid water, followed by perfect drying, and strict *quietude.*

31.—Scrofulous Ophthalmia *(Ophthalmia Strumosa)*.

Definition.—Inflammation of the conjunctiva, or mucous membrane which lines the inner surface of the eyelids and the front part of the globe of the eye, occurring in young persons advancing towards puberty and in children of scrofulous constitution, living chiefly in low, badly-drained situations.

Symptoms.—The three prominent symptoms are—extreme *intolerance of light*, so that the child obstinately holds its head down and can only open its eyes with the greatest difficulty; *spasmodic contraction of the orbicularis palpibrarum muscle*, the lids being everted by the spasmodic action; *profuse flowing of tears*, so that the skin of the cheeks is often excoriated or covered with an itching eruption. And when, at length, the eyes are opened, there is nothi[ng] to be seen at all commensurate with that dread of light [w]
patient manifests, for it is more a nervous than [
disease. These symptoms are generally accom[
others which mark the scrofulous constitution—

of the absorbent glands about the neck, sore ears, a large hard abdomen, grinding of the teeth, and general debility.

CAUSES.—As above stated, the *predisposing* cause is a strumous habit; the *exciting* causes are, undue exposure to cold, to bright light, irritating vapours, neglect of cleanliness, etc.

EPITOME OF TREATMENT.—

1. *For the inflammatory symptoms.*—Merc. Cor., Bell., Euphr., Phos. Ac., Hep. Sulph., Ars., *K*ali Bich.

2. *For the constitutional condition.*—Calc. Carb., Sulph., (See also treatment of "Scrofula," pages 197–201).

LEADING INDICATIONS.—

Mercurius Cor.—Severe acute attacks, with extreme intolerance of light. This is a most valuable remedy, and if administered early, in 2nd dec. dil., will generally cut the disease short.

Belladonna.—In less severe forms of the disease than that for which *Mer. Cor.* is prescribed.

Euphrasia.—Profuse discharge of tears. It is most useful at the commencement of the disease, but requires to be followed by some deeper-acting constitutional remedy, such as *Sulphur.*

Arsenicum.—Extremely obstinate cases, in which other remedies have been unsuccessful.

Sulphur.—Useful in every kind of inflammation affecting the various tissues of the eye; it is chiefly valuable in ophthalmia in unhealthy, strumous patients.

Calcarea Carb.—Indicated when inflammation of the eyes is accompanied by other marks of the scrofulous constitution, as swelling of the glands.

ACCESSORY MEANS.—As a lotion, warm water should frequently be applied during the acute stage, or tepid milk and water. Much comfort may also be derived from holding the eyes over the vapour from hot water. The eyes should be protected by a shade. Wholesome nourishing food, including cod-liver-oil, and pure country or sea air, are essential.

32.—Scrofulous Disease of Glands (*Morbus Strumosus Glandularum*).

DEFINITION.—In this term are included all those affections of the lymphatic glands—enlargement, induration, and suppuration—which arise as manifestations of the scrofulous cachexia.

The glands most commonly affected are those in the neck and under the jaw, the axillary, and the inguinal glands. The disease is usually confined to children and young persons.

SYMPTOMS.—The gland slowly enlarges, becomes hard, and is painless up to a certain point; afterwards there are inflammation, pain, and suppuration, the pus being curdy and ill-conditioned, probably from the growth of tubercular matter; and when the wound is healed, a marked and, frequently, protuberant cicatrix remains. In other cases, however, the gland remains enlarged, without proceeding to suppuration.

EPITOME OF TREATMENT.—

1. *Acute inflammatory symptoms.*—Bell., Hep. Sulph., Silic. Also wet compress, poultice, fomentation, etc., according to the requirements of the case.

2. *Chronic enlargement.*—Iod., Merc. Iod., Kali Iod., Phyto., Calc. Carb., Sulph. Also, nourishing diet, including cod-liver-oil, pure air, abundance of sun-light, and the general treatment recommended for "Scrofula."

38.—Phthisis Pulmonalis *(Phthisis Pulmonalis)* Pulmonary Consumption.*

Definition.—The growth in the lungs of tubercle, which undergoes various changes, and is associated with the constitutional phenomena of scrofula.

Pathology.—The nature of *tubercle* is stated in the section on Scrofula, to which the reader is referred. The frequent manifestations of this scrofulous or tuberculous cachexia in the lungs is probably owing to the great vascularity of these organs, their loose and spongy texture, and their ceaseless movements.

Symptoms.—The early symptoms, which are often obscure, may appear at any age, but most frequently from the eighteenth to the twenty-second year. The chief symptoms are, *impaired digestion*—loss of appetite, red or furred tongue, thirst, nausea, vomiting, and in rare cases, gastralgia; more or less *cough*; irregular *pains in the chest*; *dyspnœa* on slight exertion; *debility*, languor, and palpitation; persistently *accelerated pulse*; *heightened temperature*; and *progressive emaciation*.

Cough is a prominent symptom. In the early stage it is dry, short and irritative, and most troublesome in the morning, or after exertion; it is unattended with expectoration, or is simply to clear the throat, and may continue for months without aggravation or the supervention of any other symptom. In a more advanced stage, cough recurs during the day, and especially after slight exertion, being caused by the necessity for getting rid of secretions, and then may be regarded as a conservative effort to clear the tubes of the morbid deposit, the inflammatory products and disintegrated lung tissue,

* This disease is more fully considered in all its bearings in the author's work "On Consumption: its Symptoms, Signs, Causes, and Preventive and Ge[redacted]t." London: Jarrold and Sons.

which then begin to accumulate. The recognition of this different variety of cough is necessary in order to prescribe for its cure or relief, as remedies suited to one condition are inadmissible in the other. The mere existence of a cough *per se*, by no means proves that consumption is present, as it may arise from diseases of other organs than the lungs; neither does the absence of cough prove the non-existence of the disease.

Hæmoptysis frequently, but not invariably, occurs, and gives the patient the first intimation of the real nature of the malady; its occurrence either before or soon after the commencement of a cough always renders consumption probable, especially if the patient has received no injury of the chest, has no disease of the heart, or of the uterine system. The amount of blood discharged is sometimes very small in the early stage, merely streaking the sputa, or there may be a few teaspoonsful, and it proceeds only from the small vessels that are congested in the neighbourhood of the tubercles; but in the latter stages there is sometimes a copious and even fatal hæmoptysis, arising from some large vessel being opened by ulceration and rupture of an artery in a *vomica;* but this is comparatively rare, because the vessels become plugged with coagula before the ulceration opens them.

A *persistent rapidity of the pulse*, ranging from 90 to 120, or higher, is an invariable symptom of active phthisis. It is especially liable to become accelerated towards evening, and, as the disease advances, becomes more rapid and also feebler. "The nervous system has the heart for its gnomon or dial of the clock; and extreme rapidity of the heart's action, while it has a most grave import in acute disease, is also an accurate measure of the failure of nervous power in chronic affections. It is rarely under 100, and may run up from this to 140, or till it is impossible to be reckoned; and there is no more disastrous symptom" *(Pollock)*.

Shortness of breath or *difficult breathing*, although not an invariable early symptom, is a common one. In phthisis the capacity of the lungs is diminished, and enough air is not inspired to aërate the blood, sent there by the quickened action of the heart. An extensive growth of tubercle in the lungs gives rise to very great distress in breathing; this symptom becomes, therefore, a sign of the extent of the deposit. This is confirmed by the use of the Spirometer. The number of respirations in healthy, tranquil breathing, is from 14 to 18 per minute, and bears a remarkable proportion to the pulsations of the heart, that is, one complete respiration to about every five beats of the heart. In phthisis, the number of respirations is from 24 to 28, the number increasing as the disease progresses. Inspiration is generally short, limited, and speedily checked, causing uneasiness, or inducing coughing, and is quickly succeeded by expiration. The patient complains of want of breath; exercise, especially going up-hill, or up-stairs, or walking fast, exhausts him, and he often requires to rest. Such lowered respiratory power tends of itself to induce accumulations of mucus in the air-cells, and to excite inflammatory action.

Emaciation, one of the earliest symptoms, extends to nearly every tissue of the body, the adipose, the muscular, and the bony; even the intestines and the skin become thinner; it often proceeds uniformly from the commencement to the termination, and appears to bear a closer connection with the constitutional, than with the local, affection. Though liable to be increased by extensive disease of the lungs, intestines, and mesenteric glands, and by hectic fever, still, in the absence of these conditions in their ordinary intense form, *wasting* goes on to the fatal termination, the patient sustaining a total loss of from one-third to half his entire weight. *Slow and gradual emaciation*—"the grain-by-grain decay"—is far more indicative of phthisis, than a rapid or irregular diminution of weight; and emaciation is more marked, and also more dangerous, in individuals who have been previously stout. To detect the continuously progressive emaciation it is necessary to have patients accurately weighed from time to time. By this means a physician is also able to judge of the proportion of the weight of a patient to his height, age, breathing, and other functions.

Hectic Fever, at length, makes its appearance, and its coincidence with the symptoms already mentioned clenches our diagnosis of consumption. The patient is feverish and flushed in the evening, and in the morning is found drenched with perspiration. The pulse is small and weak, uniformly too high, but greatly accelerated towards evening, reaching 120 beats in the minute, or more; "the beat being performed with a jerk, as if the result of irritation upon a weakened heart." The bowels are relaxed, especially in advanced stages of the disease, the diarrhœa aggravating the effects of the sweating, and consequently the exhaustion is greater; the tongue is furred white or brown in the centre, but unnaturally red around the tip and edges, and immediately preceding the final break-up, is covered with the eruption of thrush. The urine deposits the red brick-dust or pink sediment, consisting of the urates of soda and ammonia; the skin is clammy, except during the evening exacerbation, when it is burning hot; the complexion is clear, the eyes are bright and sparkling, and there is most marked emaciation, especially as death approaches.

Finally, all the symptoms are gradually intensified: the dyspnœa becomes *very distressing*, so that the patient is unable to make any active exertion, or even to read a short paragraph without pausing; the sputa is more purulent; the pus is often expectorated pure, in roundish masses, that remain distinct in the vessel into which it is spat; the disease often spreads to other organs, as the lymphatic system and the intestinal canal, in which a deposit of tubercle takes place, similar to that in the lungs, which afterwards bursts into the intestines, leaving an ulcer; and thus the entire alimentary canal is affected, and diarrhœa produced. The respiratory mucous membrane may also be ulcerated, producing huskiness, and even loss of voice, but more frequently the former, from the thickening and increase in vascularity which it undergoes. *Aphthæ* of the mouth, pharynx, etc., or œdema of the lower extremities, ensue. It is therefore but seldom that the local affection of the lungs alone causes death.

The mind usually remains bright, often vigorous, and so hopeful that, even amidst this general wreck of the material frame, the patient dreads not the future, and thinks he "would be well but for his cough;" towards the end, however, slight delirium sometimes occurs, from circulation of venous blood in the brain, or a deposit of tubercles in its membranes.

The most characteristic symptoms are:—*undue shortness of breath* after exercise; *cough;* excessive *sensitiveness to cold air; spitting of blood; progressive emaciation; heightened temperature; rapid pulse; hectic fever;* and, lastly, *diarrhœa* and *aphthæ*.

PHYSICAL SIGNS AND THEIR METHODS OF DETECTION.—Notwithstanding the comparative conclusiveness of symptoms, a physician does not rely on them alone, but calls in the aid of other evidence. In consequence of the frequent obscurity that surrounds symptoms, or of the possibility that they admit of explanation by causes distinct from phthisis, a physical examination is necessary to remove all uncertainty; and if conducted with care, and aided by the study of natural science, the diagnosis of this disease may be rendered almost as clear as if the morbid processes beneath the chest-walls were exposed to view.

A physical examination of the chest is conducted by the following means—*Inspection*, or ocular observance of the form, size, and movements of the chest; *Mensuration*, by hich the comparative volume of the two sides of the est, and also the degree of expansion and retraction during spiration, are determined by measurement; *Percussion*, or pping the chest to ascertain the relative degree of dulness resonance; *Auscultation*, listening over the chest to discover e condition of the respiratory murmurs, either with or thout a stethescope; *Thermometry*, which indicates the mperature of the patient apart from his own sensations; d *Spirometry*, which tests the capacity of the lungs by eans of a machine for the purpose *(Spirometer)*. The ight and *height* of the patient are also considered in conction with his age and the revelations of the spirometer.

DIAGNOSIS.—The importance of the aid of the thermometer the diagnosis of phthisis will be recognized by the fact at during the deposit of tubercle in the lungs, or in any gan of the body, the temperature of the patient is always ised from 98° Fahr., the normal temperature, to 102° or 03°, or even 104°, the temperature increasing in proportion the rapidity of tubercular growth. This sign may be tected several weeks before reduced weight or other signs dicate the undoubted existence of tubercle; and, in the sence of other signs peculiar to the disease, will determine e diagnosis of consumption from *chlorosis* or *heart-disease*.

CAUSES.—The causes of consumption are the causes of rofula (see that section). The most potent causes are—*reditary taint*, and "the *impoverished nutrition* resulting from *pure air*, and an improper *quantity*, *quality*, or *assimilation f food;* and so long as misery and poverty exist on the one and, or dissipation and enervating luxuries on the other, so ng will the causes be in operation which induce this terrible isease" *(Bennett)*.

DURATION.—The average may be said to be from nine onths to two years; but in acute cases, the tubercles grow pidly through the entire substance of both lungs, and it may prove fatal in two or three months, or even in as many weeks. The influence of the digestive organs is very considerable. An irritable mucous membrane—indicated by loss of appetite, furred tongue, diarrhœa, etc.—will hurry the tubercular deposit through its stages; while a healthy digestive apparatus may prolong the stages indefinitely. Other circumstances must also be considered—age, amount of hereditary influence, hæmoptysis, fever, etc. Lastly, the type of disease transmitted greatly influences the duration.

TREATMENT.—Phthisis being a disease in which the assistance of a medical man is so necessarily required, we only give a few general indications for the sake of those to whom professional homœopathic skill is not accessible. Each case must be treated according to the individual nature and extent of the local and constitutional disease. Useful remedies may be found among those recommended for "Dyspepsia;" also "Bronchitis," "Pneumonia," and other diseases of the respiratory system, to which the reader is referred. *Preventive* treatment is of the highest importance: the section on "Scrofula" contains ample hints on this part of the subject.

EPITOME OF TREATMENT.—

1. *Tuberculous Cachexia.*—Sulph., Calc., Iod., Ars., Phos., Merc., Ferr.

2. *The Indigestion.*—Puls., Nux Vom., Calc., Lyco., Merc., Kali Bich., Ant. Crud., Carbo Veg.

3. *Cough*, etc.—Phos., Bell., Hyos. *(nightly dry cough)*, Bry. *(stitching pains in the side)*, Stannum *(profuse expectoration* and *night sweats)*.

4. *Hæmoptysis.*—Ham. V., Ipec., Dros., Arn.

5. *Dyspnœa.*—Ars., Ant. Tart.

6. *Hectic-fever*, *Night-sweats*, *Diarrhœa*, *etc.*—Phos. Ac., China, Hep. S., Samb.

7. *Various Symptoms.*—Kreas. *(sympathetic vomiting)*; Phyto., Kali Iod., Kali Bich., Kali Carb., Calc., Spig., Sulph. Ac., Merc. Cor.; etc.

Leading Indications.—

Calc. Carb.—This remedy is well adapted to those constitutions in which the digestion and assimilation of food does not lead to the formation of good blood and healthy tissues; there are obstinate acid eructations, relaxed bowels; sensitiveness to cold and damp; fatigue after slight exertion; cough; gradual emaciation; and, in females, too frequent and profuse menstruation.

Phosphorus.—Having a local affinity for the lungs, this remedy is of great utility in confirmed, as well as in incipient consumption, and especially in young girls of a delicate constitution; there are,—frequent, dry, short cough, so constant as to lead to exhaustion of strength; or moist cough with greenish fœtid expectoration from an abscess in the lungs; shortness of breath; tendency to diarrhœa or perspiration; emaciation; pain and soreness of the chest; loss of appetite; dry or hot skin; small and quick pulse; etc.

Iodium.—Consumption associated with glandular affections—enlargement or atrophy—and diarrhœa from mesenteric disease.

Ferrum.—Anæmia, diarrhœa, œdema of the lower extremities, emaciation. *Ferr.* is required in most cases, for the constitutional condition.

Pulsatilla.—This drug is adapted to that form of indigestion in which *fat*, an important constituent of a mixed diet, is distasteful; and is not taken without more or less derangement of the mucous membranes.

Lycopodium.—Useful if the chest-symptoms are associated with chronic indigestion—intestinal flatulence, constipation, etc.

Hyoscyamus.—Night-cough, especially when the cough commences or is aggravated on lying down.

Bryonia.—Tearing dry cough, as if the chest or the head would burst by the effort; stitching pains in the sides, catching the breath.

Drosera.—Severe fits of coughing, causing frequent discharges of blood.

Arsenicum.—Tightness of the chest; oppressed breathing, aggravated by lying down; chilliness in the chest; or soreness and burning from coughing; exhausting diarrhœa; rapid emaciation; depression of spirits. *Ars.* is a valuable medicine in all stages of the disease, and especially in the last.

Hepar Sulph.—For scrofulous young persons, in the early stages of the disease. The chief symptoms are, hoarse, rough, or weak voice, hollow cough, accompanied by expectoration of mucus, sometimes of blood; dyspnœa, especially on lying down; night-sweats; pain after eating the smallest quantity of food; clay-coloured or greenish stools.

Sulphur.—Very valuable for the constitutional condition, and also as an intercurrent remedy throughout the disease.

Aconitum.—This is a prominent remedy in consumption, and its occasional administration during the whole course of the disease is attended with the best results. It is especially valuable in removing congestion, and modifying inflammatory and febrile action. Physicians of the old school were formerly accustomed, and in many cases are so still, to use depletory measures—leeches, cupping-glasses, etc.—to diminish local congestion; but, thanks to Homœopathy, in *Aconite* we have a remedy which answers this purpose better than the lancet or the leech, without the consequent loss of strength.

Inhalation (see Part IV) often proves extremely useful for administering such remedies as *Iodine, Kreasote, Aconite, Bryonia, Hyoscyamus, Belladonna, Ipecacuanha*, etc., especially when the throat and large bronchial tubes are involved. Apart from remedies, the simple vapour of hot water is of great utility; it soothes the inflamed mucous membrane and assists in detaching mucus from the air-passages.

General Measures.—To describe in detail the general

treatment of consumptive patients, were to write a treatise on hygiene; we shall therefore only throw out several hints on the most important points; and refer the reader to the section on "Scrofula."

1st. *Nutritious Food.*—The diet should be nourishing, digestible, and sufficiently abundant to meet the particular requirements of each case. As a general rule, it should include animal food once or twice a day; fish, especially oysters; good home-made bread, not less than one day old; puddings of arrowroot, rice, sago, or tapioca; various kinds of green vegetables and mealy potatoes; *good milk*, eggs raw, or beaten up with a little milk; and, if the patient is benefitted by its use, a moderate allowance of beer or wine. Pork should be avoided; also veal; fish not having scales; pastry; and all articles that give rise to irritability of the stomach, nausea, eructations, or any other symptoms of indigestion.

Cod-liver oil must be considered as an item of food, and a very important one; but as it often disagrees with the stomach, the author has found *Cream* of great value as a substitute, though it is inferior. To favour its digestion a teaspoonful of French brandy, or a tablespoonful of cold, strong, black tea, may be mixed with it.

2nd. *Clothing.*—This should be sufficiently warm to maintain a vigorous cutaneous circulation; the extremities especially should be kept warm, to obviate congestion in the chest or abdomen. Flannel should be worn both in summer and winter; in the former, it neutralizes any variation of temperature, and prevents sudden cooling by evaporation of the perspiration; in the latter, it prevents loss of the vital warmth of the body. In winter, the addition of a chamois leather vest may be advantageously worn over the flannel. The notion that delicate children may be hardened by habitually exposing them to atmospheric changes, when but imperfectly clad, is erroneous in all cases; and in the instance of children of tuberculous predisposition, often leads to the worst results.

3rd. *Bathing and friction of the skin.*—Except in confirmed cases, bathing is generally beneficial; even sea-bathing may be often recommended. But on no account should the patient bathe when exhausted by fatigue, or when the body is cooling after perspiration. When sea-bathing is not admissible, sponging the chest both in front and behind, with water to which sea-salt has been added, can generally be borne and enjoyed, and when it is followed by a general glow, it is a most valuable aid in promoting the capillary circulation. Under all circumstances, vigorous friction should immediately follow the bath, as reaction is thus rendered more complete. In cases in which patients are prevented from taking exercise, friction by means of a towel or flesh-glove is the more indispensable. Bathing must be regarded as injurious if a brief immersion renders the surface cold, numb, and pale. In such cases, warm salt-baths are recommended.

4th. *Exercise.*—Next to diet, the unrestrained exercise of the muscles and lungs in the pure open air is of the greatest importance. "The more fully the lungs are judiciously used, the more is their capacity nursed; and conversely, the less they are used and expanded, the more useless are they likely to become, if not absolutely diseased. Under a judicious system of training, an undeveloped man, even although he may be feeble, narrow-chested, and sickly, may yet become active, full-chested, and healthy. It is therefore within the power of the medical officer to direct the physical training of young persons, so that the apparently sickly and the short-winded may in time be developed into the wiry and active young man, long in wind, sound in body, and lithe of limb; a result which, however, can only be attained by judicious feeding, careful exercise throughout the development of the body, and by the gradual nursing of the breathing ...vers" *(Aitken).*

If possible, exercise should be so taken as to bring all the muscles into moderate and agreeable action, and with the body in an erect posture. Walking-exercise secures these conditions to a certain extent; riding on horseback has the advantage of permitting the patient to breathe a large amount of fresh air, while it does not occasion great difficulty of breathing. Rowing, gymnastic exercises, and especially the *cross-bar swing* (described in the work on "Consumption" before referred to) are valuable aids when practised according to the patient's strength. Excessive exertion, however, either of the mind or body, should be avoided, and an interest fostered in the objects and operations of nature, such as the garden, the farm, and the hill-side.

5th. *Healthy Residence.*—The climate should be moderately warm, *dry*, and uniform, to suit the consumptive. A *voyage* sometimes wonderfully renews the constitution. The climate of, and voyage to, Victoria (Australia) is strongly recommended. Moreton Bay or Adelaide are said to be the most suitable places for patients with tubercular disease or chronic bronchitis. It is, however, only in the early stages of consumption that such a course is advisable. When removal to a foreign country is impracticable, Torquay, Undercliffe in the Isle of Wight, Hastings, Bournemouth, and Queenstown (Ireland), are places in our own isles to which consumptive patients may resort with great benefit.*

In conclusion, all excesses must be avoided, whether in the pleasures of the table, wine and liquors, exercise, or in the gratification of any passion, which over-stimulates the mind or the body. Business and intellectual pursuits should not be followed to the extent of inducing mental or bodily fatigue,

* For a description of the various health-resorts in the British Empire, and their adaptation to different classes of patients, see the papers on "Watering-Places" in *The Homœopathic World*, Vol. i.

but should be laid aside as early in the day as possible, and while there is sufficient strength remaining to permit the patient to engage in healthy exercise.

34.—Tabes Mesenterica (*Tabes Mesenterica*)—Consumption of the Bowels.

Definition.—A growth of tubercle in the mesenteric glands, which undergoes changes similar to those in the lungs, and is also associated with the phenomena of scrofula. Unless arrested, the disease results in the destruction of the glands, and, consequently, in the death of the patient, from inability to repair the wear of the tissues of the body.

Symptoms.—Swollen and tense abdomen; irregular action, or, more generally, relaxation of the bowels, with unhealthy, fœtid stools; passage of undigested food; pain in the bowels, so that the patient draws his legs up towards the abdomen; at the same time he is feverish and indisposed to activity. There is also pale and flabby skin; anxious and aged expression; inordinate or fitful appetite. The process of absorption becomes suspended, so that the quantity of nutriment added to the blood is inadequate to the requirements of the system; hectic fever sets in, with obstinate diarrhœa, extreme thirst, restlessness, and sleeplessness; the body wastes, until the degree of emaciation becomes extreme, hence the term *tabes* (to melt away); and the patient dies, in most cases, from actual starvation. If, however, treatment is resorted to before the glands are irreparably disorganised, the patient slowly recovers.

Treatment.—The remedies required in this affection are the same as those recommended in the section on *Scrofula*, a selection from which should be made according to the existing symptoms. The most important are—*Iod.*, *Ars.*, *Sulph.*, and *Calc.*

The best hope of cure is in *early* and judicious treatment; the disease, however, is so serious, that it should only be confided to a Homœopathic practitioner.

Accessory Means.—The food should be *nourishing* and simple,—goats' milk, beef-tea, *soda-water with milk*, and cod-liver oil. Warm clothing, including a flannel bandage round the abdomen, so as to guard against the vicissitudes of the weather, is a necessary adjunct. See also the accessory treatment of "Scrofula."

35.—Rickets *(Rachitis)*.

Definition.—A constitutional disease of early childhood, consisting essentially of a lack of earthy phosphates in the bones, and manifested by curvature of the shafts of the long bones, and enlargement of their cancellous extremities, so that they yield to pressure, and are liable to harden afterwards in unnatural forms.

In slight cases, the ankles may be only a little sunk, or the shins bent, or the spine curved; but, in aggravated cases, the physiognomy and general appearance are very peculiar.

The skull undergoes remarkable changes; it is *larger*, at least relatively, and often absolutely; but the change in shape is most marked; it loses its natural arched form, and becomes flat, both at the top and around; the frontal and parietal protuberances are increased; the frontal, coronal, sagittal, and sometimes even the lambdoid sutures are depressed *(Gee)*, and slow in closing. The face is small and triangular, with a narrow, sharp-peaked chin, and projecting teeth which tend to decay, or to drop out undecayed; and the first and second dentition is often delayed. The chest is narrow and prominent in front, hence the popular term, *pigeon-breast;* the spine is variously curved; the pelvis deficient, the promontory of the sacrum and acetabula being pressed together, the cavity is rendered perilously small for child-bearing; and the whole structure is stunted. The most characteristic alteration in the bones of a rickety child is *beading of the ribs.* This important element in the diagnosis of the disease can usually be detected earlier than any other sign.

Rickets generally becomes evident in children during the first year of their age; and it is probable that a child who is not idiotic or weakened by some recent acute disease, and who cannot walk at eighteen months of age, is either rickety or paralysed.

Causes.—Hereditary scrofulous disposition of the constitution. It is frequently met with in the children of parents who have suffered from syphilis, sexual excesses, unhealthy occupations, or other unfavourable conditions. It, however, often arises in children of parents who, though naturally healthy, have disregarded hygienic laws. It being strictly a disease of the nutritive processes, it will readily be perceived how such conditions as the above should tend to produce it. Dr. Jenner, in the following passage, strikingly shows the influence of improper *feeding and physicking* of children in the production of rickets.

"For the first two or three days after birth, their tender stomachs are deranged by brown sugar and butter, castor-oil and dill-water, gruel and starch-water; as soon as the mother's milk flows, they are, when awake, kept constantly at the breast. And well for them if they are not again and again castor-oiled, and dill-watered, and even treated with mercurials—for the poor have learned the omnipotent virtues of *grey-powder.*

"After the first month, bread and water sweetened with brown sugar is given several times a day, and during the night the child is, when not too soundly asleep, constantly at the breast. As soon as the little ill-used creature can sit erect on its mother's arm, it has at parents' meal-times 'a little of what we have'—meat, potatoes, red herring, fried liver, bacon, pork, and even cheese and beer daily, and cakes, raw fruits, and trash of the most unwholesome quality, as special treats, or provocatives to eat, when its stomach rejects its ordinary diet. Then, instead of being weaned when from ten to twelve months old, the child is kept at the breast when the milk is worse than useless, to the injury of the mother's health, and to the damage of its after brothers and sisters, in the hopes that thus keeping it at the breast may retard the next pregnancy. The children are sacrificed that the passions of the parents may not be restrained" (*Medical Times and Gazette, May 12th*, 1860).

Consequences of Rickets.—Softening and curvature of the bones often deprive a child of the use of his limbs; the deformity of the thorax produces difficult breathing; and the abdominal organs, especially the liver, are constantly compressed in consequence of sedentary habits. Sometimes the enlarged bones inflame, leading to local swelling, suppuration, and caries; and derangement of the digestive organs, wasting, hectic fever, etc., make their appearance, if they did not exist before. Under favourable treatment, however, and with proper care, the bones become very firm in adult life, and are remarkably strengthened by strong ridges developed on their concave sides.

Treatment.—This must be radical, and if commenced early the best results may be expected.

Phosphoric Acid.—This is an excellent remedy in scrofulous affections of the bones, with pains in the limbs, diarrhœa, and other symptoms of hectic.

Silicea.—This medicine is often indispensable in rachitis; it corrects the perspirations about the head, the sensitiveness of the surface, and the tendency to the increased growth of cartilage (*Hughes*).

Calc. Phos., *Asafœt.*, and *Sulph.*, are also recommended.

Accessory Means.—Country air, abundance of sunlight, and out-of-door exercise suitable to the case, will wonderfully aid the cure, by imparting tone to the digestive organs, energy to the nervous system, and, in short, invigorating the whole constitution. Patients not able to walk should sit or recline in the open air, warmly clad, during suitable portions of the day. This will be found far more contributory to recovery than passing the chief part of the day in the confined air of a sick-room. Further, tepid and cold bathing, especially in sea-water; also nourishing food, which should be well masticated, or if the teeth be inefficient, pounded in a mortar; the food should include milk, meat, good animal broths, and cod-liver oil. Respecting mechanical support, Mr. J. C. Forster remarks: "I am quite sure none yet invented is of any service. Splints on the outside and inside of the leg, boots, irons, etc., only add to the weight which already overburdens the feeble limb."

Cure of Pigeon-Breast.—In most instances this deformity can not only be improved but radically cured, if the following simple method be adopted sufficiently early, that is, before the cartilages of the ribs have become partly ossified. The object is to develop the muscles of the chest concerned in breathing. Pressure is to be applied by the hands of an assistant placed one on the projecting part of the breast-bone, the other between the shoulder-blades, the pressure being gentle but firm, and carefully increased as the patient takes five or six deep *in*spirations. The tendency of this pressure, if skilfully applied, combined with the inspiratory efforts, is to enlarge the sides of the chest in some measure at the expense of the projecting portion of the breast-bone. If this easy plan be followed twice a day for a few weeks an astonishing change may be effected, the unnatural form of chest giving way to one of symmetry and beauty. At the same time the muscles of the chest are to be brought into action in a special manner by varied movements of the arms and trunk of an active or passive nature. The *cross-bar swing* is also a valuable measure for increasing the capacity of the chest, and is fully described in the author's work "On Consumption," pages 59–60. The so-called chest-expanders are unnecessary and useless. The whole chest of the child should be sponged with cold water every morning and thoroughly dried by means of a towel.*

36.—Diabetes (*Diabetes*)—Diabetes Mellitus.

Definition.—A cachectic, constitutional disease, characterised by an excessive discharge of pale, sweet, and heavy urine, containing grape-sugar.

Symptoms.—Excessive debility and progressive emaciation; rough, dry skin; red and fissured tongue, and intense thirst; the bowels are costive, and the evacuations from them dry and hard. The quantity of urine is generally in great excess, amounting to ten, twenty, or even thirty pints in the twenty-four hours, inducing frequent calls to micturate day and night, and producing soreness and inflammation of the urethra. Thirty pints of urine of the specific gravity of 1·040, which is about the heaviest, contains nearly four pounds of sugar. In a few months patients will pass a quantity of sugar equal in weight to that of their own bodies.

Discharges of excessive quantities of urine, especially if associated with the above symptoms, should excite suspicion, and suggest an examination of the urine. There are various tests for diabetic sugar, but the one most readily practised is *Trommer's*, which is as follows:—Half fill a test-tube with the urine to be examined, and add about two drops of a solution of *sulphate of copper* to make it slightly blue, and then excess of *liquor potassæ* enough to clear it, by re-dissolving the precipitate which it at first produces. Let it boil up once over a flame, and if there be sugar there will appear a reddish-brown precipitate of the sub-oxide of copper; but if there be no sugar, a precipitate of black oxide of copper.

* See "Notes on Pigeon Breast," *Homœopathic World*, Vol. II.

The most certain information, however, may be obtained from the specific gravity of diabetic urine, which varies from 1·025 to 1·040 or upwards, according to the quantity of sugar it contains. Whenever the urinometer stands above 1·030, we may conclude that sugar is present.

CAUSE.—A defect in the function of digestion, so that sugar, which ought to be available for the maintenance of the body, enters the blood, and leaves it again unchanged, and is discharged in the urine. And here we refer not merely to sugar which is taken as such into the mouth, but to that which is formed out of the starch contained in food by the action of the saliva.

TREATMENT.—The Allopathic treatment of this disease by drugs is most striking for its inexactness and nearly uniform abortiveness. Almost every agent in the materia medica, and bleeding, have been fruitlessly employed to arrest the excessive quantity of sugar. Homœopathic medication, however, exerts a direct and often complete and permanent influence on the defective function.

Phosphoric Acid.—This remedy stands in the front rank as a curative agent in diabetes, and may be given in two- or three-drop doses of the dilute acid several times a day.

Uranium Nitricum is also reported to have effected cures.

Arsen., *Nux V.*, *Canth.*, or *Merc.* may be required to meet special symptoms.

ACCESSORY TREATMENT.—Amylaceous food, and every substance containing sugar, or readily convertible into it, must be avoided. Fat meat, fish, eggs, milk, good soups thickened with finely-powdered bran, cocoa prepared from the nibs, lettuces with oil, vinegar, etc., may be taken, if they agree, and be varied to suit the patient. The action of all articles must be watched, and anything that occasions indigestion avoided. As a substitute for ordinary bread, which is inadmissible, *bran bread* or *bran cakes*, or *ground almond powder* made into bread or biscuits, with eggs, are recommended. The excessive thirst of diabetic patients may be gratified, as fluids aid in the elimination of the sugar in the blood, and patients become greatly depressed if they are not allowed to drink as much water as they desire. Warm baths, wearing flannel next the skin, and a warm climate, are useful accessories in the cure of diabetes.

37.—Purpura *(Purpura)*—Land-Scurvy.

DEFINITION.—"A disease not usually attended by fever, characterised by purple spots of effused blood, which are not effaced by pressure, and are of small size, except where they run together in patches." This is the *Simple* form *(purpura simpler)*. When the disease is accompanied by hæmorrhage from a mucous surface, it is called *Hæmorrhagic (purpura hæmorrhagica)*.

SYMPTOMS.—Languor, faintness and gnawing pains in the stomach usually precede, for some weeks, the appearance of spots. The appetite is variable, the tongue yellowish, the countenance is sallow, dingy, or bloated and pale, with swelling beneath the eyelids. The spots first appear on the legs, and afterwards, without any certain order, on the thighs, arms, and trunk of the body; their presence being attended with great weakness and depression of spirits. They are first bright red, but are distinguished from flea-bites hy the absence of a central puncture; in a day or two they become purple, afterwards brown, and when about to disappear they assume a yellowish tint, and frequently have the appearance of *bruises*.

The pulse is feeble; there are deep-seated pains in the stomach, chest, loins, or abdomen. Constipation, palpitation, and irregular action of the heart, with a tendency to frequent syncope, are the most distressing and dangerous symptoms.

A peculiar danger attends this disease in the occurrence of extravasation of blood into internal organs—the lungs, the brain, the liver, or the alimentary canal *(Aitken)*.

EPITOME OF TREATMENT:—

1. *Febrile symptoms.*—Acon.

2. *Purpura Simplex.*—Acon. (sometimes alone sufficient), Bell., Arn., Merc., Sulph. Ac., Rhus. Tox.

3. *Purpura Hæmorrhagica.*—Merc., Ars., Phos.

ACCESSORY MEASURES.—The general health must be improved by simple, good food, plenty of exercise in the open air and sunlight, healthy dwelling, and other hygienic conditions.

38.—Scurvy *(Scorbutus)*.

DEFINITION.—"A chronic disease, characterised by sponginess of the gums, and the occurrence of livid patches under the skin of considerable extent, which are usually harder to the touch than the surrounding tissue."

CAUSES.—The disease arises from a peculiar state of malnutrition, supervening gradually upon the continued use of a dietary deficient in fresh vegetable material, and tending to death after a longer or shorter interval, if the conditions under which it arose remain unaltered.

SYMPTOMS.—"The condition is essentially marked by a dull leaden pallor of complexion; excessive bodily and mental lethargy; dyspnœa upon slight exertions, unaccounted for by the auscultatory signs; spontaneous effusions of blood-coloured fluid into the various tissues of the body, causing petechiæ and bruise-like patches to appear on its surface; together with (commonly) a livid, swollen, and spongy state of the gums, and a disposition for them to bleed upon the slightest irritation" *(Buzzard)*.

"There is no more interesting fact in the history of

medicine," says the writer just quoted, "than that this condition, which has been looked upon at various times as a plague, as a mysterious infliction of Divine justice against which man could only strive in vain, or as a disease inseparable from long voyages, should have been proved, by evidence of the most satisfactory character, to arise from causes in the power of man to prevent, and to be curable by means which every habitable country affords."

TREATMENT.—All that is required to cure a scorbutic patient is the supply of those articles of food—*fresh vegetables*, *milk*, and good dietary generally—which contain elements, the absence of which has led to the diseased condition. *Vinegar*, good *lemon-juice*, and other vegetable acids are also recommended. An ample supply of these acids as well as of *preserved vegetables*, should be provided for ships which are engaged in war, or have to make prolonged sojourns where fresh vegetables cannot be obtained.

39.—Anæmia *(Anæmia)*.

DEFINITION.—A condition in which the *red blood-corpuscles are deficient*, the *liquor sanguinis* watery, and the albumen poor.

SYMPTOMS.—The skin, the lips, and the mucous membrane generally, are pallid and have a bloodless appearance, and the face looks like wax; the lining of the gums and mouth is white, and the tongue is large, flabby, and pale; the pulse is feeble, thready, beats about eighty times in a minute, and is easily excited. The patient becomes very *weak* and languid, is easily fatigued and loses breath; there is indigestion, loss of appetite, flatulence, and irregular action of the bowels; scanty menstruation (in women); palpitation; the temperature of the extremities and surface is deficient, and there is, generally, œdema of the ankles or even of the feet.

There is also dejection of spirits, and morbidly heightened nervous sensibilities.

CAUSES.—Seclusion from air and sun-light, and a wrong quality of food. On these points, Dr. Pollock says, "The sufferers are the victims of our subterraneous kitchens and back shops, and of that atrocious domestic system which deprives young women in service of open-air exercise and enjoyments peculiar to their age. Secondarily, a depraved appetite arises, and tea with bread-and-butter comes to form their sole diet, as all healthy desire for meat soon vanishes. These devitalised plants, which never see the sun, languish in nervous power, and furnish our worst cases of hysteria."

Also, copious, or frequent small discharges of blood, as in hæmorrhoids, too profuse menstruation, venesection, etc. Profuse or prolonged evacuation of fluids which contain much of the organic constituents of the blood also gives rise to this condition, as in diarrhœa, dysentery, ague, etc.

ANÆMIA AND CONSUMPTION.—The diagnosis between these two diseases is easy to the physician, as the physical signs of consumption are absent in anæmia. In the latter the blood is only *impoverished*; in the former it is *contaminated* as well; in the latter the pulse is about normal; in the former it is accelerated; and, again, in anæmia the temperature is below the normal standard; whereas in consumption it is considerably higher.

EPITOME OF TREATMENT.—

1. *From loss of animal fluids.*—China, Phos. Ac.

2. *Associated with scanty or suppressed menstruation.*—Puls., Ferr.

3. *From deficient open-air exercise and sunlight.*—Ferr., and Puls. or Nux. Vom.

These remedies are prescribed only as auxiliaries to the hygienic treatment.

ACCESSORY MEANS.—Medicinal treatment alone will be of

little use in most cases. *Nourishing, digestible diet*, is needful in quantities as large as can be assimilated—milk, eggs, animal broths, and afterwards, fish, poultry, game, mutton, etc. Combined with suitable food, *moderate daily out-of-door exercise in a pure air* is a *sine qua non*; bathing, especially sea-bathing, aids the restoration of the patient.

40.—Chlorosis (*Chlorosis*).

Definition.—"A condition of general debility affecting young persons at about the age of puberty. There is anæmia or deficiency of the red corpuscles (*hæmatine*) of the blood, which gives the skin a pale, yellowish, often greenish, hue. The temperature of the body is diminished, and morbidly sensitive to cold. In females there is generally delayed, suppressed, or imperfectly-performed menstrual function. Respiration, circulation, and digestion are also disturbed; and the whole organism, physical and mental, is feeble and enervated." (*From the* "Lady's Manual of Homœopathic Treatment.")

Symptoms, *Causes*, and *Treatment* are fully pointed in the work just referred to. The best remedies are—*Ferr.*, *Calc.*, *Phos. Ac.*, *Puls.*, *Sulph.*

41.—General Dropsy* (*Anasarca*).

Definition.—A serous or watery accumulation in the areolar tissue, more or less general throughout the body, with or without effusion into the serous cavities.

Dropsy is of two distinct varieties, for besides its occurrence in the meshes of the loose tissue beneath the skin, it may

* In this section we have also included most of the *local* forms of dropsy, both for convenience of reference, and to present a more connected view of the whole subject.

take place as a *local* dropsy in any of the natural cavities or sacs of the body, and is named according to the parts involved. If the watery accumulation occur in the ventricles of the brain, it is called *hydrocephalus*; if in the membrane that lines the surface of the lungs, *hydrothorax*; if in the membrane of the heart, *hydropericardium*; if in the membrane of the intestines, *ascites*; if in the serous sacs of the joints, *hydrops articulorum*; if in that of the testicles, *hydrocele*.

Dropsy is also sometimes designated according to the cause from which it arises, as, (1.) *Cardiac dropsy*, from valvular disease of the heart; and (2.) *Hepatic dropsy*, from cirrhosis of the liver. Both these are mechanical forms of dropsy, resulting from impediment to the return of venous blood, the watery part exuding from the capillaries in consequence. (3.) *Dropsy from debility*. This is a functional dropsy, there being no organic disease, but feebleness of the circulation and tenuity of the blood. This variety occurs chiefly in delicate females who are anæmic or menorrhagic, or in persons advancing in life; it shows itself in the areolar tissue under the skin of the dependent parts, chiefly the ankles at night and the eyelids in the morning, and is often called *œdema*. (4.) *Acute renal dropsy*, sometimes called post-scarlatinal dropsy. See page 100. (5.) *Chronic renal dropsy*, from Bright's disease of the kidneys.

PATHOLOGY.—In health, there is a gentle and uninterrupted oozing forth of fluid, just sufficient to allow of the free motion of the membranes and their contained organs; if this fluid be arrested (as in inflammation), pain or adhesion may result; but if it take place in excess, or if exhalation take place more rapidly than absorption, then dropsy results. Indeed, dropsy is altogether due to the latter cause. Absorption is arrested or diminished, and the natural transudation still continuing, a collection of its products remains distending the small sacs of the areolar tissue, as well as the large serous sacs of the body. So that it is more correct to speak of dropsy as a *collection* than as an *effusion*.

CHARACTER OF THE SWELLINGS.—Dropsical swellings are soft, inelastic, diffused, and leave for some time the indentation made by the pressure of a finger. In old cases, and when the œdema is very great, the skin becomes smooth, glassy, and of a dull-red or purple colour, and where the skin is less elastic, as over the tibia, it becomes livid or blackish, and troublesome, or even gangrenous, sloughs may form.

EPITOME OF TREATMENT.—

1. *General Dropsy.*—Dig., Apis., Ars., Bry., Senega.
2. *Dropsy of the abdomen.*—Apocy., Apis., Ars., Chin.
3. *Dropsy of the ankles.*—Ferr., Chin., Ars.
4. *Dropsy of the brain.*—Hell., Merc., Bell., Apis.
5. *Dropsy of the chest.*—Bry., Dig., Ars.
6. *Dropsy of the heart.*—Dig., Spig., Ars.
7. *Dropsy of the testicle.*—Iod., Rhod., Puls.
8. *Dropsy of the joints (knee, etc).*—Acon., Puls., Iod.

LEADING INDICATIONS.—

Arsenicum.—This is a prime remedy in œdema of the face, hands, and feet, and anasarca from disease of the heart; also in ascites from enlargement of the liver or spleen. It is especially indicated when there is much general debility, rapid emaciation, and anxious depression; constriction and oppression of the chest, and a sensation of suffocation on attempting to lie down; the skin is dry and pale, or burning and itching, and sometimes peels off in large flakes; the tongue is red and parched, sometimes with excessive burning thirst; the pulse feeble and irregular, and the extremities cold.

Apis.—The action of this remedy on the kidneys is sufficient to make it most useful in acute febrile dropsy from a chill, in post-scarlatinal dropsy, in that of incipient Bright's disease, and in that which sometimes appears in the later months of pregnancy, laying the foundation of future puerperal convulsions; sometimes, also, for a time, it removes the œdema of the lower extremities symptomatic of disease of the thoracic organs *(Hughes)*. *Apis* is particularly valuable in dropsy complicated with strangury, suppression, or other urinary difficulties.

Digitalis.—This drug is useful in several varieties of dropsy—ascites, hydrothorax, anasarca, etc.; and is especially indicated by a small, feeble, and irregular pulse, pale face, livid lips, distressing dyspnœa, inability to lie on the back. It benefits dropsical affections from heart- or kidney-disease by improving the action of these organs.

Bryonia.—Œdematous swellings of joints; hydrothorax; dropsy or œdema from the retrocession of perspiration or an eruption, or associated with chest symptoms—cough, dyspnœa—or with liver-complaint, constipation, etc.

Helleborus.—Dropsical effusion in the ventricles of the brain *(hydrocephalus)*, in which it often proves most valuable.

Ferrum.—Functional œdema, especially in anæmic or chlorotic females, with pale and cadaverous skin, feebleness, nausea after eating, constipation, etc.

Sulphur.—Œdematous swellings following skin-affections or suppressed eruptions.

Aconitum.—Chiefly useful in the commencement of dropsy, and in dropsy supervening upon the sudden retrocession of a rash or perspiration, or associated with palpitation or organic disease of the heart. In the latter case, in alternation with *Digitalis.*

Accessory Treatment.—A *dry*, soft, and moderately warm atmosphere is generally most suitable, and if the dropsy be at all owing to climatic influences, or to any disease that is endemic to the place, a change of residence is necessary. A damp climate or soil is particularly unfavourable. In acute dropsy, the diet should be similar to that in acute fever; in chronic dropsy patients require very nourishing diet, but on account of extreme feebleness commonly present, all but easily digestible food must be avoided. To allay the burning thirst often experienced, cold water is the best beverage; but any other that the patient desires, if not positively injurious, may be taken. Water may be said to be a real restorative, for it increases the amount of fluids excreted to an extent greater than its own bulk; it also tends to improve the appetite and strengthen the pulse, while it diminishes the dropsical collections. It will thus be seen that the common notion that drinking water increases dropsy is quite erroneous.

Warm baths for promoting perspiration, drinking Hollands, tapping, and other palliative measures may sometimes be necessary, but the propriety of such means can only be decided by the circumstances of each individual case.

CHAPTER III.

Diseases of the Nervous System.

42.—Encephalitis (*Encephalitis*), Meningitis (*Meningitis*), and Inflammation of the Brain (*Inflammatio Cerebri*).

Definitions.—By "Encephalitis" is meant inflammation of the *brain or of its membranes*; the term being used only when it is impracticable to diagnose the *precise* seat of the inflammation. "Meningitis" signifies inflammation of the *membranes* of the brain ("*Tubercular* Meningitis" has been already discussed). By "Inflammation of the *Brain*" is meant "inflammation of the *brain-substance*, with or without implication of the membranes, usually partial, and in many cases dependent on local injury, or foreign deposit."

As these diseases require professional treatment, we only state here the ordinary symptoms which are more or less common to the various inflammations of the brain and its membranes, giving general indications for treatment, which may be of service under circumstances in which a physician's aid is inaccessible.

Symptoms.—In Encephalitis there may be premonitory pains in the head, irritability, sleeplessness, and general indisposition. But usually the disease manifests itself at once—there is high fever, much headache, vomiting, constipation, general sensitiveness both of the skin and the senses—sight, hearing, etc.—and violent delirium; after a few days the delirium is less; the patient clutches at the bed-clothes or the air, the pupils dilate and contract, and become insensible to light; there is grinding of the teeth, rolling of the head, and somnolence. The respiration is irregular; urine is retained; the bowels are still constipated; and the abdomen may become retracted. Muscular twitchings, anæsthesia, spasm or paralysis supervene, with thready pulse, and collapse and coma set in. "The pupils are widely dilated, and are insensible to light, the eyes half-open, the face sunk and ghastly, and the skin cold and clammy; the sphincters relax, the urine and fæces pass involuntarily, and the pulse becomes more frequent than before, but small, thready, and uncountable; the breathing is stertorous, and the patient at last dies in a state of complete coma" *(Ranskill)*.

In inflammation of the brain-substance only *(inflammatio cerebri)* the excitement and delirium are not so marked, neither does the pulse rise above its normal standard: indeed it frequently falls below it, and is very irregular. There is also tonic rigidity of one or more limbs, which is succeeded by permanent paralysis.

CAUSES.—Amongst the *predisposing* causes are, *age*, sex, *the abuse of alcoholic liquors*, *excessive grief*, and *mental work*. Simple meningitis may occur before birth, and is common in new-born infants, but is more rare after two years of age; the ages between sixteen to forty-five are next most liable; the disease also occurs in the proportion of three males to one female.

The *exciting* causes are—*blows* on the head, *falls*, etc.; and, in hot countries, *exposure to the sun*. The sudden retrocession of an eruption on the scalp has been known to be followed by acute meningitis.

DIAGNOSIS.—From *Tubercular meningitis* the diagnosis may be made by comparing the two diseases as described; from *Delirium Tremens* it may be recognised by the absence of headache in the latter affection, and the previous history of the patient, which "usually tells a long story of inebriations." In Typhoid-fever there is less headache, but a more frequent pulse, diarrhœa, abdominal tenderness, and after the fifth day the peculiar eruption of that disease.

Treatment.—On this point, Dr. Ranskill, a high authority on brain-diseases, writes:—"The treatment of Acute Meningitis is only successful when employed very early in the disease, and carried out with energy. It resolves itself into three great remedial measures: first, blood-letting; second, hard purging; third, application of cold water." Homœopathic treatment is simpler, safer, and more successful than that prescribed above. The principal remedies are—*Acon.*, *Bell.*, and *Bry.*; or *Arn.* alternately with *Acon.*, if the disease arises from an injury to the head. *Hyos.*, *Opi.*, and other remedies may sometimes be required: for their indications see "Typhus-fever."

Accessory Measures.—Cold applied to the head by means of a bladder containing small pieces of ice, "or a mixture of common salt and ice is an excellent mode of applying cold, because of the facility with which it adapts itself to the shape of the head." The hair should be shaven or cut close; and the extremities kept warm. Quietude is important, and, when there is *photophobia*, the room should be darkened. Beef-tea, strong broths, but no solid food, should be given. Cold water or other simple liquids may be freely given. The patient's apartment should be well ventilated; and great caution exercised during recovery.

43.—Apoplexy (*Apoplexia*).

Definition.—A condition characterised by the abrupt loss, more or less complete, of consciousness, from extravasation of blood (hæmorrhage) within the cranium.

Varieties.—(1) *Congestive* apoplexy is an overloaded condition of the vessels of the brain. (2) *Hæmorrhagic* or sanguineous apoplexy is the most frequent, and consists in the rupture of a vessel, and extravasation of blood in the substance of the brain or outside the nervous masses. The symptoms are usually sudden, and its development most rapid.

Modes of Attack, and Warnings.—Apoplexy may come on *suddenly* or *gradually*. The patient may be suddenly struck —falling, at once bereft of motion and consciousness. Such a case is termed *primary apoplexy*. More frequently, however, apoplexy is indicated by well-marked premonitions, which are, chiefly—headache; giddiness, particularly on stooping; fulness and pulsation of the blood-vessels of the head; epistaxis; retinal hæmorrhage; sleepiness, with heavy or snoring breathing; transient blindness, considerable difference in the sizes of the pupils; deafness, or noises in the ears; momentary loss of consciousness, with or without indistinctness of speech or incoherent talking; flashes, motes, etc., before the eyes; vomiting; numbness or tingling in the hands or feet; unsteady gait; partial paralysis, sometimes involving the muscles of the face, sometimes those of a limb; the patient becomes comatose, and drowsiness gradually increases to perfect *coma*. This is called *ingravescent* apoplexy, because the symptoms become worse *gradually*, and is far more serious than a primary case, because we have evidence that the cause of the symptoms is still in operation, and because such a case is always hæmorrhagic, and the brain has undergone organic and permanent changes. On the other hand, a primary case may be of a congestive variety, and the condition may pass off without any permanently injurious result.

Symptoms.—These vary according to the seat and amount of the hæmorrhage, and are sometimes so vague that cerebral hæmorrhage can only be suspected. Pain in the head, giddiness, faintness, sickness, labouring pulse, succeeded by some reaction, may only be present. In the early stage of an ingravescent case, before the patient becomes comatose, there is great depression in the circulation from the shock to the nervous system; the surface is cold, pale, and clammy, and the pulse frequent, small, and weak. As coma comes on, the pulse becomes full, slow, and laboured (passes slowly under the fingers); the surface warm, sometimes preternaturally so, and perspiring; the countenance has a peculiar bloated appearance, and is often congested; the pupils are insensible to light, and usually dilated, although one or both may be contracted; the breathing is stertorous from paralysis of the soft palate; the urine is retained from inaction of the bladder; and the bowels are sluggish.

One or several of the above symptoms may, however, occur as the consequence of indigestion. Vomiting and headache are more important as indications when they come on suddenly without any obvious cause, and not on first rising in the morning; and the vomiting, or efforts at vomiting, are continued beyond the emptying of the stomach; if these symptoms are associated with degeneration of the arteries, and albuminuria, we may suspect the existence of clots of blood in the brain.

Predispositions.—(1) *Age.* After fifty, apoplexy is one of the most frequent causes of death. This arises not so much from the years of a man's life, as from a bad constitution and tissue-depravation, not often present in early life. After the middle period of life, the capilliaries become impaired, and, as a consequence, the veins congested. "The cerebral arteries also are often diseased; the heart has often acquired an abnormal power, driving the blood with great violence, and with an increased momentum, towards the brain, while the lungs have their functions so impaired that the blood is only imperfectly oxygenated; and all these are causes of congestion, and of tendency to rupture of the

...sels of the brain" *(Aitken).* (2) Certain *habits* of life, ...ch as intemperance, excessive eating, uncontrolled passion, ...essure about the neck, and too close mental labour, or any ...abit favouring congestion to the head. (3) *Disease* affecting ...e heart, kidneys, or blood-vessels of the brain; suppressed ...æmorrhoids or menses.

APOPLEXY NOT OFTEN SUDDENLY FATAL.—A popular opinion ...current, and is to some extent shared in by the profession, ...at a fatal effusion of blood in the brain is a frequent cause ...sudden death. In stories and theatrical representations ...e characters are made to die suddenly of apoplexy; and, in ...ewspapers, accounts are often given of sudden deaths attri...uted to apoplexy. This error has also been fostered by ...nother equally common, namely, that persons with a short ...ick neck and red face are most liable to apoplexy. It is ...ue that such persons often die suddenly, but the suddenness ...the death is generally due to heart-disease. A man with ...red face has no more blood in his head than another without ...red face; and if blood is poured out into the brain it is ...ecause the diseased blood-vessel could no longer avert the ...tal mischief. It is, then, a person with diseased arteries in ...hom apoplexy is likely to occur, and this may exist in those ...ho are pale and thin and have long necks. Dr. Wilks ...ates that he once knew a gentleman who had such an ...traordinary red face that some young friends disliked to ...alk the streets with him, lest he should die of apoplexy. ...his gentleman, whose face was of a deeply purple hue, died ...heart-disease. "Although cerebral hæmorrhage sometimes ...ills *rapidly*, it does not kill *instantly*, as rupture of the aorta, ...heart-disease, sometimes does" *(Jackson).*

CAUSES.—The main cause of apoplexy is disease of blood-...essels, and hence the explanation of the increasing liability ...apoplexy with advancing age. The gradual degeneration ...ossification of arteries common to old age, renders them inelastic, and as the blood is forced on them by the action of the heart, they give way.* Hæmorrhage within the cranium is sometimes caused by the bursting of *aneurisms* involving the arteries of the brain. The idea that increased pressure on the blood-vessels of the brain, as during exertion or rapid movements of the body, is an *originating* cause of apoplexy is incorrect; there must be actual degeneration of the arteries, the process probably of years, before they can give way. The *predisposing* cause of apoplexy is a more or less general bodily unsoundness, which may be especially due to granular disease of the kidney, or hypertrophy of the left ventricle of the heart. Apoplexy is almost always the local expression of a general constitutional failure: hence it is classed as a constitutional disease.

DIAGNOSIS.—*Apoplexy and Epilepsy.*—The latter begins with a scream, is always attended by convulsions, and much frothing at the mouth, symptoms which do not occur in apoplexy. From *intoxication* or *poisoning with opium*, the history and circumstances of the patient must be considered; as whether he is likely to have been drinking, the presence or absence of the odour of spirits in the breath, or whether he has been low-spirited or in any difficulties likely to have led him to swallow poison. It is from such circumstances, considered in connection with the entire history of the case, that we must make our diagnosis, the condition of the brain, especially in the advanced stages, being nearly the same in all these cases. The importance of promptly recognising apoplexy from alcoholic or narcotic poisons arises from the difference in the immediate measures that would be taken in the one or the other case. An emetic, or the stomach-pump, might remove in the one case what, if suffered to remain, might lead to serious or even fatal results; while in the other

* For a fuller account of these vital changes, see the section on *Old Age and Senile Decay*.

case wholly different measures would be necessary. It is obviously far better to mistake drunkenness for apoplexy than apoplexy for drunkenness, and when anyone is found deeply insensible he should be carefully attended under the direction of a medical man. Even if death could not possibly be averted, it is sad that a human being should die of cerebral hæmorrhage in a police-cell. Under any circumstances, then, an unconscious person needs our care, for he may be so from a combination of causes; a drunken man may have had a blow on his head and ruptured his blood-vessels; or a drunken debauch may coincide with the breaking up of his cerebral arteries.

Epitome of Treatment.—

1. *For the premonitory symptoms.*—Nux. V., Acon.
2. *Cerebral hæmorrhage.*—Acon. *(strong tinct.)*, Bell., Opi.
3. *After-consequences (paralysis, etc.).*—Acon., Bell., Phos., Cocc., Rhus Tox.

Leading Indications.—

Aconitum.—Full, rapid, and strong pulse; dry, hot skin. This remedy is suitable for the premonitory symptoms, and for an actual attack, and both immediately and remotely is infinitely superior to the abstraction of ten, sixteen, or twenty ounces of blood, as recommended in the most recent Allopathic practice of medicine.*

Belladonna.—Red, swollen face, throbbing of the blood-vessels, convulsive movements of the face or limbs, dilatation of the pupils, loss of speech, suppression or involuntary discharge of urine, etc.

Opium.—Drowsiness, heaviness, stupor, or profound coma; irregular breathing; bloated face, stupid and besotted expression, eyes half open, pupils contracted; coldness of the extremities; etc.

* "At one time every case of apoplexy was treated by blood-letting, and statistics prove, of such indiscriminate practice, that the more freely the blood was taken away the greater was the mortality" *(Aitken)*.

Nux Vomica.—Congestive conditions of the brain favouring apoplexy. Even when effusion has taken place it is often the best remedy unless active febrile symptoms call for *Aconite*. *Nux V.* is particularly valuable for apoplexy in patients who have spent an inactive sedentary life, and indulged in rich diet and alcoholic beverages.

Phosphorus.—This remedy is an extremely valuable one for retarding or correcting the *calcareous degeneration* of the arterial blood-vessels which we have stated to be the great cause of the disease. It may be given when such a change in the arterial system is suspected, and also during recovery from a fit of apoplexy from that cause.

ADMINISTRATION.—During a paroxysm, one or two drops of the tincture in a teaspoonful of water, or on a small piece of sugar, every fifteen or thirty minutes; in *threatened* apoplexy, a dose every hour; as the symptoms are subsiding, every three to six hours.

ACCESSORIES DURING A FIT.—1. If possible, convey the patient immediately to a large apartment where the cold air can freely circulate around him. 2. Loosen the neckerchief, stays (in the case of females), and bandages of every kind, and place the patient in a warm bed, with his head moderately raised. 3. Apply warmth to the extremities and axillæ *(armpits)*, and a cold wet towel, or ice, crushed, in a bladder, to the head; also a sinapism to the epigastrium. 4. At the same time, one of the aforementioned medicines should be given, especially *Aconite* or *Belladonna*.

AFTER A FIT.—Should the patient recover from the fit,

remedial agent of high value; it tends to promote a more active circulation through the entire system, and, consequently, to diminish the pressure on blood-vessels which a little extra force might cause to give way. If active exercise cannot be taken, frictions performed by a second person by means of towels or flesh-brushes over the surface of the body and the extremities are necessary. The causes of the disease should as far as possible be avoided or modified.

PREVENTIVE MEASURES.—Undeviating temperance in eating and drinking. Physical and mental exertion and excesses of every nature; fits of passion or excitement; sudden changes of temperature, over-heated rooms, warm baths, wet feet, etc., must be uniformly avoided. Errors in diet, exposure to a too hot sun, violent emotions, etc., may excite the gravest symptoms in persons predisposed to apoplexy.

44.—Sun-stroke (*Solis Ictus*)—Insolation—Sun-fever—Coup de Soleil.

DEFINITION.—A disease of the nervous system, excited by heat, sometimes following exposure to the direct rays of the sun, particularly when to heat is added the pressure of tight and unsuitable clothing.

SYMPTOMS.—The affection is generally preceded by premonitory symptoms, such as thirst, heat, and dryness of skin; vertigo; congestion of the eyes; frequent desire to micturate; syncope follows, and is often instantly fatal; or insensibility and stertorous breathing occur, with or without convulsions. In both varieties the mortality is high, and unexampled congestion of the lungs is the most common morbid appearance observed after death.

CAUSES.—Besides the direct effects of heat, the fatigue consequent on continued physical exertion in a heated atmosphere, combined with breathing vitiated air in crowded apartments, predispose to an attack. Hence its frequency amongst our soldiers who in eastern countries are exposed to great heat, have to carry heavy accoutrements, and often sleep in crowded barracks, etc. "Two points are remarkable in the history of sun-stroke, viz., its extreme rarity in mid-ocean, and at great elevations. In both cases the effect of the sun's rays, *per se*, is not less, is even greater than on land and at sea-level; yet in both sun-stroke is uncommon; the temperature of the air, however, is never excessive in either case" *(Dr. Parkes)*.

TREATMENT.—*Glononine.*—Very severe pain in the head, particularly at the back, heavy and throbbing: or, sudden loss of consciousness.

Belladonna.—Violent dizziness, or sudden falling down as if from apoplexy; redness of the face.

Camphor.—Great depression of the pulse, and pale face, with violent distress in the head; followed immediately by a reaction—flushed face, accelerated pulse, etc.

The *after-effects* of sunstroke may usually be met by *Bell.* or *Glon.*

ACCESSORY MEAMS.—It is now generally agreed that sun-stroke results, as indeed will be seen from the foregoing remarks, from a depressed, and not, as was formerly taught, from a stimulated, condition of nervous centres. The treatment, therefore, by the lancet, which a few years since was the orthodox method, and supposed to be strongly "indicated," has been generally abolished, and that by cold douche constantly applied over the head, neck, and chest, is almost universally adopted.

PREVENTION.—Clothes should be light and loose, especially avoiding undue pressure on the veins of the neck. *Flannel* tends to prevent chills. Spirit-drinking, particularly in India, should be discontinued.

45.—Chronic Hydrocephalus (*Hydrocephalus longus*)—Dropsy of the Brain—Water in the Head.

Definition.—A local dropsy, consisting of a collection of watery fluid within the cranium, which may be congenital or acquired.

It generally occurs in infancy within the first year, before the sutures and fontanelles are closed, so that the bones yield to pressure from within. Infants are sometimes born with the disease, when it is an occasional cause of difficult labour. Instances of the disease attacking children in the seventh or eighth year have been reported, and in some extremely rare instances the disease has first appeared at a more advanced period of life.

Dr. Watson mentions the case of a young distinguished lawyer, who had one or two attacks of loss of consciousness while engaged in the Court of Chancery: by degrees he became dull, stupid, forgetful, insensible, and shortly died from watery fluid within the skull. The celebrated Dean Swift died of this complaint at the age of seventy-eight, three years after the commencement of the disease. In these instances, after the sutures are closed, the bones cannot yield to pressure, and the size of the head is natural, the collected fluid distending the cavities within the head, and causing an anæmic and wasted condition of the brain-substance. In children the bones of the skull are separate, sometimes to an enormous extent, so that the head has been known to measure twenty-four, thirty-six, and even thirty-nine inches in circumference, the quantity of fluid varying accordingly. The shape of the head is generally round, and somewhat flat on the top; rarely it assumes a sugar-loaf shape.

Symptoms.—The premonitory indications of this disease are not very distinctive: there may be squinting or rolling of the eyes if the disease be congenital, followed by convulsions and enlargement of the head.

The most marked features are—a disproportion between the size of the skull and that of the face, the fontanelles are wider than usual, and the bones feel thin under pressure of the fingers. Emaciation is generally present through non-nutrition: in some cases there is an unnatural fat condition. If an infant, he sucks well, even voraciously, and yet he does not grow; his bowels are constipated, and his motions unhealthy. The gradually-increasing head soon attracts notice: the anterior fontanelle pulsates, there is heat of the head, and the child becomes more restless than usual. Fluctuation may be felt by applying the hand to the top of the head; the hair ceases to grow as usual; the face appears small and triangular; the countenance is dull, having an aged appearance; and the patient wants to lie down continually. In unfavourable cases (and recoveries are rare) the senses become impaired; paralysis sets in; and the patient dies either from exhaustion, convulsions, or spasmodic croup, to which such children are liable.

The duration of the disease varies from one to eight, or even ten years. Should effusion be arrested, the accumulation of serum already present is never absorbed, but remains.

Causes.—Chronic Hydrocephalus is usually associated with the scrofulous cachexia; sometimes it follows scarlatina, hooping-cough, or measles. The most common exciting causes are—undue exposure to heat or cold, injuries of the head, suppressed eruptions, or extended inflammation of the ear. "One warning may be learned from this disease, namely, that it is said to be most common in the children of parents addicted to drunkenness, and from this cause it often runs in families" *(Aitken)*.

Treatment.—The best remedies for this disease are those adapted to the constitutional cachexia: these are—*Calc.*,

Sulph., *Ferr. Iod.*, *Silic.*, etc., the indications for which will be found in the section on "Scrofula."

Hell., *Dig.*, or *Merc.*, may be required as adjuncts.

The *Accessory Treatment* is the same as that recommended in the section just mentioned. Tapping the skull is admissible in some cases.

46.—Paralysis *(Paralysis)*—Paralytic Stroke.

Definition.—Paralysis or Palsy, is a condition in which there is loss of motion, to a variable extent, associated with disease of the brain or spinal cord, from injury to, or pressure upon, a nerve-trunk, or from the action of a poison.

There are many different forms of paralysis, some of which, with their chief causes, are as follows:—

Hemiplegia is that form of paralysis in which one lateral half of the body is affected from disease of the opposite half of the brain, the parts generally involved being the upper and lower extremities, the muscles of mastication, and the muscles of one side of the tongue, and the patient is said to have had a "paralytic stroke."

Hemiplegia may be very partial, as when it affects the third nerve only, causing dropping of the upper eyelid, to which that nerve sends branches, so that it cannot be raised except by the hand. This condition is termed *Ptosis*. The eye is also sometimes turned outwards or inwards *(squinting)* from a similar affection.

The chief *causes* are—cerebral hæmorrhage *(apoplexy)*, obstruction of the blood-vessels of the brain, and cerebral softening. The general pathology and treatment are the same as pointed out in the previous section.

Facial Paralysis.—This is a local paralysis of the *portio dura* nerve, from cold, and must be distinguished from Hemiplegia, being quite independent of disease of the brain, and is probably due to swelling of the investing membrane of the bones through which the nerve enters.

The features are drawn up to the opposite side; but there is still sensibility of the skin of the cheek, and the muscles of mastication act.

PARAPLEGIA is a form of paralysis, more or less complete, of the *lower half* of the body, in which the legs, and perhaps also the muscles of the rectum and bladder are implicated. It is caused by disease of the spinal marrow, or of its membranes, or of the vertebræ, so that the marrow is either pressed upon or disorganized. It may also arise as one of the symptoms of chronic cerebral disease.

Other forms of paralysis may be named:—*General Paralysis* or paralysis of the insane; *Wasting Palsy; Locomotor Ataxy; Infantile Paralysis;* Palsy from *Lead* or other poisons; or from specific disease, as *Diphtheritic Paralysis.*

EPITOME OF TREATMENT.—

1. *Facial Paralysis.*—Baryta C., Caust., Bell., Acon.

2. *General Paralysis.*—Phos. *(from degeneration)*, Baryta C. *(of old persons)*, Merc. Cor., Cocc., Coni., Plumb. *(with wasting)*.

3. *Hemiplegia.*—Nux V., Arn., Phos. *(Tabes Dorsalis)*.

4. *Paralysis of the upper eyelid (Ptosis).*—Gelsem., Spig., Bell. *(and of the face)*, Stram.

5. *Rheumatic Paralysis.*—Rhus Tox., Arn., Acon., Sulph.

6. *Diphtheritic Paralysis.*—Gelsem., Coni.

7. *Paralysis of Painters.*—Opi., Iod.,, Cup., Ars.

ACCESSORY MEANS.—1. *Electricity*, or *galvanism*, judiciously employed, after the acute inflammatory symptoms have subsided, is an agent of great value. 2. The cold *douche*, bathing with salt water, or, if the patient be capable of the effort, sea-bathing, tends to promote the nutrition of the spinal marrow. 3. *Regulated exercise*—active when the patient is capable of it, passive when he is not—is of great utility in overcoming muscular rigidity, and restoring the functions of paralyzed limbs. 4. *Well-directed frictions** and *shampooing* tend to obviate the injurious results of continued pressure from lying on the paralyzed parts.

47.—Tetanus (*Tetanus*)—Lockjaw.

Definition.—A disease characterized by a contraction of voluntary muscles, general or partial, alternating with relaxation more or less complete, arising from an excited state of the spinal cord and medulla oblongata.

Causes.—Tetanus may be *idiopathic*—from some disorder of the blood or nervous system; or *traumatic*—from a wound which produces local nervous irritation. It may occur at all ages, but is probably most common in the young, and males are more subject to it than females. Sudden atmospheric changes from heat to cold, seem to have considerable influence in producing the disease.

Symptoms.—There may be premonitory indications of an attack, such as fear, or sense of impending danger, or a disturbed state of the digestive organs. But the unmistakable symptoms soon appear, namely,—inability to open the mouth fully *(lockjaw)*; painful expression of the countenance, convulsed or fixed features, the corners of the mouth being drawn up *(risus sardonicus)*. When fairly set in, the spasms of the voluntary muscles are of the most violent character, with much pain, and partial remissions. The pain is of that kind which attends ordinary cramp in the muscles, as of the legs, and is usually very severe. The breathing becomes loud and sobbing; if the muscles of the trunk are affected, the body is jerked forwards *(emprosthotonus)*, or backwards *(opisthotonus)*, or is perfectly rigid *(tonic spasm)*, like a piece

* See "The Anatriptic Art," reviewed in *The Homœopathic World*, Vol. i, pp. 191–3.

of wood. The mind continues clear; and, if death ensue, as is most frequently the case, it is from exhaustion consequent on the frequency of the tetanic spasms (*Erichsen*).

EPITOME OF TREATMENT.—

1. *Idiopathic Tetanus.*—Acon. (*from exposure*), Cham., or Cina (*from worms*).

2. *Traumatic Tetanus.*—Nux Vom. (or Strychnia), Acon., Bell., Hydroc. Ac.

The remedy should be given in low dilution, and administered every few minutes as soon as the first indications are noticed. Surgical measures are sometimes necessary.

48.—Hydrophobia (*Hydrophobia*)—Rabies.

DEFINITION.—A disease resulting from the bite of a rabid dog, or from its licking an abraded portion of the skin,* the chief characteristics of which are,—severe constriction about the throat; spasmodic action of the diaphragm; a peculiar difficulty of swallowing, and, consequently, dread of fluids; anxiety and restlessness; followed by exhaustion, delirium, and death.

SYMPTOMS OF RABIES IN THE DOG.—According to Youatt, the earliest are,—sullenness, and frequent shifting of posture; loss of appetite; lapping his own urine; disposition to lick cold surfaces, to eat straws, *excrementitious* matter, and other rubbish; and fighting with his paws at the corners of his mouth. A very early and constant symptom is *change of voice*, every sound uttered being more or less changed.

* The following accident, narrated by Mr. Lawrence, shows the impropriety of permitting caresses from a dog. "A lady had a French poodle, of which she was very fond, and which she was in the habit of allowing to lick her face. She had a small pimple on her chin, of which she had rubbed off the top; and, being ignorant of the dog's state, allowed him to indulge in his usual caresses; he licked this pimple, of which the surface was exposed, and thus she acquired hydrophobia, of which she died."

The amount of *ferocity* varies; some show extreme fondness; whilst others bark, and rush to the end of their chain to meet an imaginary foe; or, if loose, rush out, biting every one they meet. There is *no dread of water*, as in human beings, but, on the contrary, great thirst; and the saliva becomes viscid, and adheres to the mouth. In the last stages of the disease, the eyes become dull; the hind legs, and afterwards the muscles of the jaw, are paralyzed; and the poor dog dies exhausted, in from four to six days. Next to the dog, probably the wolf, the fox, the jackall, and the cat, are most liable to hydrophobia.

Symptoms in Man.—These are not manifested till a period after receiving the infection, varying from a few weeks to one or two years; the wound having probably healed, and the scar presenting no remarkable appearance. Twitching and itching sensations are sometimes felt in the vicinity of the wound prior to an attack. Sometimes there is stiffness, or numbness, or partial palsy; or the wound may be red and swollen; there is an indistinct feeling of uneasiness and anxiety, with giddiness, chills, heats, and a general feeling of being unwell. The special symptoms are arranged by Mr. Erichsen under three heads; consisting (1) of a *spasmodic affection of the muscles of the throat and chest*: the act of swallowing commonly exciting convulsions, makes the patient afraid to repeat the attempt; hence that horror of all liquids which is so remarkable a feature of the disease. (2) *An extreme degree of sensibility of the surface of the body*. (3) *Mental agitation and terror* frequently mark the disease throughout. To these symptoms we may add, extreme thirst; the secretion of a remarkable viscid saliva, the effort to swallow which brings on the convulsive fits; the convulsions increase in frequency and violence; the lips and cheeks become livid, and perpetually quiver; till, at length, one fit lasts long enough to exhaust the remaining strength.

CAUSE.—A bite from an animal already affected with hydrophobia.* It is asserted and generally believed in India, that rabies never originates in dogs, but can always be traced to a mad jackall or wolf entering a village or town, and biting the dogs. Close confinement, want of fresh water, unwholesome food, etc., may have some influence in developing the malady.

TREATMENT.—*Immediately* after a person has been bitten by a suspected animal, the wound should be sucked with all the force the patient can command; and if he is too much alarmed or otherwise unable to do it himself, a friend should do it for him.† As soon after this as possible, a surgeon should excise‡ the wounded part, care being taken to remove every portion touched by the animal, and to obtain a clean raw surface. The wound must then be washed by a stream of warm water, and, afterwards, the nitrate of silver freely applied.

The chief Homœopathic remedies are:—*Belladonna*, *Stramonium*, and *Scutellaria Lateriflora*. These medicines are on no account to supersede the local means just pointed out, but are to be used as additional preventives, or as palliatives.

Belladonna, according to Hahnemann, is the most sure

* "The susceptibility of the human subject to this poison is by no means universal, for only ninety-four persons are known to have died out of one hundred and fifty-three bitten, making the chances of escape nearly as three to two" *(Aitken)*.

† No danger attaches to the person thus sucking the wound so long as the poison does not come in contact with any abraded or otherwise imperfect surface of the mouth or other part of the body.

‡ Youatt objected to *excision* because he said the point or blade of the instrument used was apt to be touched by the virus and thus infect the sound parts. He recommended the free use of caustic, which decomposed the virus, and formed a sort of cake enveloping it. He had himself been bitten many hundred times by rabid dogs without infection, having always used caustic; nor did he think it scarcely ever too late to take this precaution.

preventive; and certainly no other drug has the power of simulating hydrophobia to the same extent. Several very interesting cases of genuine rabies, said to have been cured by this drug, are quoted in Hempel's "Materia Medica."

Scutellaria.—In his "New Remedies," Dr. Hale proves that this drug has caused nervous derangements similar to those of hydrophobia, and cites cases of cure of the disease by this remedy.

In his last edition of "The Science and Practice of Medicine," Dr. Aitken shows that after experimenting with nearly two hundred different drugs, in massive doses, *scientific medicine* has signally and totally failed, and adds: "All that remains is to mention the most leading experiments, with the hope that, as they have not been successful, they may not be wantonly repeated. . . . . In all probability no prophylactic medicine exists in nature, and the administration of any potent substance by way of prevention is worse than useless."

It is refreshing to contrast the above with Dr. Hughes' remarks in his recent work on Homœopathic "Therapeutics." After referring to the cases cured by *Belladonna*, he says: "I think you will feel inclined, if any one whose life you value has been bitten by a suspected dog, to keep such an one under the influence of *Belladonna* until the utmost limit of incubation has been reached. . . . . And if *Belladonna* has cured a single case, it has done more than all the resources of traditional medicine have been able to accomplish."

Precaution.—After a person has been bitten by a *suspected* dog, the animal should on no account be killed, for after all it may turn out that it was not really mad; by shutting it up and allowing it to live, the non-malignant character of the affection may be ascertained, and the patient's mind relieved of a most harassing fear, that might otherwise have tormented him for months or years.

49.—Infantile Convulsions (*Membrorum distentio infantilis*)—Fits of Infants.

Infantile convulsions are the most frequent of the cerebral affections of children, and are usually from some eccentric cause, as teething, but sometimes are forerunners of hydrocephalus.

Symptoms.—In slight cases, the child suffers from twitchings of the muscles of the face, some difficulty of breathing, rolling of the eyes, etc. In severer cases, he suddenly becomes insensible, and the muscles of the head, neck, and extremities, are convulsed; the eyes are insensible to light, and turned rigidly up and to one side; the face is usually congested, but sometimes pale; the lips are livid, and there is frothing at the mouth; the hands are generally firmly clenched, and the thumbs turned inward, with the fingers on them; the feet are turned together, with the great toe bent into the sole, from the greater irritability of the flexor muscles. After one or two minutes the convulsions cease, either altogether, or recur again in a short period.

Causes.—Irritation of the brain from pressure of a tooth upon an inflamed gum, or anything which over-excites the nervous system; disease of the brain; an insufficient supply of blood to the brain, as in badly-fed children; an impure supply of blood, as in the eruptive fevers; the irritation of worms; fright; powerful emotions of the mother; suppressed eruptions; indigestion. The remote causes are, hereditary constitutional taint, too early or too late marriage of the parents, etc.

Treatment.—*Belladonna.*—Convulsions with determination of blood to, or inflammation of, the brain, *hot, flushed face*, especially in stout children, who start suddenly in sleep, and stare wildly. It should be given early, and repeated every fifteen minutes for several times. A drop of the tincture in a teaspoonful of water, or one or two pilules on the tongue.

Chamomilla.—Spasmodic twitching of the eyelids and muscles of the face, one cheek red and the other pale. It is especially suitable for irritable children, and in fits from indigestion. True brain symptoms require *Bell.*

Opium.—Convulsions from *fright*, followed by *stupor*, laboured breathing, and confined bowels.

Cuprum.—Red, bloated face; shrieking before an attack; *convulsive* movements, the paroxysm resembling an epileptic seizure.

Cina or *Ignatia.*—Convulsions from thread-worms.

Aconitum.—Fever—restlessness, flushed face—and for *threatened* convulsions (in turns with *Bell.*).

ACCESSORY TREATMENT.—Loosen all clothing about the neck, chest, and body; raise the head, sprinkle the face with water, and admit plenty of fresh air. A warm bath, however, at a temperature of 98° Fahr., is generally advisable, as it tends to withdraw the blood from the brain to the general surface of the body. See "Warm Bath," Part IV.

50.—Epilepsy *(Epilepsia)*—Falling-Sickness—Fits.

DEFINITION.—Sudden and complete loss of consciousness and sensibility, with spasmodic contractions of the muscles, lasting from two to twenty minutes, recurring without any typical regularity, and followed by exhaustion and deep sleep.

"This disease has been known from the earliest antiquity, and is remarkable as being that malady which, even beyond insanity, was made the foundation of the doctrine of possession by evil spirits, alike in the Jewish, Grecian, and Roman philosophy" *(Aitken)*.

SYMPTOMS BEFORE A FIT.—In the majority of cases the premonitory symptoms are too brief to allow the patient to remove to a convenient place, or even to give an intimation of what is about to happen. In other instances, an approaching seizure is clearly indicated for many minutes, or even hours, before its actual occurrence. The kind of warning is variable in different cases, often consisting of such symptoms as headache, giddiness, indistinctness of vision, irritability, gloomy mood, spectral illusions, etc. Dr. Gregory, of Edinburgh, was informed by a patient that in his case an attack was always ushered in by an illusion in which he saw a little old woman in a red cloak advance towards him, and strike him a blow on the head, on receiving which he immediately lost all recollection and fell down. But the most striking premonition is that called the *aura epileptica*, a sensation compared to a stream of warm or cold air, to the trickling of water, or to the creeping of an insect, which commences at the extremity of a limb, and gradually runs along the skin towards the head; or, occasionally, it gets no further than the pit of the stomach; and, as soon as it stops, the fit occurs. A knowledge of these circumstances is important, as, in some instances, time is afforded to interpose remedies that may avert the paroxysm, or to secure the patient's safety during a fit.

An Epileptic Fit.—The patient utters a loud shriek or scream, and falls suddenly to the earth, convulsed and insensible. The cry is peculiar and often terrifying. "On one occasion," Dr. Cheyne states, "a parrot, himself no mean performer in discords, dropped from his perch, seemingly frightened to death by the appalling sound." The convulsive movements, especially of the head and neck, are often very extreme, one side being frequently more affected than the other; there is violent closure of the jaws; the tongue is liable to be bitten; a foam issues from the mouth, often coloured by blood; the eyes quiver and roll about, or are fixed and staring; the hands are firmly clenched, and the thumbs bent inwards upon the palms; urine, etc., sometimes escape involuntarily; the breathing is impeded by spasm of the larynx, and performed with a hissing sound; the cheeks and lips become purplish and livid, the veins of the neck and forehead are greatly distended, the heart acts tumultuously, and death seems inevitable. Gradually, however, the symptoms remit, and the patient is left insensible and apparently in a sound sleep.

Symptoms following a Fit.—Some few patients recover perfectly in a few minutes; some regain consciousness and then sink into profound sleep; but more frequently consciousness is not immediately recovered, the slumber succeeding the struggles without any lucid interval. On emerging from the slumber, the patient may merely feel languid and inert, or like a person stunned, or in a state bordering upon idiocy, unconscious of what has passed.

Consequences of Epilepsy.—"Every successive attack strengthens the *habit*, and renders the individual more obnoxious to future seizures" *(Sieveking)*. Repeated attacks of a severe kind are liable to enfeeble the memory, impair the intellectual faculties, and, in some instances, terminate in irremediable imbecility. It is the liability of such a termination as this that invests the disease with such painful interest.

Causes.—These are very varied, but the most common is hereditary tendency. That epilepsy is often hereditary is proved by the fact, observed in medical practice, that two or more cases of epilepsy occur in the same family far more frequently than they would as mere coincidences. Injuries of the skull; local irritation, as a splinter or shot under the skin, or the local cause may be in some internal organ; tumours; inflammations; parasites in the brain; malformations of the skull, as one half being unlike the other; osseous deposits within the cranium, especially spiculæ of bone formed on the inside of the *dura mater*. In *post-*

mortem examinations, the bones of the head are sometimes found thickened or otherwise diseased. It is well known that epilepsy is most frequent in confirmed lunatics and idiots, as the result of some malformation of the brain. The most frequent *exciting causes* are—derangement of the nervous or sexual systems; immoderate sexual indulgence; self-abuse; and prostration of nervous power from any cause.

"The most powerful predisposing cause of any, not congenital, is masturbation—a vice which it is painful and difficult to allude to in this manner, but still more difficult to make the subject of inquiry with a patient. But there is too much reason to be certain that *many* cases of epilepsy owe their origin to this wretched and degrading habit; and patients have voluntarily confessed to me their convictions that they had thus brought upon themselves the epileptic paroxysms for which they sought my advice" *(Sir Thomas Watson)*.

Fright, fits of rage, gastric disorders,* the irritation of worms, menstrual difficulties, repelled eruptions, especially those about the head, and the sight of other epileptics, are also exciting causes.

TREATMENT DURING A FIT.—The patient's tongue should be put back into his mouth, and a cork or linen pad fixed between his molar teeth; he should be laid on a couch or rug, fresh air freely admitted around him, his head slightly raised, and all ligatures relaxed that interfere with circulation and respiration. Throwing cold water on the face appears to do no good; and restraint should not be exercised beyond

* As an illustration of the manner in which gastric disorder may become an original exciting cause of epilepsy, the following case may be cited:—A boy was injured in his head by the kick of a horse, and thus he probably acquired a predisposition to the disease; but no symptom of it appeared until one day he ate an enormous quantity of cherries, including many of the stones, and an epileptic fit followed; this was succeeded by others, first at intervals of a few months, then of one month, and then more frequently. They were preceded by an *aura* from the stomach to the head. He was obliged to give up his occupation, and at length was found drowned in a shallow ditch into which [redacted]llen in a fit.

what is necessary to prevent exposure or to guard against injury. In epilepsy preceded by the *aura*, a firm ligature applied above the part where the sensation is felt, is said to prevent the attack. After the fit, the patient should be allowed to pass the period of sleep which usually follows without disturbance.

TREATMENT BETWEEN THE FITS.—In addition to the administration of any remedy indicated, an endeavour should be made to discover, and then if possible to remove, the cause of the malady. But a cure is not always possible; and the obscurity which often surrounds the etiology of epilepsy should tone down our prognosis of cure. Still, in reference to cure, Homœopathy contrasts most favourably with Allopathy; even when cure is out of the question, the striking relief afforded is worth all the pains taken to obtain it.

EPITOME OF TREATMENT.—

1. *Recent Epilepsy.*—Ign., Hydroc. Ac., Kali. Iod.
2. *Chronic.*—Bell., Cup. Met., Calc., Sulph.
3. *From worms.*—Cina.
4. *From abuse of alcohol.*—Nux V., Opi., Cocc.
5. *From onanism, sexual excesses, etc.*—Phos., Phos. Ac., China, Ferr., Sulph. Ac.
6. *From fright, and for fits in sleep.*—Opi.
7. *Additional remedies sometimes required.*—Stram., Agar. Mus., Plumb., Ars., Hyos., Cicuta, Zinc., Zizia.

LEADING INDICATIONS.—

Belladonna.—Cerebral congestion, evidenced by sparkling of the eyes, dilated pupils, intolerance of light, flushes of heat in the head, and redness of the face; startings at the least noise; tumours, etc.; also when the disease occurs during teething (see *Chamomilla*, below, and the section on "Infantile Convulsions"). If administered as soon as the indications of an attack are noticed, it may ward it off, or mitigate its severity. Dr. Hughes suggests *Glon.* for this purpose.

Cuprum.—This remedy is indicated in preference to *Bell.* by *paleness* of the face, and by the extreme severity of the convulsions. Epilepsy is sometimes cured by this remedy.

Cina.—If the affection be associated with the irritation of worms. An interesting case of cure is recorded in the first volume of the *Homœopathic World*, page 51. The fits were very frequent, the nights restless and disturbed by moans, and worms were often noticed in the evacuations. The child was cured by *Cina* given alternately with *Cuprum.*

Chamomilla.—Epilepsy in irritable children; the attacks are often preceded by colicky pains, sour vomitings, and paleness of one cheek and redness of the other.

Kali. Iod.—Dr. T. K. Chambers recommends this drug as curative in recent cases of epilepsy, and ameliorative in chronic, and gives in his lectures interesting illustrative examples.

Sulphur.—Epilepsy connected with a suppressed eruption or discharge; or in scrofulous persons, and when the disease is chronic. When the two latter conditions exist, *Calcarea* is also a valuable remedy.

Accessory Means.—Hygienic treatment, especially such as the causes of the disease suggest, is of great importance. Regular healthy exercise is beneficial, but it should never be carried too far, as fatigue often excites an attack. Epileptic patients require much rest. Should fright, disappointment, anxiety, or other mental influences, tend to keep up the disease, a thorough change is necessary, including change of residence, companions, and habits. All ambitious intellectual exertion, especially rapid and discursive reading and writing against time, should be absolutely prohibited. But moderate employment of the thoughts, especially on familiar and interesting hobbies, is useful in preventing that stagnation or concentration of the mind upon itself, which is so hurtful in all chronic complaints (*Chambers*). The food should be plain, nourishing, and taken regularly and in moderate quantities. All violent emotions, excesses of every kind, more especially sexual, must be strictly avoided. The treatment of epilepsy occurring in children during teething, is precisely similar to that recommended in the section on "Infantile Convulsions," and is almost uniformly successful.

51.—Chorea *(Chorea)*—St. Vitus's Dance.

Definition.—A disease characterised by convulsive movements of the limbs, occasioning ludicrous gesticulations, arising from incomplete subserviency of the muscles to the will. It has been wittily termed *insanity of the muscles.*

Causes.—Fright, irritation from dentition or worms, onanism, deranged uterine functions, hysteria, and descent from nervous, hysterical women. A frequent cause is "contagion of the eye," that is, patients seeing others suffering from the disease are liable to contract it.

Stammering and stuttering are local manifestations of chorea, and are frequently the result of seeing or imitating others having the same defect.

Epitome of Treatment.—

1. *From fright.*—Acon., Ign.

2. *From worms.*—Cina, Ign., Spig.

3. *From scrofula or other cachexia.*—Iod., Ferr., Ars., Sulph. See also the accessory treatment under "Scrofula."

4. *From causes not traceable.*—Cup., Bell., Agaricus, Stram., Hyos., Zinc.

General Measures.—The most important part of the treatment of chorea consists in the use of moral influence, especially when the disease does not occur from any appreciable cause. (1) There must be removal from too sympathising friends; the patient being placed under the care of a kind but firm guardian. (2) He must be encouraged to exercise his will in the control of the muscles: if the hands be affected, he should be required to carry crockery or other fragile articles; or if the lower limbs, to walk on short stilts, etc.; if the muscles of speech be implicated, inducing stammering or stuttering,* "the best way is for the person to humble himself to the infant state, and be taught anew the use of language from those ingenious instructors who teach the deaf and dumb, and systematically learn to shape slowly and deliberately his mouth into the form requisite for definite enunciation. By practising thus at leisure, and before a looking-glass, he may gain great control over the articulating muscles" *(Chambers)*. (3) The patient must not be allowed to associate with others similarly affected; nor should his disease be enlarged upon in his presence; but his attention must be diverted from it as much as possible. (4) Where the constitution is feeble, hygienic measures must be adopted.

Forcible control of the muscles only increases the disease.

52.—Hysteria *(Hysteria)*.

DEFINITION.—A functional disorder of the nervous system, not exclusively confined to women, and, therefore, not of necessity uterine, but occurring in persons of excessive impressionability of the nervous centres, and in whom there is

* This form of imperfect speech must not be confounded with the stammering which arises from a habit of excited speaking, in which the patient's words splutter out of his mouth in hurried confusion, with an occasional hesitating interruption, leaving the hearer to arrange them as best he may. This may have been primarily induced by a nervous excitability, and may be overcome by the patient exercising control, and speaking each word *slowly and deliberately*. Some persons, after uttering a few words, suddenly stop, and the hearer must patiently wait for the next moiety of the speech; for if impatience be manifested, the interruption is only prolonged. This impediment may be controlled by learning anew the use of language in the manner above indicated.

ot that equilibrium between the nervous and other parts of he organisation which usually exists.

An opinion was formerly current that hysteria was directly ue to disorders of the womb; but this we know to be incorrect, for it exists in women in whom all the functions of the vomb are healthily performed, and even in women born vithout a womb; again, it is also occasionally met with in he *male* sex; men of exalted impressionability, under the nfluence of some powerful emotion, coupled perhaps with xcessive bodily fatigue, break down under their feelings and lay the part of women. We "look to see what organ is iseased, but find none; the machinery is good, but it is working irregularly; it is the engine with the fly-wheel gone."

Symptoms.—Hysteria is remarkable for the wide range and indistinctive character of symptoms, and the multitudinous diseases it may mimic; we may mention especially,—loss of voice, stricture of the œsophagus, laryngitis, a barking cough (more annoying to the hearer than to the patient), pleurisy, heart-disease, difficulty in urinating, neuralgia, disease of the spine or joints, and many inflammatory diseases. In these cases the patient deceives herself, and by extreme statements of her sufferings misleads others. In some cases there is indigestion, a more or less definite affection of the head, chest, or abdomen, or other condition of impaired health or constitutional delicacy.

In the *hysteric fit*, the patient screams or makes an incoherent noise, appears to lose all voluntary power and consciousness, and falls to the ground. On closely watching a case, however, it will be noticed that there is not absolute loss of consciousness; the patient contrives to fall so as not to injure herself or dress; an attack does not occur when she is asleep or alone; the countenance is not distorted as in epilepsy; the eyelids may quiver and the eyes be turned up, but the eyes are not wide open, nor the pupils dilated, as in epilepsy, and the patient may be observed to see and to look; the breathing is noisy and irregular, but there is no such absolute arrest of breathing as to cause asphyxia; the fit continues for an indefinite period, followed by apparent great exhaustion, but not by real stupor.

Epitome of Treatment.—

1. *The hysteric fit.*—Camph., Mosch.

2. *Between the fits.*—Ign., Plat., Cimic. Rac., Aurum.

3. *Undefined cases.*—Asaf., Bell., Puls., Staph., Valer., Cocc., Hyos., Nux Vom., Nux Mosch.

4. *Accessories.*—(1) Occupation and recreation. (2) Removal from injudiciously-kind friends. (3) The shower-bath.

The above is abridged from the author's "Lady's Manual of Homœopathic Treatment," third edition, where the disease is fully described, together with its causes and treatment: the reader is therefore referred to that work.

53.—Neuralgia *(Neuralgia).*

Definition.—Severe darting, stabbing, or burning pain in the trunk or branches of a nerve, recurring in paroxysms at regular or irregular intervals, the periods of intermission being, in recent cases, free from any suffering, but in chronic cases with traces of persistent local mischief, from some morbid condition of the nerves of sensation, the consequence of a local, or more frequently of a general, affection.

Varieties.—The chief *superficial* neuralgias are the following: (1) *Facial neuralgia*—the branches of the fifth pair of nerves are the seat of the pain; any one, or in rare cases, all three, of its divisions may be involved; it is commonly recognised as *Tic-douloureux.* (2) *Hemicrania* or *brow-ague*—the seat of pain being just above the eye-brow. (3) *Inter-*[illegible] (between the ribs) *neuralgia*—often associated with an eruption of clustered vesicles *(herpes zoster)*. (4) *Sciatica*—neuralgia affecting the sciatic nerve from the *nates* (buttocks) to the knee, and sometimes to the ankle.

Of the *visceral neuralgias* we may mention *Gastrodynia*—the disease being located in the nerves of the stomach; *Angina pectoris*—the cardiac nerves being involved; *Hepatic*—the nerves of the liver; *Ovarian*—those of the ovary; *Testicular*—those of the testicle.

Of all the varieties of neuralgia, those described as *Tic-doloureux* or trifacial neuralgia, and *Sciatica*, are the most frequent.

SYMPTOMS.—Darting or shooting pain in the course of a nerve, of different degrees of intensity, at times almost unendurable; the severe form generally comes on suddenly, and is of a sharp, darting, or tearing character, coursing along the trunk or ramifications of the affected nerve. Sometimes there is spasm in the muscles that are supplied by the nerve thus affected; in others, heat and redness of the surface, with augmented secretion from the neighbouring organs, as a flow of saliva or tears when the nerves of the jaw or eyes are implicated; in some cases, and this is very common, especially in chronic cases, there are "*tender spots* at various points where the affected nerves pass from a deeper to a more superficial level, and particularly where they emerge from bony canals, or pierce fibrous fasciæ" *(Anstie)*. In many cases a paroxysm of neuralgia is preceded by *anæsthesia* or diminished sensibility of the nerves of feeling. A frequent, if not an invariable, concomitant symptom is general or local *debility*. It is true, neuralgia is sometimes supposed to be associated with muscular vigour or robustness, but a close examination will almost uniformly reveal evidences of deterioration in the nervous system. This is confirmed by the very common observation, that depressing agents—as bodily fatigue, or mental anxiety—act as exciting causes of neuralgia, or aggravate an existing attack.

The duration of neuralgia is very uncertain; an attack may pass off after a few paroxysms, or it may persist for many days or months, with a well-marked, or irregular, intermittent, or remittent character.

CAUSES.—These are various, and may be of an *hereditary*, *constitutional*, or *local* nature. Neuralgia is distinctly hereditary, occurring in particular families, and appearing in successive generations. It is well known, also, that such neuralgic families are liable to severer derangements of the nervous system included in this chapter—paralysis, epilepsy, hypochondriasis, and even softening of the brain and insanity—suggesting some congenital imperfections in the formation of the nerve-cells and fibres. This seems to be proved by the fact that, though a precisely similar accident occur to a hundred persons, not more than two or three will experience any neuralgia; and these will probably be found to belong to a neuralgic family.

Constitutional causes are—Impairment of the constitutional health; *depressing influences*, whether mental or physical; hæmorrhage and consequent debility; affections of the alimentary, or urinary organs; exposures to wet and cold; a gouty, rheumatic, or syphilitic taint; decay or loss of teeth; malaria, now a less frequent cause in consequence of improved drainage and cultivation; and, lastly, organic degeneration at the decline of life, the most severe and intractable form presented to the physician. The great majority of patients is found among the hard-working, the poor, and the badly-nourished classes.

Local causes may be—wounds; lodgement of a foreign body in the substance of a nerve-trunk; gun-shot wounds, or other injuries; tumours, especially cancer; spiculæ of bone pressing on the nerve (an occasional cause of facial neuralgia); carious teeth or stumps. Even neuralgia from injury is aggravated by any impairment of the constitutional vigour.

Treatment.—In many cases, this must be both local and general. The first includes the detection, and if possible the removal, of any source of local irritation of the nerve, either at its source or in any part of its course. The second includes the medicinal and general measures afterwards pointed out. A clue to the treatment may be gathered from the causes, for as these are various, it cannot be expected that any single drug, or any one plan of treatment, will be effective in every case.

Epitome of Treatment.—

1. *Facial neuralgia.*—Bell., Ars., Acon., Coloc., Spig.
2. *Hemicrania or brow-ague.*—Chin., Nux V., Bell., Kali Bich.
3. *Gastrodynia and Enteralgia.*—Nux V., Coloc., Kali Bich.
4. *Neuralgia of the heart.*—Bell., Cact. Grand., Spig.
5. *Sciatica.*—Ars., Coloc., Acon., Rhus Tox.
6. *Pleurodynia (pain in the walls of the chest).*—Ranun. Bulb., Arn., Acon., Ars.
7. *From loss of animal fluids.*—Chin., Phos. Ac.
8. *From mechanical injuries.*—Arn., Acon.
9. *From malaria.*—Chin. or Quinine.

Leading Indications.—

Arsenicum.—Burning or tearing pains, of an intermittent character, having a tendency to periodicity; the pains are aggravated by the continuous application of cold; increased at night or during rest, but lessened during exercise, and generally first occur on the left side, it may be of the face, involving the same side of the head, the eye, and the ear. There are generally associated with this form of neuralgia, excessive restlessness and anguish, a general exhausted or debilitated condition, small pulse, cold extremities, etc. Influenza, malaria, overwork, or, more generally, some constitutional cachexia, may have caused the disease.

The judicious employment of this potent mineral is often attended with the most marked success in neuralgic affections. The homœopathic law, indeed, leads us to expect that it would be so, for immoderate doses of *arsenic* cause true neuralgia. Persons who have attempted to poison themselves with the mineral are said to suffer excruciating pains along the course of the nerves.

Belladonna.—Acute, throbbing, and intermittent pains, accompanied by *redness of the affected part*, and unusual sensitiveness to light, noise, and movement. Neuralgia of the fifth pair of nerves, and Hemicrania, are the varieties chiefly curable by *Bell.* In most cases the appearance of the patient strongly contrasts with that described under *Ars.*, the habit being plethoric.

Aconitum.—Facial neuralgia from cold, anxiety, or night-watching; the pains are severe, recur in paroxysms, are worse at night; and are accompanied by congestion in the head, lungs, or heart. Recent acute sciatica.

Colocynthis.—Severe paroxysms of *cutting* pains, chiefly on the left side of the body; the lancinations are sudden, violent, and often extend from the point of origin to a distance. Facial neuralgia, enteralgia *(colic)*, and sciatica, having these symptoms, are curable by this remedy.

China or *Quinine.*—Neuralgia from malaria, or from loss of blood or other animal fluids. Brow-ague from these causes comes within the range of this remedy.

Spigelia.—Neuralgic headache and faceache, especially when the eye is affected; the pains are jerking and tearing, and are aggravated by movement and stooping.

Rhus Tox.—Chronic sciatica, especially if associated with rheumatism, stiffness, and lameness; the pains are worst on first moving the affected part, and at night.

Rhododendron Chrys.—Neuralgia of the extremities.

EXTERNAL APPLICATIONS.—When the pain is excessively severe, and does not yield promptly to internal remedies, an *Aconite lotion* may be tried, and is often quickly successful. It is prepared by adding about a dozen drops of the strong tincture of *Aconitum* to four tablespoonfuls of water. It may be applied hot or cold, as is most agreeable to the patient, by means of two or three folds of linen. Or *Bell.* may be used in the same way.

Chloroform liniment is also recommended as a local remedy.

ACCESSORY MEANS.—The *Diet* is an important part of the treatment, and should be as nutritive and abundant as the condition of the digestive organs will permit. It is especially necessary that animal fats should enter largely into the diet, and any aversion to them on the part of the patient, or inability to digest them, should be overcome; well-directed efforts of this nature are nearly always successful. The particular form of fat is not important, and that variety may be adopted which can be best tolerated. *Cod-liver-oil*, butter, cream, or even vegetable olive-oil, should be used in quantities as large as the digestive organs can bear. "In some way or other, fat must undoubtedly be applied to the nutrition of the nervous system if this is to be maintained in its organic integrity; since fat is one of the most important, if not the most important, of its organic ingredients. . . . To Dr. Radcliffe belongs the merit of having been chiefly instrumental in bringing forward this therapeutical fact in this country, and it is one which I have had repeated occasions to verify. It is a very singular circumstance, also pointed out by Dr. Radcliffe, that neuralgic patients have, with rare exceptions, a dislike to fatty food of all kinds, and systematically neglect its use. And it has several times occurred to me to see patients entirely lose neuralgic pains, which had troubled them for a considerable time, after the adoption of a simple alteration in their diet, by which the proportion of fatty ingredients in it was considerably increased" *(Dr. F. E. Anstie)*.

Protection from cold is another important element in the treatment. Exposure to a cold, damp atmosphere, with insufficient clothing, often acts as an exciting cause of neuralgia, and should be avoided, as every recurrence of the disease tends to develop the constitutional cachexia and to strengthen its hold on the system. Warm clothing, including flannel, is a great protection from atmospheric changes, and should be adopted by all neuralgic patients. *Bathing*, including salt-water baths, sponging followed by friction, or the manipulations of a clever *shampooer;* moderate and regular out-of-door exercise, sufficient to favour nutrition without causing fatigue. A change of air, and sometimes entire change of habits are necessary to ensure a cure.

Division of the affected nerve, as a means of curing neuralgia, is alike unscientific and useless. The *subcutaneous injection of morphia* is often a most valuable palliative, but is generally rendered unnecessary by the administration of homœopathic remedies.

54.—Hypochondriasis *(Hypochondriasis)*.

Definition.—Disturbance of the bodily health, attended with exaggerated ideas or depressed feelings, but without actual disorder of the intellect.

Symptoms.—The patient imagines himself, without sufficient ground, the subject of some serious disease, and is often haunted with the dread of insanity or of death. Frequently, at first, the patient considers himself dyspeptic from the fact that he is troubled with flatulence, has a furred tongue, foul breath, irregular appetite, and generally obstinate constipation. After a time he complains of a gnawing or burning pain, of uneasinesss at the pit of the stomach, or of some more serious disease. He has great hope of getting rid of his malady, and strong faith, notwithstanding repeated failures, in treatment. Afterwards, from attention being directed to particular organs, functional disturbances arise,—flushes, palpitation, suppression of bile, or bilious diarrhœa; symptoms which tend to confirm the belief that organic disease exists.

CAUSES.—Hereditary influences are potent and common: a taint of insanity, or other grave nervous disease, may be generally traced in near or remote ancestors. The development of the disease is usually in connection with the conditions of middle life, especially indolence and luxury; or, on the other hand, with anxiety and conscious failure in efforts to provide for relations and dependents. Severe shocks of a moral or emotional nature may give rise to the malady. The patient's complaints may, however, be not merely *fanciful*, but due to actual disease. Organic diseases of the liver or stomach are especially likely to evoke the symptoms of hypochondriasis, or they may arise, or be excited into new action, by a concurrent morbid process. The statements and symptoms of a hypochondriac should therefore be carefully examined. It is often said that *reading medical books* frightens laymen, and even, rarely, doctors, into the disease. This cause, must, however, be very limited and trifling compared with the more potent and general operation of such influences as grief, fatigue, the failure of efforts, or the miserable and heart-wearying habits of an idle life.

TREATMENT.—*Nux Vomica.*—Hypochondriasis associated with affections of the liver, irritability, and fractious disposition.

Aurum.—Hypochondriasis with melancholy, which nothing seems to affect; loathing of life, or a suicidial tendency; religious melancholy; uneasiness, apprehensiveness, sullenness, and indisposition to conversation.

Arsenicum.—Melancholy, with debility; also for the *burning pains* sometimes complained of.

Ignatia.—Dejection caused by the death of friends, pecuniary losses, disappointments, or any other depressing circumstances.

Pulsatilla.—Patients inclined to weep, and of a quiet and gentle disposition, the reverse of the *Nux Vom.* temperament.

ACCESSORY MEANS.—The weary mind should be relieved, and vigour of body and cheerfulness of spirits secured by a course of out-door exercises, physical training, bathing, and suitable dietetic arrangements. Horse-exercise is particularly advantageous. Exercise should be employed in such a manner as shall be amusing to the patient, and to the extent of the healthy action of the muscles, but never to an extent sufficient to produce severe fatigue. If indigestion exist, the article on that subject should be consulted. Hypochondriasis from sexual vices requires the aid of a physician.

CHAPTER IV.

DISEASES OF THE EYE.

55.—Catarrhal Ophthalmia *(Ophthalmia cum catarrho).*

OPHTHALMIA is a general term for inflammation of the conjunctiva—the mucous membrane which lines the eyelids and the front part of the eyeball. Formerly, when the eye and its diseases were less understood than they are at present, nearly all inflammatory affections of the organ were included under this term. There are several varieties of ophthalmia, the most frequent being those described in this and the following sections. First, *Catarrhal Ophthalmia.*

SYMPTOMS.—A pricking pain, especially on moving the eye, compared to sand or a little fly under the lid; sensitiveness of the membrane to cold air; watering of the eyes, and a secretion of mucus, gluing the lids together in the morning; bright redness of the conjunctiva, owing to its superficial vessels being enlarged and tortuous *(blood-shot).* The most marked symptoms are—*redness*, an *increased discharge*, and *pricking pain.* This last symptom is no doubt due to the irregular distension of the vessels, which disturbs the part mechanically, just as dust or a fly might.

CAUSES.—Vicissitudes of temperature, easterly and north-easterly winds, cold and damp, and especially draughts of cold air.

TREATMENT.—*Acon.*, *Bell.*, *Euphr.*, *Mercurius.* For the symptoms pointing to these remedies, see "Leading indications for some Ophthalmic Medicines," pp. 227–9.

ACCESSORY MEANS.—The patient should avoid exposure to currents of air, cold and damp, and if the weather is inclement during an attack, he should remain in a room of uniform temperature. A piece of lint, wetted in tepid or cold water, as may be most agreeable to the patient, should be laid over the eye, and covered with oiled-silk on retiring to bed. If the lids be agglutinated in the morning, they should on no account be opened without being first well moistened with tepid water; but any gumming together may be prevented by smearing the lids at night with a little cold-cream or olive-oil, or by covering them with the lint and oiled-silk just recommended. The food should be simple, nourishing, and digestible.

PREVENTIVE MEANS.—Persons predisposed to ophthalmia should guard against all needless exposures during the prevalence of *easterly* and *north-easterly* winds. The habits should be regular and early; and bathing practised as directed in the article on that subject, pages 50-3.

56.—Purulent Ophthalmia (*Ophthalmia purulenta*).

DEFINITION.—By this term is meant the purulent ophthalmia occurring in adults.

SYMPTOMS.—These are more violent and destructive than those of either *catarrhal* or *strumous* ophthalmia. The tingling sensations first experienced are soon followed by acute pains, which extend through the eyes to the temples and brain itself; the flow of tears is changed into a profuse secretion of pus, the lids are swollen, and there is almost total loss of vision. There are also constitutional symptoms, such as headache, nausea, quick pulse, hot skin, etc.

CAUSES.—Sudden extreme alternations from heat to cold; the irritation of sand in the eyes; *metastasis* of measles, [scar]latina, small-pox, etc.; also endemic and epidemic influences, as crowding together of persons in ill-drained, dirty, badly-ventilated, and insufficiently-lighted dwellings.

Egyptian or *contagious ophthalmia* arises when people are crowded together in filthy habitations, and was first brought into this country from Egypt by our troops, early in the present century; hence its name. There are, however, many local influences which render the disease endemic in places besides Egypt. It is very common among the Irish poor.

TREATMENT.—*Hep. Sulph.*, *Rhus Tox.*, *Nit. Ac.*, *Phos.*, *Sulph.*

PREVENTION OF THE SPREAD OF PURULENT OPHTHALMIA.—As the matter from an affected eye applied to a healthy one will produce a similar disease—as by the use in common of towels, basins, etc., and even by infinitesimal particles dissolved in, and propagated by, the air—the healthy should be separated from the diseased, and each person use his own towel, sponge, etc. Discharged soldiers affected with purulent ophthalmia have often been the means of propagating the disease among civilians.

57.—Purulent Ophthalmia of Infants *(Ophthalmia infantium purulenta)*—Ophthalmia Neonatorum.

SYMPTOMS.—The eyelids become red and swollen at their edges, and are gummed together during sleep; the discharge being removed, the conjunctiva is seen to be swollen, and so vascular as to resemble crimson velvet; the cornea looks smaller than natural, and as if sunk in the bottom of a pit. The infant is very restless and feverish. The symptoms usually occur within three days after birth, although occasionally not for two or three weeks.

CAUSES.—The most common is contact, in the vaginal passage during birth, with leucorrhœal or gonorrhœal discharge. Possibly irritation of the eyes from neglect of cleanliness, or exposure of the eyes to a too bright light or a strong fire, may be a cause in other cases.

TREATMENT.—*Arg. Nit.*, *Merc.*, *Acon.*, *Sulph.*

The best results may be expected from early and judicious treatment. If, however, proper treatment be not commenced early, the eyes are often materially injured, if not destroyed, by the ophthalmia of new-born infants; in other cases, the eyes may be left in a weak condition, and susceptible of disease for some time.

PREVENTION.—The disease is *contagious*, and care should be taken to prevent the matter from the infant's eyes accidentally coming in contact with the eyes of other children, or even of grown-up persons. It also spreads by *infection*, and may be propagated through the air of a badly-ventilated apartment from one infant to another. At the same time, a suitable temperature should be combined with good ventilation, and pure air not confounded with cold air or a draught.

58.—Gonorrhœal Ophthalmia *(Ophthalmia Gonorrhoïca)*.

This arises from the accidental contact of gonorrhœal matter with the eye, and not, as some have supposed, from a metastasis of the disease from the organs of generation to the eyes. In this way the matter may be accidentally applied to the eye of a healthy person through the medium of clothes, towels, etc. Even children are sometimes thus contaminated. The disease presents similar symptoms to the purulent, and to the ophthalmia neonatorum.

In this form, as also in the purulent or contagious variety, there is great danger that the conjunctiva should swell extremely and overlap the margin of the cornea, and lead to its sloughing, apparently by strangulation of the vessels by which it is nourished. When this condition occurs, it is called *Chemosis.* Gonorrhœal ophthalmia is a most dangerous affection of the eye, and often rapidly fatal to the sight.

TREATMENT.—*Arg. Nit., Bell., Merc., Sulph.*

ACCESSORY MEANS.—Assiduous bathing, fomentations, etc.; astringent *collyria* (eye-waters), and, sometimes, surgical measures. See also "Prevention" in the previous section.

LEADING INDICATIONS FOR SOME OPHTHALMIC MEDICINES.

Belladonna.—Pain, redness, and swelling; throbbing pains in the temples; flushed cheeks, glistening eyes, and great intolerance of light. Half-a-dozen drops of the tincture may be mixed with as many table-spoonfuls of water, and a spoonful given during the acute stage every hour, and afterwards every three to six hours. This medicine is often required in alternation with *Aconitum* if there be much heat and dryness of the skin, thirst, etc.; or one or two doses of *Acon.* may precede *Bell.*

Mercurius Cor.—In the most violent forms of acute ophthalmia with extreme dread of light, or in *chemosis*, the 1st or 2nd dilution of this remedy will often cut short the attack.

Mercurius Sol.—Ophthalmia marked at first by a copious discharge of watery fluid, which afterwards changes to mucus and pus; agglutination of the lids; smarting heat and pressure, with aggravation of the pains when moving or touching the eyes. There is not much fever present, but considerable itching and irritation.

Argentum Nit.—This remedy is especially valuable in the *purulent ophthalmia of children*, which it cures rapidly and completely, without the local use of the nitrate. It is also valuable in chronic ophthalmia.

Aconitum.—Ophthalmia with febrile symptoms—quick pulse, dry skin, and thirst; and when arising from cold.

Euphrasia.—This is a valuable remedy in catarrhal ophthalmia, with profuse secretion of tears, sensitiveness to light, and catarrhal inflammation of the frontal sinuses and of the lining of the nose. In simple catarrhal inflammation, profuse lachrymation being the chief symptom, it is often sufficient to cure without the aid of any other remedy.

Arsenicum.—Obstinate ophthalmia in weak and nervous patients, particularly if the secretion be of an acrid, corroding character, with burning, tearing, or stinging pains in the globe and lids, aggravated by exposure to light.

Phosphorus.—Chronic and obstinate cases of ophthalmia which have resisted the usual remedies. There are—sensitiveness to light, heat and itching of the eyes, sudden attacks of blindness, black spots floating before the eyes, and secretion of viscid mucus.

Nit. Acid.—Purulent ophthalmia; swelling and redness of the mucous membrane and lids; secretion of viscid mucus or pus; burning and smarting in the eyes; photophobia; nightly agglutination; and pains in the bones and parts around the eyes. *Nit. Acid.* is indicated in cases originating in syphilis, or aggravated by mercurial preparations.

Hepar Sulph.—This is an excellent remedy in similar cases, and may follow or be alternated with *Nit. Acid.*

Arnica.—All inflammations affecting either the mucous membrane, or the deeper structures of the eye, from *mechanical injuries.* In addition to its internal administration, the eye should be bathed with a lotion made by adding twelve drops of *Arnica* ϕ to four table-spoonfuls of water. After being well bathed, a piece of lint or linen should be saturated with the lotion, applied to the eye, covered with oiled-silk, and secured by a handkerchief.

Other remedies may be required,—*Sulph.*, *Gels.*, *Sil.*, *Puls.*, *Lyc.*, *Aur.*, *Rhus Tox.*, *Spig.*, etc.

ACCESSORY MEASURES.—In the treatment of the various forms of ophthalmia, and weak and imperfect vision generally, the causes of the disease should, if possible, be correctly ascertained, so that they may, as far as possible, be obviated and guarded against. Patients in crowded and unhealthy towns should remove to the country, at least for a time, where they may take daily out-door exercise, and enjoy a pure and bracing air. Frequent careful tepid washing of the eyes to prevent accumulations of matter; a spacious well-ventilated apartment; and avoidance of all causes likely to keep up the inflammatory process. The food should be plain and nourishing, avoiding coffee and fermented drinks; the habits early and regular, and frequent bathing should be practised. A small *wet compress*, covered with oiled-silk or india-rubber, worn over the nape of the neck, is a valuable counter-irritant when the more violent inflammatory symptoms have been subdued; it is also useful in obstinate cases which resist the usual treatment. See also "Accessory Measures," previously pointed out, especially under "Catarrhal Ophthalmia."

59.—Iritis *(Iritis)*.

Definition.—Inflammation of the *iris*. It may be necessary to explain that the *iris* is a movable curtain, having a circular aperture nearly in its centre, and occupies the space between the *cornea* and *crystalline lens*. Its use is to regulate the amount of light admitted into the eyes; for this purpose its inner circumference is capable of dilating and contracting, in obedience to certain influences, whilst its outer circumference is immovably fixed.

Symptoms.—The iris changes its colour and becomes dull; the pupil becomes contracted and irregular in shape, and, if the disease be neglected or mistreated, closed or obstructed; and the rays of light being intercepted on their way to the retina, sight is prevented; a radiating zone of vasculur redness surrounds the cornea; matter forms; there are burning pains of a neuralgic character in the eye, and severe aching in the supra-orbital region, which come on in paroxysms, and are aggravated at night.

Varieties.—*Traumatic iritis* generally occurs in artisans, such as engineers, blacksmiths, etc., from injury, as a stab, cut, or blow. It has been called *common iritis*, because it is a cause of *common inflammation*, without any specific or constitutional taint.

Rheumatic iritis arises from cold or is the consequence of rheumatism, and is the most frequent form of the disease; it is very painful, because the *sclerotic*, which is an unyielding membrane, is so much implicated. Unless skilfully treated, it has a great tendency to recur at intervals, so that a person may have an attack once or twice a year during the remainder of his life.

Arthritic iritis is associated with the gouty diathesis.

Syphilitic iritis generally occurs about the middle period of secondary syphilis, after the patient has suffered from sore throat, etc., but before the periosteum and bones become affected. It chiefly differs from the traumatic variety in the comparative absence of pain, except during the night, and in its being a more subacute or chronic disease.

Scrofulous iritis is connected with scrofula.

Epitome of Treatment.—

1. *Traumatic Iritis.*—Arn. *(both internally and externally)*, Acon. *(febrile symptoms)*, Bell.

2. *Rheumatic.*—Merc., Bell., Acon.

3. *Arthritic.*—Cocc., Coloc., Spig., Sulph.

4. *Syphilitic.*—Merc. Sol., Cinnabar, Clematis, Merc. Iod., Bell., Aur.

5. *Scrofulous.*—See treatment of "Scrofulous Ophthalmia," Section 31.

For *Leading Indications*, see Sections 55–58 and 60.

ACCESSORY TREATMENT.—This must be varied according to the nature or cause of the disease, and may include fomentations, poultices, *collyria*, and, perhaps, surgical measures. Sudden changes from heat to cold, much exertion of the eyes, and indigestible food should be avoided.

60.—Amaurosis (*Amaurosis*)—Weak Sight—Blindness.

DEFINITION.—Impairment or loss of vision from imperfect nervous power.

The word *amaurosis* is derived from the Greek, and means obscure or dark; for it may be of various degrees, from the slightest defect of vision to complete blindness.

In *partial amaurosis* the patient sees dimly, as through gauze (*amblyopia*), or sees only part of the object (*hemiopia*), or sees doubly (*diplopia*), or sees only when the eye is in a certain position with respect to the object. The patient finds himself incapable of estimating distances, so that he misses his aim when attempting to thread a needle, or pour water into a glass.

In *complete amaurosis* the patient cannot distinguish day from night. "The transparent parts of the eye, the several media, so skilfully and exquisitely adjusted for the due refraction and collection of the rays of light into an image of the object from which they flow, may all be perfect and in order; but the beautiful apparatus is useless, for the patient cannot see with it. The fault is in the *nervous* matter, that should receive and transmit the impression, and render it an object of perception to the mind" (*Watson*).

SYMPTOMS.—These are very various and inconstant. Approaching amaurosis is indicated by pain in the forehead and temples, diminishing as the disease advances, and ceasing when it becomes complete. The patient sees best in a bright light, and objects usually appear perverted, being only partially seen, or of an unnatural colour, or double; or dark bands cross the field of vision, or floating dark spots (*muscæ volitantes*), or flashes of light. If there be complete loss of vision, the pupil is dilated, fixed, insensible to light, but beautifully black and clear; hence the disease has been called *Gutta serena*.

Amaurosis is not peculiar to any age, but occurs at almost any period of life, and may come on either rapidly or gradually.

VARIETIES.—Amaurosis may be *organic* or *functional*. This is a very important division, because the latter form is easily curable if its cause be ascertained and appropriate treatment adopted. On the other hand, the organic variety is generally incurable, and the patient is liable to die of disease of the brain. The diagnosis is now greatly assisted by the use of the *ophthalmoscope*.

CAUSES.—*Organic* amaurosis arises from disease of the retina, optic nerve, or brain, or of some neighbouring structure interfering with those parts. It may also arise from fractured bone, extravasated blood, tumours, etc. In elderly persons amaurosis is a symptom of senile decay, and generally comes on gradually.

Functional amaurosis arises from various causes:—excessive use of the eyes on too bright or too minute objects; constitutional derangement or debility, such as anæmia from great losses in child-bed; from prolonged nursing; excessive sexual indulgences, etc.; abuse of stimulants; the excessive use of tobacco;* too much sleep, or other circumstances which produce

* From the poisoned state of the blood caused by *Tobacco*, inflammatory affections of the eye from occasional causes generally take on a troublesome form and often lead to the destruction of sight. If the habit of smoking must be indulged in, it should be in the open air, or at least in a well-ventilated room, with a long pipe, and when resting from work. But from a healthy point of view, *it is far better not to smoke at all*.

determination of blood to the head, and over-stimulate and exhaust the retina, but do not primarily damage the structure of the nervous apparatus of the eye. These causes, if in long-continued operation, may lead to irremediable blindness.

EPITOME OF TREATMENT.—

1. *Amaurosis from debility.*—Ferr., Phos. Ac., Euphr., Chin.

2 *From over-straining the eyes.*—Euphr., Gels., Nux V., Arn., Ruta, Staph.

3. *Organic.*—Merc. Cor., Bell., Phos., Cann.

LEADING INDICATIONS.—

Belladonna.—Excessive photophobia; redness of the eyes and face, threatened amaurosis, with headache, bright flashes before the eyes, and a sense of weight and pressure in those organs. It is particularly suited to stout, plethoric persons; also if the disease has been caused by inflammation or congestion of the optic nerve, retina, or some part of the brain.

Merc. Cor.—This is one of the most efficient remedies in amaurosis; even when the disease arises from organic changes it will be of service; its chief indications are—contraction of the pupil, mistiness of sight, dread of light, *muscæ volitantes*, sensitiveness of the eyes to the glare of the fire, and a scrofulous or syphilitic taint.

Nux Vomica.—Intermittent obscuration of vision; stupefying headache; or temporary loss of sight which occasionally accompanies intermittent diseases. This remedy is further indicated in amaurotic complaints traceable to too close confinement within doors, excessive mental labour, indigestion, or indulgence in stimulants.

China or *Quinine.*—Indistinct vision, sudden obscuration of sight, great general debility, and in all cases in which the disease is due to profuse discharges of blood or pus, or prolonged nursing. In some cases *China* may require the aid of *Bell.*, or some other remedy.

Phosphorus.—The pupils and eyes are of a natural appearance, and distant objects are seen as if enveloped in mist; black spots appear before the eyes, and there is diminished vision. It is especially indicated when the disease occurs in aged or enfeebled persons; or when self-abuse, etc., has led to it. *Phos. Ac.* is also useful in these latter cases.

Gelseminum.—A prominent indication for the use of this remedy is—*desire for* light, thus contrasting with *Bell.* Diplopia, confusion of sight, pain in the orbits. Affections of the sight from over-exertion of the eyes are much relieved by *Gels.*, as are also those arising from over-doses of *Quinine.*

Ruta Graveolens.—Also valuable in over-fatigue of the eyes.

Euphrasia.—Excessive discharge of tears; also when the disease is traceable to catarrh.

Arnica.—Aching of the eyeballs when reading; amaurosis from external injuries; and from gastric irritation, with contraction of the pupil.

Suggestions on the Preservation of the Sight.—All habits likely to produce amaurosis should be strictly avoided. Some of these are referred in this section, under *causes*, and when impaired vision is connected with exhaustion or debility, pure country- or sea-air, nourishing diet, tepid or cold bathing, and other favourable hygienic conditions are necessary. A few additional general hints, however, on (1) the improper exercise of the eyes, and (2) on the most favourable kinds of light, may be useful.

Unfavourable conditions for exerting the eyes.—The eyes should not be exercised directly after a full meal; when the body is fatigued; late at night, when sleepy; when in a recumbent or stooping posture; when dressed in tight clothing, especially tight cravats, tight stays, or even tight garters or boots; in badly-ventilated rooms lighted by gas; during recovery from severe or exhausting disease. These are some of the conditions in which, if reading or other close exercise of the eyes be persisted in, the sight will suffer, and partial or complete amaurosis ultimately ensue. The danger to the sight is very great during *convalescence* from prolonged exhausting disease, when patients are apt to read a great deal; to the weakness of vision is then often added that of a bad posture, as recumbency, or even artificial light, rendering such a use of the eyes extremely prejudicial.

It should be remembered that the reading of a novel is more hurtful than that of a scientific book, because it is read faster, and the eyes are more severely exercised. A broad page is also obviously more fatiguing to the eyes than a narrow one. On the eyes becoming dim after too long exertion they should *rest*, and on no account should an attempt be made to persist in reading by increasing the light.

Conditions of light favourable to the eyes.—Daylight, owing to its mildness, uniformity, and steadiness, furnishes the kind and degree of illumination best suited to the function of vision. With all our scientific improvements, artificial light is but an imperfect substitute for the clear light of day; being often too powerful or too feeble, or flickering or wavering; at the same time the air is often injuriously heated, and deteriorated by the combustion of its oxygen. To enjoy daylight to its fullest extent, involves an observance of the excellent and healthy habit of *early rising;* which, therefore, on this account, as well as on other considerations, we heartily recommend.

If it is necessary that work should be done by artificial light, that kind should be selected which requires least exertion, as writing rather than reading for the student, and sewing lighter and coarser work instead of fine and dark-coloured for the seamstress. Light must not be too strong or it is apt to dazzle the eyes, cause a rush of blood to the head, and excite a discharge of tears: on the other hand, a weak light is equally injurious; and if the eyes are used when the light is declining, so that it becomes necessary to hold the book or work nearer in order to see, the sight is sure to suffer. An unsteady light, as from imperfect gas; or using the eyes when the waves of light are moving about, as under a tree, or when riding, is highly detrimental, as the eyes are severely exercised in continually re-adjusting themselves.

Eye-shade.—An *eye-shade*, of brown or slate-coloured paper, covered with green or gray silk, and secured by a tape or piece of elastic, answers the purpose well for protecting the eyes from gas, etc., in-doors. For protection from the rays of the sun out-of-doors, a wide-brimmed hat answers admirably. An eye-shade should be worn when there is unnatural sensibility to light.

In all attempts for general protection of the eye, good ventilation and a healthy temperature must not be forgotten.

Eye-Douche.—Much benefit often results from a cold douche-bath, a stream of water being directed on the closed eye and adjacent parts. Surgical instrument-makers sell instruments specially adapted for this purpose. In the absence of one of these, water may be thrown by the hand against the closed eyes when holding the face over a basin of water.

61.—Muscæ Volitantes (*Muscæ Volitantes*)—Spots before the Eyes.

Definition.—An appearance before the vision as of black motes; or of thin gray films, like the wings of a fly; or half transparent gray threads, like spiders' webs; or if viewed against a clear and near object, as a white wall, they appear as one or a number of small circles with a central aperture.

Causes.—The exciting causes of these ocular spectres are chiefly the following,—excessive use of the eyes especially in artificial light, or in badly ventilated rooms; insufficient sleep; certain fevers, as typhus and typhoid; deranged digestion; hypochondriasis; morbid sensibility of the general system from business or family cares, or mental distress. A hypochondriacal person having once detected muscæ, takes such frequent notice of them that they become a subject of great anxiety.

Muscæ volitantes may, however, arise from organic causes, and are frequent precursors of amaurosis or of cataract. Muscæ are more serious, as indicating organic changes in the organs of vision, when associated with real impairment of vision, and when the motes are not *floating* but *fixed*. Fixed muscæ are generally associated with amaurosis (see Section 60).

Treatment.—*Hyos.*, *Bell.*, *Cocc.*, *Coni.*, *Merc.*

Accessory Means.—As floating muscæ are due to morbid sensibility of the retina, the treatment must be mainly directed to detecting and removing the exciting cause. If the eyes have been overstrained, *rest* is essential (see the preceding section); entire or partial relief from ordinary daily duties; daily moderate out-of-door exercise in country- or sea-air; a regulated, nourishing diet; and bathing of the eyes, closed, with cold water, for two or three minutes, several times daily.

62.—Cataract *(Suffusio)*.

Definition.—An opacity in the crystalline lens, or its capsule, or both, causing obscuration, or total loss of vision.

Varieties.—Several are described, such as *hard* cataract *(Suffusio dura)*, of a brownish colour and almost peculiar to old people; *soft* cataract *(Suffusio mollis)*, the lens being of a white glossy appearance, having a wider circle; *fluid cataract (Suffusio liquida)*, which may be recognised by being seen to move with different positions of the head. The last two forms occur chiefly in young people, but the hard is the most frequent, for it is one of the changes incident to old age.

SYMPTOMS.—The opacity comes on in a gradual manner, first affecting one eye, but afterwards both, and is often discovered by accident only. The lens becomes of an amber or grayish colour and somewhat less, and the central part first becomes opaque. Objects appear to the patient as if seen through a mist or gauze, and a flame is observed surrounded by a halo. Vision is less affected in a weak light, such as twilight, or when the patient has his back to the window; for, under such circumstances, the pupil dilates widely, and the light enters at the circumference of the lens, which is less opaque than the centre. The patient also sees better in an oblique than in a straight direction, because the lens, being shrunk, does not completely cover the vitreous humour. From the gradual way in which the disease comes on, the patient has a natural, easy manner, and very different from the fixed, vacant stare which marks complete *amaurosis*. Indeed, the patient never becomes so blind but that he can distinguish day from night, the position of the window, the shadow of passing objects, and find his way about his own house with little difficulty.

CAUSES.—Exposure of the eyes to irritating vapours; mechanical injuries; congestion of blood to the eyes from exercise in the hot sun, or before hot and bright fires; chemical and mechanical irritants; long-continued use of the eyes in looking at too minute objects; hereditary predisposition. Cataract is sometimes found to exist in several children of the same family, evidently pointing to some peculiarity in the constitution of the parents. The children of parents of first cousins not unfrequently suffer from cataract and other congenital defects.

Epitome of Treatment.—Bell. (*after inflammation of eyes*), Cann. (*specks on the cornea*), Calc. (*in strumous persons*), Sulph. (*after cutaneous eruptions*), Silic., Euphr., Phos., Puls.

Operations.—Often cataracts are amenable to medical treatment, but some varieties require such surgical assistance as *couching* or *extraction*. Any operation, however, should be deferred so long as the patient has useful vision with one eye, lest an operation should produce inflammation, which might extend to the other, and thus both eyes be lost.

63.—Inflammation of the Eyelids (*Inflammatio Palpebrarum*)—Sore Eyes.

Symptoms.—Redness, soreness, and swelling of the eyelid, along the margin, whence it spreads over the whole lid.

Treatment.—*Aconitum.*—When the affection has arisen from exposure to cold; and when febrile symptoms are present.

Belladonna.—Bright redness of the part, with dread of light.

Apis.—Much swelling (*œdema*).

Rhus Tox.—When the disease has an erysipelatous character, and small vesicles form.

Hepar Sulph.—Should the disease be neglected till suppuration is set up.

Accessory Treatment.—Bathing the eyelids with lukewarm milk-and-water; and avoidance of exposure to cold draughts of air.

64.—Hordeolum (*Hordeolus*)—Stye on the Eyelid.

Definition.—A stye is a small, painful boil, with slight inflammatory symptoms, projecting from the margin of the eyelids.

CAUSE.—Scrofula or debility.

TREATMENT.—*Pulsatilla.*—This is the principal remedy, and should be the first administered, alone, or in alternation with *Acon.* If given very early, *Puls.* often disperses the stye.

Aconitum.—Inflammation, pain, and restlessness.

Sulphur.—A dose night and morning, for a few days, for preventing a recurrence of the disease.

Calcarea and *Sulphur.*—These medicines are chiefly valuable in frequently-recurring styes, and especially in patients of a scrofulous constitution. They should be administered for a week each in succession as follows:—*Calc.*, morning and night, for a week; then wait two or three days, and afterwards administer *Sulph.* in the same manner, repeating the course as often as necessary.

AUXILIARY TREATMENT.—If there is much inflammation, the stye should be fomented with lukewarm water, and a bread-and-water poultice applied over it at night. If the stye is tedious in breaking, it should be opened with a lancet, or punctured with a needle, and the matter gently pressed out.

65.—Entropium *(Entropion)*—Inversion of the Eyelid; and Ectropium *(Ectropion)*—Eversion of the Eyelid.

DEFINITION.—*Entropium* is a growing inwards of the eyelid and lashes, so as to occasion great disfigurement, and constant irritation of the globe of the eye, often leading to chronic ophthalmia. It generally occurs amongst the lowest ranks of society, especially the Irish.

Ectropium is an *eversion* of the eyelid. It may result from burns on the face, or from thickening of the conjunctiva from tarsal ophthalmia. Both conditions require surgical treatment.

ACCESSORY MEANS.—Great benefit will arise from frequent cold or tepid baths, and occasionally employing *Calendula* lotion (ten drops of *Calendula* φ to two table-spoonfuls of water). If the deformity result from a cicatrix on the cheek, such as from a burn or abscess, and surgical measures have to be adopted for its removal, this will be an excellent topical application.

66.—Tarsal Ophthalmia *(Ophthalmia Tarsi)*—Granular Eyelid.

DEFINITION.—A thickened condition of the conjunctiva, and enlargement of its *villi* (little elevations or processes), with disordered secretion of the meibomian glands, causing irritation similar to that from foreign bodies. It is a chronic inflammation, and is sometimes called *granular ophthalmia*.

SYMPTOMS.—The granulations are rough and uneven, and may sometimes be detected by the touch; there is an abundance of pus secreted, so that the eyelids stick together, and become encrusted with dried mucus during sleep. It is chiefly confined to the upper lids, but sometimes extends to the lower.

CAUSES.—A strumous constitution, or debility arising from disorders of the digestive and other organs. It occurs chiefly in the young, and is popularly called *blear-eyes*, but is much less seen now than formerly.

TREATMENT.—This must be both local and constitutional. The chief internal remedies are—*Hep. Sulph.*, *Sulph.*, *Clematis erect.*

Clematis erecta.—Chronic inflammatory state of the borders of the eyelids, with soreness and swelling of the meibomian glands, such as often occur in scrofulous patients. See also Sections 31 and 55.

Accessory Treatment should include frequent bathings with lukewarm milk-and-water, and avoidance of indigestion, cold winds, etc.

67.—Strabismus (*Strabismus*)—Squinting.

Definition.—A condition in which the axis of one eye is not parallel with that of the other; there is not loss of movement, but only of *harmonious* movement of the eyes, and if the unaffected eye be closed, the squinting one looks straight.

Varieties.—If the squint is directed towards the mesial line, it is called *convergent;* if outwards, *divergent.* The inward or convergent is the most common.

Causes.—These are sometimes obscure. Sometimes it arises from an unequal use of the eyes, as from imitating others who squint, or looking at spots on the nose or face; sometimes as a consequence of scarlatina or measles; from irritation, as of worms, teething, indigestible food; from passion; from disease of the brain (see Section 30); and from general ill-health. Sometimes it is congenital. In aged persons the condition is due to partial paralysis of the internal rectus,—the inner muscle of the eye.

Epitome of Treatment.—

1. *Squinting from cerebral irritation.*—Bell., Stram., Hyos., Sulph., Gels. These remedies are adapted to cases following the eruptive fevers, teething, etc.

2. *From the irritation of worms.*—Cina. See the Section on "Worms."

3. *From causes not traceable.*—Phos., Spig.

Corrective Treatment.—The careless or irregular use of the eye should be guarded against. An attempt may also be made to correct the deformity by closing the unaffected eye for a short time every day, when the other will look straight. This, however, must be done intelligently, or while curing the one, the affection may be set up in the other.

CHAPTER V.

DISEASES OF THE EAR.

68.—Inflammation of the Ear *(Inflammatio auris)*—Ear-ache.

DEFINITION.—Acute or chronic inflammation of the external meatus *(outer canal)*, or of the tympanitic membrane *(in the middle portion of the ear)*. When the latter is the seat of inflammation, the pain is much more intense.

SYMPTOMS.—Pain in the ear, with feverishness; the meatus swells and becomes red, and a thin discharge follows. Or, if the membrana tympani is affected, the pain is sudden and severe, even excruciating, worse at night; there is tenderness and a sense of fulness; unnatural noises are heard by the patient; there is either deafness or unusual sensitiveness to noise; and considerable fever. If the disease be neglected, suppuration occurs; and in very bad cases the inflammation extends to the brain, and may prove fatal.

CAUSES.—Exposure to *cold;* irritation from gastric disorder or teething; scrofula; improper syringing, or the introduction of probes into the ear; fevers; rheumatism; etc.

TREATMENT.—*Aconitum.*—Excessive pain and soreness, with throbbing in the ear; sensitiveness to noise; red, shining swelling of the meatus; and fever. Two drops in a little water every half-hour till relieved.

Belladonna.—In alternation with *Acon.* when the head is much involved, and the patient shows signs of delirium. When the meatus only is affected, *Bell.* may be given alone.

Pulsatilla.—In less acute forms of the disease than those which indicate *Acon.*, and are slow to disappear. The remedy should be continued several days after the pain has ceased.

Sulphur.—Chronic inflammation, and when the disease is very apt to recur. In these cases, and in scrofulous patients, *Sulph.* should be alternated with *Bell.* twice a day and continued for some time.

Chamomilla is sometimes of great service to children, and *Bryonia* to rheumatic persons.

Accessory Treatment.—Fomentations with moderately hot water, the application of a bran poultice, or the *Aconite* lotion, hot, in the early stage, will be found very soothing. If there be any discharge, the ear should be washed clean with warm water, and thoroughly dried afterwards.

69.—Disease of the Mucous Membrane of the Ear (*Morbi membranæ mucosæ auris*)—Otorrhœa—Running from the Ears.

Definition.—A chronic inflammation of the mucous membrane of the ear, accompanied by a milky, purulent, or bloody discharge.

Causes.—It is commonly met with in scrofulous children, and, in such constitutions, is likely to follow the eruptive fevers, or any exhausting illness.

Treatment.—*Mercurius.*—*Thick*, bloody, and fœtid discharge, accompanied by tearing pains in the affected side of the head and face, and swelling and tenderness of the glands about the ear. Also when the disease has followed small-pox.

Hepar Sulph.—Discharge of pus and blood; and when the patient has been dosed with *mercury*.

Pulsatilla.—Discharge of a thin, watery character, and when it follows *measles*.

Mur. Ac. is said to be a good remedy in affections of the ear consequent on scarlatina.

Arsenicum.—Excoriating discharge, in *feeble* constitutions.

Calcarea and *Sulphur.*—Tedious cases; and in scrofulous patients; the former may be administered morning and night for a week, to be followed, after a couple of days' interval, by the latter.

Nit. Ac., *Iod.*, *Aurum*, *Merc. Iod.*, or *Kali Iod.*, may also be required in some cases.

For the treatment of acute attacks the previous Section should be consulted.

General Measures.—The intractable character of this affection is often, in great measure, due to the neglect of that strict cleanliness which is so necessary to be observed. The irritating discharge, if allowed to accumulate within the meatus, undergoes decomposition, and gives rise to changes in the deeper structures of the ear, the nature of which may be inferred from the irritation and excoriation so often existing in the external orifice. A little fine wool, frequently changed, may be put into the ear when the discharge is declining, to protect it in cold weather; but even this should be done with great caution, particularly if the discharge smells offensively, for nothing can be more prejudicial than stopping the ear with cotton-wool to prevent its escape.

The *use of the syringe* by non-professional hands, is probably productive of more harm than good, and had therefore better be discarded; at least, it should only be used with great *caution and gentleness* once or twice a day, to cleanse the ear, which should be carefully dried immediately afterwards. To correct the *fætor* of the discharge, which is often very great, a lotion of *Sir Wm. Burnett's Fluid* should be used, mixed as directed on page 301.

The *improvement of the general health* of the patient is a point of great importance; for this purpose, change of air, and, in the autumnal months, sea-air, is often attended with marked beneficial results. In the absence of sea-air, country-air, in a bracing district, is of great advantage. See the *Accessory* and *Medicinal Treatment* in Section 29.

70.—Deafness (*Surditas*).

Varieties and Causes.—

a. Functional or nervous deafness.—This variety depends on constitutional debility; the same conditions which weaken and relax the general muscular and nervous systems act injuriously upon the ear, of which it is a part. Functional deafness is painless; it is better when the digestive organs are unimpaired, the spirits exuberant, and the weather fine.

b. From disease.—Under this head we may mention,—organic changes in the brain; obstruction of the internal ear; ulceration and perforation of the tympanum; paralysis of the acoustic nerve; various acute or chronic inflammatory affections, and disease of the throat (*throat-deafness*).

c. Deaf-dumbness.—This is due to congenital malformation of the ear, and is irremediable.

Other causes not mentioned above are,—sudden loud noises; blows on the head, or fracture, which lead either to concussion or rupture of the auditory nerve; swelling of the lining membrane; accumulation of ear-wax, exfoliated scarf-skin, or other substances lodged in the ear-passage, may cause deafness by obstruction. The deafness that results from catarrh is often but an aggravation of pre-existing deafness—all the share the cold has in the production of the disease being that of reducing the hearing power a little further, and so rendering the defect more obvious.

Prognosis.—In forming an opinion as to the chances of recovery, or of amelioration, the following circumstances should be duly taken into account:—age of the patient;

y tendency to deafness, or the association of the with any constitutional disease, or with cerebral s, or with the nervous temperament. If a patient us with deafness who has suffered from scrofulous ent of the tonsils, chronic catarrh, rheumatism, secondary syphilis, our hope of a favourable result greatly diminished. Deaf persons sometimes state can hear well under exceptional circumstances, as ise of a railway carriage, a crowded thoroughfare, t the whirl of busy machinery; these and similar which suspend the hearing of healthy persons, furnish egree of abnormal stimulation as to excite the dull unwonted quickness of hearing. The inference from ealthy condition of hearing must be regarded as able for the prospect of recovery.

MENT.—The cure of deafness of course depends on val of the cause; in many cases this is practicable; t is not. In most cases, however, skilful treatment sful, and it is very rare indeed after a course of thic remedies for a patient not to find his hearing- ecidedly and permanently stronger. *Recent* cases urse most hopeful. But long-standing cases, even th ears are affected, are generally benefited to a r less extent.

E OF TREATMENT.—

m debility of constitution, struma, etc.—Phos., Iod., , Spong., Ars.

m cold.—Acon. or Puls. (*recent*); Merc. or *Kali* nic); Dulc. *from damp*; Bry. (*with rheumatism*).

r fevers, etc.—Bell., Puls., Phos. Ac.

s suppressed eruption about, or discharge from, the ph., Hep. S.

m enlarged tonsils (*throat-deafness*), *etc.*—Merc. Iod., , Merc. Cor., Iod.

[illegible]

[illegible]

(1.) *Wet or damp ears.*—A frequent cause of disease of the ear is the unphilosophic practice of leaving the head and ears of children imperfectly dry after bathing or washing. The danger is the more necessary to be guarded against if there already exist any discharge from the ear. After bathing, or the ordinary morning or evening wash, the greatest care should be taken to dry the hair and ears thoroughly. As a further precaution, a piece of fine linen or blotting-paper should be twisted into a roll, and introduced into the cavity of the ear, to absorb any remaining moisture.

(2.) *Boxing the ears.*—Parents, governesses, and others who have the care of children, should be aware of an accident very liable to occur from blows on the head or boxing the ears, namely, laceration of the *membrana tympani*, a membrane which closes the bottom of the meatus, and is stretched something like the parchment of a drum. The accident may be recognised by a sense of shock in the ear, deafness, and slight discharge of blood from the orifice; and if examined by an ear-speculum, the rent may be seen. There should be *complete rest* for several days, and a weak *Arnica lotion* used.

(3.) *Deafness not stupidity.*—Another point of considerable importance, is the case in which a child, from being slightly deaf, has been thought to be stupid or obstinate. "Very sad is it to think how often a child is thus punished for his misfortune, and, it may be, irremediable injuries inflicted on the mind or temper of this poor victim of unintentional injustice. It is hardly necessary to insist upon the care which is requisite in examining the state of the hearing-power in a child, or to refer to the fact that children will often say, and doubtless think, that they hear a watch when they do not" (*J. C. Foster*).

(4.) *Wet compress.* A small wet compress, covered with oiled-silk or tissue, worn over the nape of the neck, as recommended for ophthalmia, is equally applicable in affections of the ear, especially when of an obstinate nature; and if persevered in steadily for some time will frequently relieve deafness.

(5.) *Dilutions of the medicines.*—Lastly, a remark may here be appropriately made, bearing on the treatment of the diseases of the ear. In all *chronic* affections of this organ, the higher dilutions (6 to 12) of the different medicines are generally more efficacious than the lower (1 to 3).

CHAPTER VI.

Diseases of the Nose.

71.—Ozœna (*Ozæna*).

Definition.—Ozœna (from a Greek word signifying a *stench*) is a disease in which there is ulceration of the mucous membrane of the nose, from which fœtid, purulent, or sanious matter is discharged. There is often lachrymation from obstruction of the ducts leading from the lachrymal glands to the nose.

Causes.—Uncured catarrh; fevers; syphilis; or it may arise from an unknown cause. A strumous constitution no doubt predisposes to the disease.

Treatment.—The disease, especially if chronic, is not easily cured; but in most cases will be benefited by one or more of the following remedies.

Aurum.—Pain above the nose; heat and soreness of the nostrils; discharge of yellowish-green, fœtid pus.

Kali Bich.—The discharge is *thick*, tenacious, in the form of "elastic plugs," and may be bloody.

Iodium.—Great fœtor; the Schneiderian membrane undergoing putrid ulceration.

Mercurius Biniod.—Sanious discharge; destruction of the septum and bony structure of the nose.

Nitric. Acid.—Syphilitic ozœna; and when the patient has been drugged by large doses of *mercury*.

Arsenicum.—Ichorous, fœtid, and malignant discharge, particularly if the constitution is much shattered.

Sanguinaria Canadensis is said to be a good remedy.

Zinc. Met.—The nose swells, and is sore; there is also loss of smell, dryness, and lachrymation.

Accessory Measures.—Perfect cleanliness of the nasal passages is imperative; the nose may be syringed with a lotion of the last-named remedy in the form of *Sir Wm. Burnett's Disinfecting Fluid* (chloride of zinc). Add thirty drops to eight ounces of warm water; or of the tincture of *Iodine*, two drops in eight ounces of water, and inject with a *large* syringe. This may be done daily.

72.—Epistaxis *(Epistaxis)*—Bleeding from the Nose.

Causes.—A blow on the nose or some part of the head; the hæmorrhagic diathesis; congestion of the head, from passion, over-exertion, stooping, apoplexy, etc. In women it sometimes occurs as vicarious of the menstrual function (See "The Lady's Manual of Homœopathic Treatment," article, "Vicarious Menstruation.")

In simple cases no treatment is necessary; that suggested below is for cases in which the bleeding is excessive, long-continued, oft-recurring, or in which it arises from a debilitated state of the constitution.

Epitome of Treatment.—Arn. *(from a blow)*; Acon. *(from passion, and whenever there is arterial excitement)*; Hamam. *(from a hæmorrhagic diathesis)*; Bell. or Nux Vom. *(from cerebral congestion)*; Secale *(during fevers, etc.)*; China *(afterwards, if the bleeding have been excessive)*.

Accessory Means.—The upright posture; application of cold water or ice to the forehead, neck, or back; frequently, raising the arms above the head, and holding them so for a short time, promptly arrests hæmorrhage.

If, in spite of these means, the bleeding continue so long as to appear to endanger life, the nostrils should be plugged by means of linen rags rolled together so as to form two plugs. Sufficient length of the linen should be left outside by which to withdraw them when the hæmorrhage has ceased.

Plethoric persons predisposed to epistaxis or to congestions, should lead a temperate life, avoid stimulants, use frequent ablutions of cold water, and take moderate exercise daily in the open air. Immoderate exertion and much stooping are injurious. On the other hand, delicate persons, of spare habit, are benefited by nourishing food.

73.—Polypus Nasi *(Polypus Nasi)*—Polypus of the Nose.

Varieties.—Polypi are of two kinds, and are generally located either in the nose, ear, throat, womb, or rectum.

a. Gelatinous polypi are composed of the elements of the mucous membrane; they are pear-shaped, of yellowish colour, and consist of several soft, pedunculated, pendulous tumours, streaked with a few blood-vessels. Their texture is so spongy as to imbibe atmospheric air, which renders them larger in damp weather than in dry. Polypi of the nose are usually numerous and of various sizes; and sometimes extend to the fauces, causing great obstruction in breathing. After removal they are apt to return.

b. Fibrous polypi are much less common; they are often of a malignant character, and the cause of much suffering.

Symptoms.—A nasal sound in the voice; the patient acquires the habit of keeping his mouth open to facilitate breathing; difficulty of swallowing liquids; the nose is enlarged externally on the affected side; and on looking up the nostril the polypus may be seen. In consequence of the stuffy symptoms which a polypus occasions, it may at first be mistaken for a cold in the head. But on the nose being violently blown, the polypus descends and appears near the orifice, causing the obstruction to return, contrary to the usual result of such an operation.

TREATMENT.—*Calc.*, *Merc. Iod.*, *Kali Bich.*, *Phos.*, *Teucrium*, *Thuja*, *Sang. Can.*, and *Opium* have proved the most successful remedies.*

In the choice of one of the above remedies, reference should be made to the general constitution of the patient, and it should be used locally in a more concentrated form, as well as internally.

In most cases it is necessary to remove these growths by surgical means.

74.—Loss or Perversion of the Sense of Smell— *(Odoratus perditus vel perversum).*

This condition is generally consequent on some other affection, especially chronic catarrh.

TREATMENT.—When *recent*, and dependent on a catarrhal cold, or rheumatism, *Aconite* in a low dilution will be readily curative. We have cured *chronic* cases, from similar causes, with *Puls.* or *Merc.*, according to the condition present. *Sulph.* is also valuable in *perverted* smell.

Gels., *Sang. Can.*, and *Calc.* have been recommended.

* Mr. Bryant, in the *Lancet*, recommends *tannin* to be blown up the nostril as a snuff through a quill daily, and cites six cases in which this treatment has been completely successful.

CHAPTER VII.

DISEASES OF THE CIRCULATORY SYSTEM.

75.—Diseases of the Heart and its Membranes
(Morbi cordis et membranarum ejus).

Diseases of the heart command much attention in the present day, not only on account of the frequency of their occurrence, and the serious consequences they often involve, but also as the result of our more perfect acquaintance with the organ both in its healthy and morbid conditions.

CAUSES.—The most common causes of heart-disease are—rheumatic fever in the young (see Section 21); over-work of mind and body, anxiety, and too little rest in middle life; and kidney-disease in older persons. The potency and frequency of the second class of causes are obvious. Life is too frequently one round of perpetual excitement, business-haste or competition, and railway-speed pursuit, both of pleasure and gain. The demands thus made on the ever-active organ lessen its nutrition, impair its structure, and imperil its action.

Speaking of diseases of the heart, we may at once state that all affections so characterized, are not *organic*, but merely due to temporary causes, as palpitation from debility, indigestion, etc. On the other hand, cases of sudden death have frequently occurred, supposed to be due to apoplexy, which were consequent on heart-disease.

TREATMENT.—Organic affections of the heart may be greatly relieved and life considerably prolonged by judicious treatment. Professional judgment and experience are, however, specially necessary. Remedies are suggested for heart affections from rheumatic fever, page 169. For affections of the heart consequent on over-exertion and insufficient rest, *Arnica* is an excellent remedy. Other remedies, for affections from other causes, are pointed out in the following sections.

76.—Angina Pectoris *(Angina Pectoris)*—Breast-pang.

Definition.—Sudden, severe paroxysms of pain, or spasm of an enfeebled or diseased heart, with a constricted, burning sensation, and intense anxiety, chiefly occurring in elderly persons, or past the middle period of life.

Symptoms.—The patient is seized with a sudden dreadful pain, which centres in the heart, and extends over more or less of the anterior portion of the chest, up the shoulder and down the arm. There is an agonizing sense of anxiety, faintness, fear of instant death, palpitation and dyspnœa, so that if walking he is compelled to stop and to fix on the first object that offers support, and so remains, pale and covered with a clammy perspiration. The paroxysms may terminate in a few minutes, or last for hours, and are liable to recur with increased severity, till at length one proves fatal.

Causes.—*Disease of the heart*, or obstruction of the coronary arteries, in consequence of which the muscular fibres of the heart become impaired. Under such conditions a paroxysm may be brought on by over-exertion, flatulent distension of the stomach, mental excitement,* or even a frightful dream.

* John Hunter, the celebrated surgeon, suffered greatly from this disease; he considered his life in the hands of any person or circumstance which acted powerfully on his mind, and at last died in St. George's Hospital, from strong but suppressed feelings on a point in which he was interested.

EPITOME OF TREATMENT.—

1. *For the diseased condition.*—Naja, Ars., Dig.

2. *For the paroxysm.*—Hydroc. Ac., Acon., Cactus, Spig., Samb., Chloric Ether.

LEADING INDICATIONS.

Aconitum.—Recent cases, and for plethoric patients; there is great sense of suffocation, anxiety, and throbbing.

Digitalis.—Cases in an advanced stage, the paroxysms recurring frequently and suddenly.

Veratrum.—Slow, intermittent pulse, cold extremities, cold perspirations.

Arsenicum.—Extreme dyspnœa, increased by the slightest movement, marked debility, pale and haggard face, feeble and irregular pulse, and dread of immediate death. *Ars.* is also valuable as an agent for warding off the paroxysms of this painful disease.

Cactus Grand.—A characteristic indication for this remedy is "a feeling as if the heart were grasped and compressed as with an iron hand" (i.e., spasm).

Sambucus.—Violent dyspnœa, awaking from sleep with a suffocative sensation, and dreadful anguish about the heart.

Nux Vomica.—Indigestion, the attacks being attended or followed by flatulence.

ACCESSORY TREATMENT.—Brandy or some other diffusible stimulant,* in frequent small doses; a large hot bran poultice over the region of the heart; and warmth to the extremities.

* Dr. Anstie, in *Reynold's System of Medicine*, recommends *Sulphuric Ether* in the purely nervous form of angina pectoris, and mentions a case under his care, which he is sure would have long since ended fatally in one of the agonizing attacks of spasmodic heart-pain, but for the discovery that by taking a spoonful of ether immediately on its commencement, the patient can greatly mitigate the attack, and has continued to do so with undiminished effect for the last three years (1868). Vol. ii., p. 749.

77.—Syncope *(Defectio animæ)*—Fainting-Fit—Swooning.

DEFINITION.—A loss of volition and muscular power, with partial or complete loss of consciousness, due to defective nervous power.

CAUSES.—*Debility* from constitutional causes, or from loss of blood or other animal fluids; emotional disturbances—fright, sudden joy, grief, etc.; hysteria, etc. Many persons faint on seeing blood or a wound, or from the sight of operations, etc.

TREATMENT.—Reference must be had to the constitutional state which causes fainting from trifling circumstances, in order to correct the tendency.

EPITOME OF TREATMENT.—

I. *For the fit.*—Camph., Mosch., Ammon. Carb., or Acon. If the patient be unable to swallow, any of the above remedies in strong tincture, especially the first two, may be administered by olfaction. At the same time all tight clothing should be loosened, the patient exposed to cool air, and cold water dashed on the face. The invariable tendency to the horizontal posture is a conservative one, and should not therefore be interfered with.

2. *For the debility.*—China, Ars., Iod., Verat.

3. *Fainting from affections of the heart.*—Mosch., Dig.

4. *Hysteric fainting.*—See Section 52.

78.—Palpitation and Irregularity* of the Action of the Heart *(Palpitatio et tumultus cordis)*.

In a perfectly healthy condition, we are scarcely sensible of the heart's action; when, however, its pulsations become

* INTERMITTENT PULSE.—This variety of irregularity of the heart's action requires a distinctive notice. By the term intermittency is meant an absolute loss of the normal beats of the pulse, covering the time of a natural stroke, or in extreme instances, of two, three, or even more pulsations;

much increased in force or frequency, or both, the unpleasant sensation known as "palpitation" is experienced.

PALPITATION AND DISEASE OF THE HEART.—We infer palpitation to be the consequence of functional disorder, as of indigestion, when it occurs only occasionally, and when the action of the heart is uniform during the intervals. In medical practice the fact is often observed, that patients with serious organic disease of the heart rarely suspect anything radically wrong until the disease has made considerable advances; while *patients with mere functional disorder* of that organ frequently *entertain the gravest apprehensions*. Most cases of palpitation are from functional disorder and not from structural disease, and are consequently quite curable. Sometimes, from nervous irritability, some of the great arteries, particularly the abdominal aorta, takes on an inordinate action, which might be mistaken for aneurism.

probably from temporary failure of the left ventricle of the heart. The pulsation following the intermission is heavier and fuller, showing that the ventricle is contracting on an extra volume of blood after the momentary pause, like a smith who, striking at the forge a number of strokes in regular succession, until tired of the action, changes it for a moment to give a more deliberate blow, and then rings on again in regular time.

As to its *cause*, it is not supposed to be due to indigestion, or to any affection of the lungs, liver, kidneys, or other secreting or excreting organ, but to *deficient nervous force*. "I have never met with a case," says Dr. B. W. Richardson, "in which it has not been traceable to some form of cerebral excitement with succeeding depression. Grief from the deaths of friends; shock from failures of business; disappointments; violent outbursts of passion; remorse; degradation; and, most fruitful cause of all in this madly striving age, overwork of brain—these are the outside influences leading to the changes on which the phenomenon of intermittency of the pulse most frequently depends."

In the *treatment* of this affection, we fully concur in Dr. Richardson's recommendations of change, sufficient rest and sleep, and the avoidance of excitement and stimulants; but our *Materia Medica* supplies us with remedies—such as *Dig.*, *Phos. Ac.*, *Acon.*, *Bell.*, *Spig.*—which are greatly superior to his depletive measures, purgatives, and opiates.—See *The Homœopathic World*, Vol. iii.

In the following Table, abridged from Aitken, the chief characters of palpitation from structural disease of the heart are placed in contrast with those from functional disorder.

TABLE OF THE CHIEF DIFFERENCES BETWEEN ORGANIC AND FUNCTIONAL DISEASE OF THE HEART.

ORGANIC.	FUNCTIONAL.
1. Palpitation usually comes on slowly and *insidiously*.	1. Palpitation generally sets in *suddenly*.
2. Palpitation, or distressed action, though more marked at one time than another, is *constant*.	2. Palpitation is *not constant*, having perfect intermissions.
3. Percussion elicits *increased extent* and degree of *dulness* in the region of the heart.	3. Dulness in the region of the heart is *not extended* beyond the natural limits.
4. *Lividity* of the lips and cheeks, congested countenance, and anasarca of the lower extremities, are often present.	4. There is *no lividity* of the lips and cheeks, countenance often chlorotic, and, except in extreme cases, there is no anasarca.
5. The action of the heart is not necessarily quickened.	5. The action of the heart is generally quickened.
6. Palpitation often *not much complained of* by the patient, but occasionally attended with *severe pain extending to the left shoulder and arm*. (See "Angina Pectoris.")	6. Palpitation *much complained of* by the patient, often with *pain in the left side*.
7. Palpitation is *increased by exercise*, stimulants and tonics, but is relieved by rest.	7. Palpitation is increased by sedentary occupations, but *relieved by* moderate *exercise*.
8. Is more common in the *male* than the female.	8. Is more common in the *female* than the male.

CAUSES.—The *predisposing* are—a nervous temperament; hysteria; a full habit; and disease of the heart. The *exciting* causes are—excessive joy, grief, fear, and other mental emotions; severe or prolonged exertions; profuse discharges;

menstrual derangements; disorders of the stomach; etc. *The excessive use of tea* has been known to give rise to various irregularities of the heart's action; in such cases, a cure can only be expected on discontinuing that beverage.

TREATMENT.—The subjoined has reference to the treatment of simple palpitation, unconnected with any organic disease.

EPITOME OF TREATMENT.—

1. *Palpitation from emotional causes.*—Acon. *(from excitement)*; Ign. *(from grief)*; Coff. *(from joy, with wakefulness)*; Cham. *(from passion)*; Opium or Verat. *(from fright or fear)*.

2. *From over-exertion.*—Arn.

3. *From congestion.*—Acon., Bell.

4. *From indigestion.*—Nux Vom., Puls. (see Section 105).

5. *Nervous palpitation.*—Mosch., Spig., Bell., Acon., Cac. G., Ars.

LEADING INDICATIONS.—

Aconitum.—Palpitation from the least excitement, with anxiety, chilliness, numbness of the extremities, or a sensation as if the heart ceased to beat; short and hurried breathing; *hot and flushed face.* It is specially adapted to patients of a *plethoric habit.*

Belladonna.—Oppression, tremor, pain about the heart; *throbbing in the neck and head; redness of the face.*

Pulsatilla.—Hysterical symptoms; and in females suffering from deranged period.

Administration.—During a sudden attack, a dose should be administered immediately, and repeated every thirty to sixty minutes; afterwards thrice daily for a few days if necessary.

ACCESSORY MEASURES.—Gentle exercise in the open air, and agreeable society, will usually moderate an attack, however severe. The patient must avoid mental excitement, stimulants, coffee, sleeping-draughts, indigestible food, etc.

Pure air; cold water, used internally and externally; regular exercise in the open air, short of inducing fatigue; a contented and tranquil disposition, with light and nourishing diet, are excellent auxiliaries in the treatment of this affection.

79.—Aneurism *(Aneurysma)*.

Definition.—A tumour formed by the dilatation of an artery, or one communicating with an artery, and containing blood. In its first stage, the tumour contains fluid blood, and pulsates; in its second stage, it contains coagulated blood, deposited in numerous thin layers, like the leaves of a book.

Aneurism may be *idiopathic*, or *traumatic:* the latter is caused by an injury to the artery. The disease is more common in men than women, and is said to be the cause of death, in England, annually, of 300 to 400 persons.

Varieties.—The *fusiform* (spindle-shaped), sometimes called *true* aneurism, consists of an unnatural dilatation of an artery; *sacculated* aneurism is a partial dilatation of all the *coats* of an artery; and *diffused*, implies a sac formed by the surrounding tissues. The last variety has been mistaken for a purulent sac, and opened accordingly, to the imminent peril of the patient.

Treatment.—An aneurism usually requires surgical measures. Cases beyond the province of surgery are generally much benefitted by *Aconite*. It prevents arterial excitement, and removes all excuse for abstraction of blood.

Rest, a favourable posture, and a light unstimulating diet, are favourable adjuncts to the treatment.

80.—Phlebitis (*Phlebitis*)—Inflammation of the Veins.

Two varieties exist of this not very common disease:—

a. Adhesive, generally arising from exposure to wet and cold, and affecting one of the large veins of the lower extremities.

b. Suppurative, which is a more serious form, frequently an aggravation of the adhesive variety, and sometimes caused by wounds.

Phlegmasia dolens (milk-leg or white-leg) is an inflammation of the veins, peculiar to nursing women, presenting symptoms and requiring treatment similar to phlebitis.

SYMPTOMS.—If the affected vein is near the surface, it appears reddish-purple; it is hard, swollen, and knobbed; severe pains may dart through the limb, especially on movement, and there is stiffness, with more or less œdema of the part. If suppuration occur, it may be by means of an abscess; or it may remain under the surface, producing purulent infection. Professional treatment is absolutely necessary for this form of the disease.

EPITOME OF TREATMENT.—Acon. (*febrile disturbance*), Ham. (*with varices*), Puls. (*with disordered menstruation*), Phos., Lach.

ACCESSORY MEASURES.—*Rest*; fomentations of warm water; *Aconite lotion* if there be much pain; *Hamamelis lotion* (see next Section) if the veins are varicose.

81.—Varicose Veins (*Varices*).

NATURE.—This condition is one in which the veins are dilated so that their valves, which cannot undergo a corresponding enlargement, cease to be efficient.

The disease occurs most frequently in the superficial veins of the lower extremities, and not usually in the deep-seated ones, because they are supported by the muscles and *fasciæ*. When in the veins of the spermatic cord, it is called *Varicocele;* when in those of the anus, it constitutes a form of *Piles*.

Symptoms.—The affected veins are dilated, tortuous, knotted, of a dull-leaden or purplish-blue colour, with much discoloration of the parts, and some œdema of the limb. If a great many small cutaneous veins are alone affected, they present the appearance of a close network. The enlarged veins and local swelling diminish after taking the horizontal posture.

Causes.—The cause of varix may be generally stated to include such conditions as induce more or less permanent distension of the veins. Strains, or over-exertion of a part, may cause an afflux of blood into them and lead to their distension; standing occupations favour the gravitation of blood to the lower extremities; and, further, the length of a vein, such as the *internal saphenous*, may lead to its undue distension in consequence of the long column of blood it contains. Obstacles to the return of venous blood, such as tight garters or stays, a tumour, the pregnant uterus, or even impacted fæces, by pressing upon one of the large venous trunks, may occasion its permanent distension as well as that of its branches. In other instances, varices seems to be due to an hereditary predisposition, altered condition of the blood, or deficiency of tone in the active organs of circulation, leading to an enfeebled and relaxed condition of the walls of the veins.

Consequences.—(1) Severe aching pain, with a sense of weight and fatigue, especially after long walking, or remaining for some time standing in one position. (2) The vein may burst by injury, and occasion severe and dangerous hæmorrhage. (3) Ulcers may arise from the imperfect circulation and nutrition of the skin, usually on the lower part of the

subsequent bleeding. Excoriations or tender spots about varicose veins should have early attention, to obviate the formation of ulcers.

82.—Goitre* (*Bronchocele*)—Derbyshire-Neck.

DEFINITION.—Enlargement of the thyroid gland, endemic in certain mountainous districts, but not limited to them.

The swelling is unattended with pain or danger, until it acquire a size sufficient to produce deformity, and, by its pressure upon the trachea and œsophagus, interferes with respiration and swallowing. Women are more subject to it than men, the proportion being about twelve to one; and the right lobe is more often enlarged than the left. It is most commonly met with in chalky districts and mountainous countries, and in the latter is often associated with cretinism.†

CAUSES.—The habitual use of water which percolates

* In the "New Nomenclature of Diseases," *Goitre* is classed as one of the "Diseases of Ductless Glands;" it is, however, more convenient in this manual to introduce it here.

† "Cretinism is a strange disease, a sort of idiocy, accompanied by deformity of the bodily organs, which has a close but ill-understood connection with goitre. Most cretins are goitrous; but the latter may exist without the former. The cretin is found principally in the valleys of the Alps, the Pyrenees, and the Himalaya mountains. Idiotism of the lowest grade is often his lot; sometimes he is deaf and dumb, or blind; and in short, if neglected, he more resembles an animal than a human being. I say, if neglected, for the humane Dr. Guggenbühl has proved, that by pure mountain air, exercise, a nourishing diet into which milk largely enters, and moral and mental training, much may be done for these apparently hopelessly-wretched beings" (*Tanner*).

We regret to learn from a visitor to the sanitary establishment founded some years since for cretins by Dr. Guggenbühl, that this valuable institution is changed into the Hotel Bellevue and Pension. The Doctor has died and the children are dispersed to their homes.

through magnesian limestome rocks or strata, and which holds in suspension the soluble salts of lime.

In some parts of England—Yorkshire, Derbyshire, Nottinghamshire, Hants, and Sussex—where the disease prevails, there is a ridge of magnesian limestone running from north to south through the centre of the district. All along that line goitre prevails to its greatest extent; and, diverging to either side, the disease is found to diminish *(Inglis)*. In a goitrous district in Switzerland, there are some waters issuing from certain rocks and trickling along crevices in the mountains, the drinking of which will produce *goitre*, or increase goitrous swellings, in eight or ten days; while the inhabitants who avoid these waters are free from the disease.

Most persons who have goitre find it enlarge during any derangement of the health, especially uterine; difficult labours, strains, twists of the neck, etc., are also apt to increase the swelling.

TREATMENT.—*Iodium* or *Spongia.*—One of these remedies may be administered morning and night for two or three weeks; then, after pausing a few days, the course may be repeated so long as it proves beneficial.

Mercurius Iodatus.—In cases of long standing, and when the previous remedies have failed to prevent the tumour from enlarging, we have used this remedy with excellent results.

Kali Iod., *Bromine*, *Calc. Carb.*, and *Sulph.* have also been suggested.

The external application of the same drug as that given internally has, in our hands, frequently facilitated the cure.

An entire removal of the swelling is not always possible; still, much is gained if the tumour be lessened, or its further enlargement prevented. Any impairment of the digestive or uterine functions should, if possible, be corrected, for under such disorders a bronchocele is much more likely to attain inconvenient and even alarming proportions.

Auxiliary Measures. The most essential point in the treatment is the *removal of the patient from the district where the infection occurs.* The necessity for this may be inferred from the fact that persons taking up their residence in affected localities soon acquire goitre, while others affected with goitre, soon lose it on leaving such localities. A dwelling on the coast, and sea-bathing, are advantageous, and under such circumstances the remedies prescribed may be employed with much greater hope of success.

Water used for domestic purposes should be boiled or distilled. Next to removal from a goitrous locality, this is the most essential point in the treatment.

Exophthalmic Bronchocele is an "enlargement, with vascular turgescence, of the thyroid gland, accompanied by protrusion of the eyeballs, anæmia, and palpitation."

Its *cause* is *nervous exhaustion.* This may be induced in females by leucorrhœa, menorrhagia, etc., or by hæmorrhoids in males.

Its *treatment* is simple, depending much on hygienic means, which may be assisted by such remedies as *China* (loss of animal fluids), *Ferrum* (anæmia), *Puls.* or *Nux Vom.* (gastric irritability), etc. The "Accessory Means" suggested for "Anæmia" (pp. 228–9) are absolutely necessary here.

[redacted]

[redacted]

[redacted]

[redacted]

producer. Inhalation should always be employed during an attack. The cold shower-bath, the Turkish-bath, and the use of a respirator, are also recommended under different conditions.

84.—Croup *(Angina Trachealis)*—Inflammatory Croup; and Laryngismus Stridulus* *(Laryngismus Stridulus)*—Spasmodic Croup—Child-Crowing.

Definition of Croup.—A peculiar inflammation of the mucous membrane of the *larynx* and *trachea*, the vessels of which exude a fibrinous or albuminous material, which concretes and forms a false membrane.

Symptoms.—The disease usually begins as a catarrh, the first indication being *hoarseness* in the voice or cry of the patient, with a peculiar barking cough, or sore throat; after one or two days, or even without any premonitory indisposition, *usually at night*, the symptoms become aggravated, the sleep being interrupted by paroxysms of *hoarse* coughing, the child throwing its head back to put the windpipe on the stretch. A metallic ringing sound is heard in the inspiration and in the cough which has been compared to the crowing of a young cock, or to the barking of a puppy; and although the respiratory efforts are great, it is evident, from the turgescence of the face and neck, and the carrying of the child's hands to its throat, that an insufficient quantity of air enters the lungs. After the fit has continued for a time, varying from a few minutes to an hour or more, there is an interval of relief usually of several hours duration. The pulse is frequent and wiry; and there is loss of appetite, thirst, and great distress.

* This disease is classified as a "Functional Disease of the Nervous System" in the New Nomenclature; but it is more convenient for us to treat of it in this place.

When a case is about to prove fatal, the breathing becomes so greatly impeded that the blood is but slightly oxygenated; the lips and cheeks become livid, cold, and covered with clammy sweats; the eyes red and sunken; the entire organism prostrated, and, unless speedily relieved, the child expires in a state of suffocation; or coma and convulsions ensue, and end the struggle.

DANGERS.—An attack may prove fatal in two to four days, from exhaustion, suffocation, convulsions, or the formation of a coagulum in the heart. If the local symptoms are very severe, and the paroxysms recur frequently, the prognosis is unfavourable. The tendency to death is by *apnœa* (privation of air), the false membrane contracting the naturally narrow passage at this part. One attack, if recovered from, acts as a strong predisposing cause to subsequent ones.

CAUSES.—The *predisposing* cause of croup may undoubtedly be explained by the anatomical fact that the trachea is very small in infants, and does not enlarge in the same proportion as other parts of the body till after the third year; after this period, the calibre of the trachea enlarges rapidly, and the liability to croup diminishes accordingly.

The *exciting* causes are—cold; dark, damp, and unhealthy localities; sudden changes of temperature; wet feet; poor or scanty food, especially the adoption of improper diet when a child is weaned; insufficient clothing, or previous illness.

Like most diseases of the respiratory organs, croup is most fatal in the winter and spring. *Low* and *moist* districts are its most favourite localities. Towns situated near the banks of rivers have an extra share of it; and it has been noticed to prevail in such places, especially among the children of washerwomen, clearly showing the relationship of cause and effect. Dr. Alison observed it often occasioned by children sitting or sleeping in a room *newly washed*, and noticed its frequent occurrence on a Saturday night—the only day in the week it was customary for the lower classes in Edinburgh to wash their houses.

Laryngismus Stridulus or Spasmodic Croup is a far more common disease, and occurs only in children before the end of the first dentition.

It is usually due to nervous irritation, especially from teething; and, except when premonitory of disease of the brain, is easily cured.

Symptoms.—It comes on *suddenly*, usually in the night, with spasm of the muscles of the throat, so that the child struggles to get its breath, making a choking or *crowing* noise, and the lips become livid.

Epitome of Treatment.—

1. *At the commencement.*—Acon., in alternation with Spong.

2. *Fully developed croup.*—Iod., Spong., Kali Bich., Brom., Hep. S.

3. *During convalescence.*—Phos. *(cough, with soreness of the chest)*; Spong. *(dry, hard cough)*; Carbo Veg. or Hep. S. *(hoarseness, with wheezing cough)*; Sulph.

Leading Indications.—*Aconitum.*—*Spasm of the larynx*, inducing *difficult breathing;* febrile symptoms. In urgent cases, a dose every ten, fifteen, or thirty minutes. *Acon.* is of priceless value in spasmodic croup, and often cures without the aid of any other remedy. If there be doubt as to the true character of the malady, it is advisable to alternate with *Spong.* Even in true croup, the remedy chosen should be alternated with *Acon.*, as spasm frequently occurs during the course of the disease.

Spongia or *Iodine.*—One of these may be chosen if there be a hard, barking, or whistling cough, and the breathing is very laboured. *Iod.* should have the preference in scrofulous patients.

Kali Bich.—Cough, with tough expectoration; and when the formation of a false membrane is feared or has taken place.

[illegible]

Hepar Sulphur.—[illegible]

[illegible]

Spongia and *Hepar* [illegible] recommended by M. Teste, [illegible]

Administration.—In very severe cases, every fifteen or forty minutes; in less severe cases, or as improvement occurs, every one, two, or four hours; during recovery, thrice daily.

Accessory Measures.—During the treatment everything should be avoided that would be likely to excite or irritate the patient. A partial or complete warm bath; sponges squeezed out of hot water and applied to the throat; the feet and general surface of the body should be kept warm, and the air of the apartment raised to about 65° Fahr., and this temperature uniformly maintained by day and night; watery vapour should be thoroughly diffused therein by keeping a kettle of water constantly boiling on the fire, or over the flame of a spirit-lamp, and fixing a tin or paper tube to the spout to convey the vapour near to the patient. In very severe cases, a tent should be formed over the patient's bed, and steam conducted under it by a tube from boiling water, to which a few drops of *Iodine* have been added; or, should a membrane have formed, *Kali Bich.* should be used in preference. This method of administering medicines by inhalation is a most valuable one in croup.

The operation of *Tracheotomy* is an important one; but as

is exclusively a professional subject, any further refe
it here would be out of place.

During cold weather, or in very susceptible patients
metimes desirable to keep the child in a large apart
e air of which is made artificially warm and moist, fo
fourteen days.

DIET AND REGIMEN.—During the attack, water is a
e only article admissible, and may be given in
antities. During recovery, milk-and-water, arrov
uel, etc. In the case of delicate children, or if great
es suddenly occur during the course of the disea
ay be necessary to support the patient by essence-of
d wine-and-water, which should be administered in
antities, at regular and frequent intervals. In the ca
infant at the breast, the mother should adopt the di
ggestions contained in the section on "Dyspepsia."

PROPHYLAXIS.—It may scarcely be necessary to re
at when cold and cough are noticed in a young
pecially with *hoarseness and loss of voice*, he shoul
dulously watched, and guarded against influences like
cite or aggravate inflammation, including protection
ld and *damp*, and a carefully-selected, light diet. If
verish symptoms exist, *Aconitum* should be administ
the absence of fever, *Hepar Sulph.*

85.—Coryza *(Gravedo)*—Catarrh *(Catarrhus)*—Cold in the Head; and Bronchial Catarrh *(Catarrhus bronchiorum)*.

The condition expressed under the above different ter
very common occurrence, and often the precursor of
rious affections. It consists of inflammation of the mu
embrane of some portion of the air-passages. It is c
ryza when the mucous membrane of the nose is affe

Bromium.—"Is probably best suited to the asthenic form of the disease, such as occurs in unhealthy neighbourhoods" *(Hughes)*.

Hepar Sulphur.—Loose cough, with a ringing or brassy sound, and constant rattling in the respiratory organs, during which the patient tries in vain to get relief by expectoration.

Phosphorus or *Arsenicum*, according to the symptoms, may be required if debility be very great and the disease take on a typhoid character. One of these remedies may be alternated with some other having more affinity to the local lesion.

Ipecacuanha and *Bryonia* are recommended by M. Teste, as curative in croup. The medicines are to be given in turns, as neither alone is sufficient.

Administration.—In very severe cases, every fifteen or thirty minutes; in less severe cases, or as improvement ensues, every one, two, or four hours; during recovery, thrice daily.

ACCESSORY MEASURES.—During the treatment everything should be avoided that would be likely to excite or irritate the patient. A partial or complete warm bath; sponges squeezed out of hot water and applied to the throat; the feet and general surface of the body should be kept warm, and the air of the apartment raised to about 65° Fahr., and this temperature uniformly maintained by day and night; watery vapour should be thoroughly diffused therein by keeping a kettle of water constantly boiling on the fire, or over the flame of a spirit-lamp, and fixing a tin or paper tube to the spout to convey the vapour near to the patient. In very severe cases, a tent should be formed over the patient's bed, and steam conducted under it by a tube from boiling water, to which a few drops of *Iodine* have been added; or, should a membrane have formed, *Kali Bich.* should be used in preference. This method of administering medicines by inhalation is a most valuable one in croup.

The question of *Tracheotomy* is an important one; but as

it is exclusively a professional subject, any further reference to it here would be out of place.

During cold weather, or in very susceptible patients, it is sometimes desirable to keep the child in a large apartment, the air of which is made artificially warm and moist, for ten or fourteen days.

Diet and Regimen.—During the attack, water is almost the only article admissible, and may be given in small quantities. During recovery, milk-and-water, arrowroot, gruel, etc. In the case of delicate children, or if great weakness suddenly occur during the course of the disease, it may be necessary to support the patient by essence-of-beef and wine-and-water, which should be administered in small quantities, at regular and frequent intervals. In the case of an infant at the breast, the mother should adopt the dietetic suggestions contained in the section on "Dyspepsia."

Prophylaxis.—It may scarcely be necessary to remark, that when cold and cough are noticed in a young child, especially with *hoarseness and loss of voice*, he should be sedulously watched, and guarded against influences likely to excite or aggravate inflammation, including protection from cold and *damp*, and a carefully-selected, light diet. If any feverish symptoms exist, *Aconitum* should be administered; in the absence of fever, *Hepar Sulph.*

85.—Coryza *(Gravedo)*—Catarrh *(Catarrhus)*—Cold in the Head; and Bronchial Catarrh *(Catarrhus bronchiorum)*.

The condition expressed under the above different terms is of very common occurrence, and often the precursor of very serious affections. It consists of inflammation of the mucous membrane of some portion of the air-passages. It is called *coryza* when the mucous membrane of the nose is affected.

If the *trachea* (windpipe) and large bronchial tubes,—*bronchial catarrh*.

Symptoms.—Coryza usually commences with lassitude, slight shiverings, a feeling of weight in the head, sneezing, watery eyes, and obstruction of one or both nostrils, with a discharge of thin, colourless fluid. If it be a severe cold, the foregoing symptoms are soon followed by a dry cough, hoarseness, sore throat, dryness, tenderness and swelling of the nostrils, pains and soreness of the limbs, general weakness, more or less fever, quick pulse, thirst, loss of appetite, etc. Under a vigorous condition of the constitution, or as the result of judicious treatment, the symptoms soon subside. In other cases, the complaint may assume the form of Bronchitis, Pneumonia, Quinsy, Erysipelas, Toothache, Neuralgia, or even excite Consumption in a predisposed person.

Causes.—Exposure to draughts of cold air; wet boots or clothing; deficient warmth or insufficient clothing when the body is *cooling after having been heated*. It is not when the body is *hot*, but when it is *cooling*, that it is most susceptible. When the body has been heated or exhausted by exercise, the frame is not able to *re-act*, and then the application of cold increases the depression. *Partial exposure* to a cold atmosphere, as in a close carriage with the windows open, is more injurious than a general exposure; probably because the balance of the circulation is less disturbed, and the lungs are better supplied with oxygen. Wet feet or wet clothes do not ordinarily result in a cold if the individual changes his clothes for *warm, dry ones*, immediately after ceasing from active exercise, and avoids any further exposure. But if a person perspires after he has been exerting himself, and then gets chilled, he will be very likely to take cold, and to exhibit some of its internal morbid effects.

Treatment.—*Camphor.*—This remedy is only suited to the *chill* or cold stage, when its prompt administration, in two-drop doses, repeated several times, every thirty or forty minutes, will often terminate the disease in the first stage. It should be chosen in preference to any other remedy when the patient has still to be exposed to atmospheric changes. It is of little or no use except in the incipient stage.

Aconitum.—This remedy undoubtedly surpasses every other at the beginning of a cold, or in the precursory stages of diseases resulting from a cold. If promptly administered it generally removes all the consequent morbid symptoms, and so obviates the necessity for any other medicine; a dose every second or third hour. If the cold have advanced or run into any other disease, *Aconitum* may be alternated with, or substituted by, some other remedy.

Arsenicum.—Abundant discharge from the nostrils of *thin, hot mucus,* which *excoriates* the parts over which it flows; *burning sensations* in the nostrils; flow of tears from the eyes; lassitude and *prostration.*

Pulsatilla.—Loss of appetite; impairment of taste and smell; thick fœtid discharge from the nose; heaviness and confusion in the head; aggravation of the symptoms in the evening or in a warm room; sharp pains in the ears and sides of the head, frequently changing from one place to another.

Mercurius.—Constant *sneezing,* with soreness of the nose; thick discharge of mucus; alternate heat and shivering; *profuse perspiration; sore throat;* aggravation of the symptoms towards evening. It is often useful in alternation with *Nux Vomica.* This last named remedy is valuable for a "stuffy cold."

Dulcamara.—Cold from *getting wet,* or from checked perspiration. This medicine should be had recourse to on the first appearance of the symptoms of catarrh following exposure to *wet;* it is also recommended as a preventive when after exposure it is feared a cold may result.

Euphrasia.—Acrid fluent coryza, with involvement of the lining membrane of the eyes, and *profuse lachrymation.*

Kali Bichromicum.—*Chronic catarrh*, and chronic affections of the respiratory mucous membranes generally, with hoarseness, *tough stringy sputa*, chronically inflamed or ulcerated throat, cough, etc. An additional indication is a concurrent affection of the digestive mucous membrane—yellow-coated tongue, etc.

Accessory Means.—The *hot-foot-bath*, as described in Part IV; if the directions are promptly and efficiently carried out, cold may generally be arrested in its incipient stage. If the catarrh be established, the most essential measure to ensure a rapid recovery is to avoid exposure to atmospheric vicissitudes, until the attack has passed away. In all serious cases the patient should remain in bed for two or three days. As a rule, light food, and a very sparing use of meat should be adopted at the commencement of a cold.

To Diminish Excessive Sensibility to Cold.—Persons extremely sensitive should consult a homœopathic physician, who will be able to prescribe both hygienic and medicinal measures suitable to individual cases. The two following measures are, however, recommended for general adoption. 1st.—*Free exposure to the open-air, daily.* Familiarity with the atmosphere has a wonderful influence in diminishing the sensibility of the skin, and enabling the body to resist the invasion of cold. A striking contrast, in this respect, is presented by farmers, shepherds, coachmen, sailors, and others who live much in the open air, to tailors, shopmen, lawyers, women, and others whose occupations are pursued within doors! The sensibility of the former is blunted by habitual exposure, while the latter are liable to cold from every vicissitude of the weather. The pure air breathed by the out-door labourer, together with his active life, lead to a rous condition of health, contrasting most favourably with the condition of one occupied within-doors. 2nd.—*The morning cold bath.* Cold-sponging over the entire surface of the body, the plunge-bath, or the shower-bath, is an invaluable method of protecting the body against injury from exposure to changes of temperature. Taken regularly in the morning, the cold bath inures the surface of the body to a greater degree of cold than it will probably encounter during the remainder of the day; at the same time promotes a vigorous capillary circulation, which is essential to the harmonious and healthy working of the system. For hints on the use of the bath, see pages 50–3.

86.—Aphonia (*Aphonia*) Loss of Voice—Hoarseness.

Aphonia is generally the result of an acute or sub-acute inflammatory condition of the mucous membrane lining the larynx and the wind-pipe, and is a frequent accompaniment of a common cold; also of several other diseases. It is rather a symptom than a disease *per se*.

SYMPTOMS.—The voice is hoarse and husky; at times almost or entirely inaudible; there is tickling, dryness, or irritation, and perhaps soreness in the throat, with a short dry cough.

EPITOME OF TREATMENT.—

1. *Simple Hoarseness.*—Phyto. (*also complete or chronic loss of voice*); Hep. S. (*wheezing*); Phos. (*paralysis of the vocal cords*); Carbo. Veg. (*chronic*).

2. *With cold in the head or chest.*—Acon., Caust., Merc., Spong., Phos., Dulc.

3. *From over-exertion of the voice—clergymen, singers, etc.* Caust., Arn., Baryta C., Kali Bich.

Leading Indications and *accessory means* are pointed out in the preceding Section; also in that on "Sore Throat."

87.—Bronchitis (*Bronchitis*).

a. ACUTE BRONCHITIS is acute inflammation of the mucous membrane of the *bronchi*, the air-tubes of the lungs. It is a diffused disease, extending more or less through both lungs, and accompanied by hoarseness, cough, heat and soreness of the chest, the mucous secretion being at first arrested, but afterwards increased in quantity. The disease is most common in elderly persons, although it is not infrequent in children.

SYMPTOMS. At first there is fever, with headache, lassitude, anxiety, and other symptoms of a common cold. There is also a sensation of tightness or constriction in the chest, especially of the upper front part; oppressed, hurried, anxious, laboured breathing, with wheezing, severe cough, which is at first dry, but is afterwards accompanied with viscid and frothy expectoration, sometimes streaked with blood; subsequently the sputa becomes thick, yellowish, and purulent. The pulse is frequent and often weak; the urine scanty and high-coloured; the tongue foul; there is throbbing in the forehead and aching in the eyes, aggravated on coughing, with other febrile symptoms. In favourable cases, the disease begins to decline between the fourth and eighth day, when the breathing becomes easier, and the expectoration thicker, less frothy and stringy; and the complaint soon entirely disappears, or assumes the chronic form.

In cases about to terminate fatally, the skin becomes covered with *cold* perspiration; the cheeks and lips pale and livid; the extremities cold; there is rattling and a sense of suffocation in the throat, the breathing being nearly suspended by the morbid secretion which chokes up the bronchial tubes and their ramifications, and which the patient has no longer power to cough up; at length, extreme prostration and complete insensibility end in death.

Morbid Anatomy.—On examination of the body after death, we find the trachea, the bronchi, and their divisions and subdivisions, completely blocked up by a frothy, adhesive mucus, resembling that which had been expectorated during life.

b. Chronic Bronchitis is a somewhat different disease, and is very common in advanced life. In mild cases there is only habitual cough, shortness of breath, and copious expectoration. Many cases of winter cough in old people are examples of chronic bronchitis. It is often insidious in its approach, although it sometimes succeeds to acute bronchitis, when that disease has been neglected or has not been properly treated.

Causes.—Similar to those of common cold:—exposure to cold draughts of air, to keen and cutting winds, sudden changes of temperature, scanty clothing, or undue exposure of the throat and neck after public speaking and singing. Bronchitis often follows cold in the head.

From recent statistics we learn that the mortality from bronchitis has increased from 135 per million of population in 1838, to 1968 per million in 1866! This enormous increase of figures is *partly* due to a practice which has been adopted for obvious reasons of late years, of returning deaths from consumption under the name of bronchitis. But, altogether apart from this, bronchitis has become alarmingly common and fatal. Besides hereditary influence, certain "social indiscretions" are fertile causes. Among these are classed the habits of our business-men, "who after a hurried early breakfast, hasten to catch the train or 'bus to the city, where they work all day on little or no food, and start on the homeward journey in the evening with the vital powers depressed, and in a condition most favourable to the inroad of disease. The ladies are also shown to be 'indiscreet' in the exposure of themselves to draughts of cold air, in the hinnest and scantiest clothing, in halls or passages, or even n the open street on the way between their carriage and the lace of public gathering. Thin boots and too late resort to vinter habiliments, are also well-recognized sources of danger; s is, also, inattention to the fact, that those advanced in ears require warmer clothing than the middle-aged."*

Winter cough, often regarded with indifference, is, in many ases, but a precursor or symptom of this common disease. When an epidemic of cholera sweeps away its *hundreds*, public ttention is attracted, and fear induces attention to precautions itherto despised. Bronchitis sweeps away its *thousands nnually*, and is surely deserving of more general attention han is ordinarily given to a mere 'winter cough.'"

Epitome of Treatment.—

1. *Acute Bronchitis.*—Acon., Kali Bich., Bry., Ipec.

2. *Chronic.*—Ant. Tart. *(much loose mucus)*; Kali Bich. *(tough, stringy phlegm)*; Carbo Veg. or Ars. *(great debility)*; Ammon. Carb. *(incessant cough, with sensation as if there were wool in the larynx)*; Merc. *(purulent expectoration)*; Silic., Phos., Sulph.

3. *In children.*—Acon., Phos., Bry., Puls. *(loose cough)*; pec. *(spasmodic cough)*; Ant. Tart. *(accumulation of mucus)*.

4.—*Remedies sometimes required.*—Bell., Coni., Senega, Nit. Ac., Spong., Iod.

Leading Indications.—

Aconitum.—This remedy should commence the treatment of all cases of bronchitis with the usual febrile symptoms. If administered early and frequently it will materially shorten the attack, and perhaps be alone curative. *Acon.* is also ndicated by a short, hard cough, excited by tickling sensations in the windpipe and chest, inducing frontal headache, and burning and sore pain in the chest.

* From *The Homœopathic World*, Vol. II. See also Vol. IV., p. 102.

Dr. Hughes has found the maximum of advantage in *acute* adult bronchitis in the use of *Acon.* and *Kali Bich.*

Acon. is also a valuable occasional remedy in chronic bronchitis.

Bryonia.—Violent cough, chiefly affecting the upper part of the chest, under the breast-bone, with copious expectoration of thick yellow mucus, sometimes streaked with blood. In advanced stages of bronchitis, this remedy will often be found valuable in alternation with *Phosphorus.* *Bryonia* is also useful in the acute attacks of children with suffocative cough, great agitation and anxiety.

Kali Bich.—This is one of the best remedies in bronchitis, with irritation in the larynx and chest, inducing paroxysms of cough which are severe and long-continued, owing to the difficulty of detaching the phlegm, which is *tenacious and stringy.* A yellow-coated tongue, with loss of appetite, are also indications for the use of *Kali Bich.* It is very serviceable when catarrh runs on into bronchitis, and in chronic bronchitis, with the above symptoms.

Antimonium Tart.—Severe paroxysms of *suffocative* cough with loose expectoration, wheezing respiration; the whole chest seems to be involved; frequently also there is palpitation of the heart, pain in the loins and back, headache, thirst, etc. In the chronic form of the disease it is sometimes very useful in promoting expectoration.

Ipecacuanha.—Spasmodic cough, with or without expectoration of blood, often with sickness and vomiting, and great difficulty of breathing. As an expectorant, it is often of great service.

Phosphorus.—Useful in chronic cases, and whenever the lungs are involved.

Arsenicum.—Chilliness in the chest; a suffocative sensation on lying down; anxious, painful, laboured breathing; or when the lungs no longer permit the free entrance of oxygen into the air-tubes, and thus are incapable of expelling the morbid secretions. *Ars.* is well indicated in aged or feeble persons.

Carbo Veg.—Chronic bronchitis in aged persons, with profuse expectoration, or profuse mucous accumulation, which the patient is unable to remove; and there is blueness of the nails, coldness of the extremities, etc.

China.—Useful in sustaining the constitution under the heavy discharges of mucus, and may be administered occasionally alone or in alternation with another remedy.

ADMINISTRATION.—In acute cases the remedy should be given every two to four hours; in chronic, thrice daily for a week or two.

Kreasote Inhalations.—In chronic bronchitis, with excessive expectoration, the inhalation of the vapour of *Kreasote*—three or four drops in a pint of boiling water—checks the secretion. It also corrects fœtid sputa.

ACCESSORY MEANS.—In acute bronchitis the diet should be light and liquid, including gum-water, barley-water, gruel, jelly, beef-tea, etc. Throughout the disease the air of the patient's apartment should be maintained at a temperature of about 65° to 70° Fahr., and it should be kept *moist* by the evaporation of hot water from shallow dishes near the bed, as directed in the section on *Quinsey*. Congestion of the lungs may be relieved by covering the chest with large hot linseed-meal poultices. If there is great prostration, nutritious liquid diet and stimulants are necessary; if they cannot be taken by the mouth, they should be administered in the form of enemata.

PREVENTIVE MEANS.—The first and most important is cold bathing in the morning, that particular form of bath being adopted which is found most useful or convenient. (See Bathing, pages 50–3). Susceptible patients may wear a good respirator whenever exposed to night air, or during inclement weather; but *such exposure should be avoided* as much as possible.

Another preventive in the case of males is the *Beard*, which protects the respiratory passages against the effects of sudden changes of temperature. We may regard the beard as a kind of *natural respirator*, the shaving off of which is a frequent cause of acute and chronic bronchitis. Can we doubt the wisdom and beneficence of the Creator in giving this ornament to the *male* sex, so frequently exposed to atmospheric vicissitudes, and withholding it from the *female*, who, as the *keeper at home*, requires no such appendage? Hair is an imperfect conductor of both heat and cold, and placed round the entrance to the lungs, acts like a blanket, which is used for warmth in cold weather, or to prevent the dissolving of ice in hot weather. In many instances, the beard would protect lawyers, clergymen, and other public speakers, as well as singers from the injurious effects of sudden variations of the atmosphere, from which professional men often suffer. It has been observed that the Jews, and other people who wear the beard, rarely suffer from bronchitis or analogous disorders; and so may be considered as examples of the utility of the beard.

Other preventive measures may be inferred from the perusal of the paragraph on "Causes."

88.—Asthma (*Asthma*).

Definition.—Asthma is a spasmodic disease, characterized by paroxysms of difficult breathing, with great wheezing, and a dreadful sense of constriction across the chest; each paroxysm terminates by the expectoration of a more or less abundant quantity of mucus.

Pathology.—The air-tubes of the lungs are encircled by minute bands of muscular structure, which, like other muscular fibres, are liable to be affected with spasm, as is proved by the phenomena presented in this disease. The spasm constricts the air-tubes, and the wheezing and difficult breathing are caused by the air being forced through these contracted channels. The spasmodic character of the disease is further proved by the fact that post-mortem examinations of the lungs of some asthmatic patients have been made without presenting scarcely any traces of disease, either in the lungs or heart, except that the air-cells are dilated, and the entire lungs are puffy and anæmic.

SYMPTOMS.—A fit of asthma generally occurs in the night, particularly from midnight to early morning—the patient wakes suddenly with a sense of suffocation, springs up in bed, and assumes various postures; or he even rushes to the opened window, where he leans forward on his arms, employing the assisting muscles of inspiration; and, wheezing loudly, from the great obstruction to the entrance and exit of air, labours for breath like one struggling for life. The countenance bears evidence of great distress; the eyes protrude; the skin is cold and clammy; the pulse small and feeble; the perspiration stands in large drops on the forehead, or runs down the face; and he often looks imploringly, sometimes impatiently, at his medical attendant for relief from his misery. At length, after an uncertain time, one to three hours or longer, there comes a remission; cough ensues, and with it expectoration of mucus, and the paroxysm ceases, permitting the sufferer to fall into the long-desired slumber.

The attacks are unattended with fever, but are generally preceded by some disturbance of the digestive organs; they are often periodic and sudden, and attended with distressing anxiety.

PHYSICAL SIGNS.—On *percussion* during a fit, the chest is resonant, showing that the lungs are distended with air; but *on applying* the stethescope little or no respiratory sound is heard, as if the air were imprisoned or in a state of stagnation in the air-cells; and it is probable there is a spasmodic contraction of the muscular fibres at the base of the trachea which stops the respiratory murmur.

DIAGNOSIS.—The physical conditions of the chest just pointed out, the abruptness and violence of the symptoms, and the comparative good health enjoyed between the attacks, are sufficient to distinguish the disease.

CAUSES.—Irritation of the nerves of respiration resulting in most cases from *deranged digestion*, from the intimate nervous connection existing between the digestive and the respiratory organs; it may also be produced by hygrometric changes of the atmosphere; or, again, by the introduction of some poisonous but subtle material floating in the atmosphere, and brought by inspiration into contact with the respiratory surface, such as the minute particles, or the mere odour, which passes off from powdered ipecacuanha or hay (see Section 83); or the vapour of sulphur. Asthma is often associated with the gouty or rheumatic diathesis. Excessive exertion and mental emotion frequently bring on a paroxysm. After it has once occurred, asthma is easily reproduced by indigestion, especially after *late dinners* or *suppers*. A frequent repetition of the fits leads to a dilated state of the air-passages and air-cells of the lungs, dilation of the right cavities of the heart, and the general displacement of that organ which uniformly exists in persons who have *long* suffered from this disease. The disease may also be hereditary, it being one of those maladies, a disposition to which is transmitted from parents to children.

EPITOME OF TREATMENT.—

1. *For the attack.*—Acon., Ipec., Cup., Lob. In., Hydroc. Ac.
2. *Asthma of children.*—Samb., Ipec.
3. *From suppressed eruptions.*—Graph., Sulph., Zinc.
4. *Chronic asthma.*—Ars., Nux Vom., Sulph., Arg. Nit., *Cocc., Plumb.*

LEADING INDICATIONS.—

Ipecacuanha.—A tight sensation in the chest, panting and rattling in the windpipe, which feels as if full of phlegm; coldness, paleness, anxiety, and sickness; troublesome cough. A dose every ten or fifteen minutes during an attack; afterwards every three or four hours.

Aconitum.—The striking power of this great remedy in affections of the pneumogastric nerve, characterised by imperfect and laboured breathing, has suggested its use in spasmodic asthma, during the paroxysms of which we have often administered it with marked and speedy relief. It is especially indicated by oppressive anxiety, dyspnœa, and laboured action of the heart.

Lobelia Inflata.—Pure nervous asthma, with a constrictive, suffocative sensation; spasmodic cough; vomiting; giddiness, etc.

Cuprum.—Also useful in attacks of nervous asthma.

Nux Vomica.—Probably the best anti-asthma remedy. It is homœopathic to that condition of the digestive system which is the most common cause of the irritation which results in bronchial spasm. Again, "after the paroxysm subsides, it leaves a condition of the digestive organs for which *Nux Vomica* is the great remedy. The tongue is coated with a thick, yellow fur; there is often slight nausea, flatulence, and constipation. Besides, the breathing is seldom quite right; generally there remains a sort of physical memory of the struggle. The patient feels that no liberties must be taken, either of diet or exercise. Out of this secondary state of bondage nothing will liberate so effectually as *Nux Vomica*" *(Russell).*

Arsenicum.—Short, anxious, and wheezing breathing; aggravation of the sufferings at night on lying down, and upon the least movement; periodic, suffocative attacks, with pale or bluish face. It is especially useful in chronic asthma, and when the disease occurs in old persons, or in feeble constitutions, and is attended with burning heat of the chest, cold sweats, general debility, etc.; also in asthma complicated with heart-disease, or following bronchitis or catarrh.

Veratrum.—Violent paroxysms of spasmodic asthma, with great prostration, coldness of the nose, ears, and feet, and cold perspirations.

Sulphur.—Chronic asthma apparently connected with gout, eruptions on the skin, or some other constitutional taint; also after other medicines have but partially succeeded.

ACCESSORY MEANS.—During a fit, striking relief may often be obtained by putting the feet and hands into hot water. Smoking *Stramonium* at the commencement of a fit, is said to remove it like a charm in some; in others, however, it fails altogether; the inhalation (see Part IV) of *Aconite-vapour* is much more certain and efficacious. Tobacco-smoking, and other such measures, are of no ultimate utility, and are, moreover, rendered unnecessary by homœopathic treatment. Relief is often obtained by the fumes of burning nitre on a plate, which is effected by placing some pieces of blotting-paper, about the size of the hand, previously saturated in a solution of the nitrate of potash; one of these pieces being ignited, the fumes are diffused throughout the room, and their influence is soon made evident. At the same time, ventilation must not be neglected; the windows should be regularly thrown wide open to renew the air of the apartment.

PROPHYLACTIC MEASURES.—Persons who are predisposed to asthma should strictly avoid all its exciting causes, more especially indigestible food and heavy suppers; wet feet, damp clothes, and sudden changes of temperature. The "plan of dietary" we have sketched in the first chapter of this volume (pages 25–8), should be adhered to; for, as may be inferred from what has already been stated, the slightest disorder of the stomach may occasion an attack. Pastry, highly-seasoned dishes, too great a variety or too great a quantity at one meal, coffee, and heating beverages, should be avoided. "More is to be done for asthmatic patients on the side of the stomach than in any other direction." In some cases the diet should be weighed, the hours of meals fixed, and rigidly adhered to. An important point is to take the last solid meal at such an hour as shall allow time for its complete digestion before retiring to bed.

A most valuable and potent agent to fortify the body against asthma is the *shower-bath;* the sudden application of water improves the tone of the whole system, and renders the body less sensitive to atmospheric changes. Out-of-door exercise is also useful, either walking or riding; but it should never be taken within one or two hours after a meal, or to such an extent as to occasion fatigue.

89.—Pneumonia *(Peripneumonia)*—Inflammation of the Lungs.

Definition.—Acute inflammation of the true lung-tissue, in contra-distinction to that which affects the air-tubes of the lungs *(Bronchitis)*, and that of the investing membrane of the lungs *(Pleurisy);* the febrile symptoms are severe, appear very rapidly, and, in favourable cases, as rapidly disappear between the fifth and tenth days, while the products of the inflammation still remain.

If one lung only be involved, it is termed single pneumonia; if both, double. The latter form occurs in about one out of every eight cases; and in the single variety two cases out of every three are pneumonia of the right lung. The portions of the lung chiefly involved are the lower posterior and the base.

The disease frequently co-exists with pleurisy, when, if pneumonia forms the chief disease, the double affection is called *pleuro-pneumonia.* If, however, pleurisy predominates, it has been termed *pneumo-pleuritis.*

SYMPTOMS.—Pneumonia generally comes on insidiously, with restlessness and febrile disturbance, and sometimes has made great progress before the true character of the disease has been discovered. There is deep-seated, dull pain, referred to the scapulæ, or felt as an oppression under the sternum; a great feeling of illness; frequent, short cough, with expectoration of viscid matter of a green, yellow, or pale colour, sometimes tinged with blood, which forms such tenacious masses that inversion of the vessel containing them will not detach them. The breathing is hurried and difficult; the skin hot, especially in the regions of the ribs and arm-pits; there is no moisture in the nostrils, and the eyes are tearless; there exists great thirst; interrupted, hesitating speech; the pulse is variable, being sometimes rapid and full, at other times hard and wiry, or quick and weak; the urine is scanty, red, and sometimes scalding; and the patient lies either on the affected side or on his back. If the disease is unchecked, the face often exhibits patches of redness and lividity; the blood-vessels of the neck become swollen and turgid; the pulse weak, irregular, or thready; and the patient may sink, either from exhaustion, or from obstruction of the lungs.

PHYSICAL SIGNS.—On percussing the chest of a person in health, a hollow resonant sound is returned, proving the presence of air. If we also apply a stethescope to the chest, we may hear, as the patient breathes, certain sounds produced by the air entering the air-cells, which are described as the "*vesicular murmur,*" and have been compared to the breeze among the leaves or the cooing of doves. In pneumonia these sounds become changed; instead of resonance there is dulness on percussion; and, in the first stage, by auscultation, *minute crepitation* may be heard, which has been compared to the sound produced by the rubbing a look of hair between t finger and thumb close to the ear. In the next stage, t sound just described cannot be heard, for as the inflammati proceeds, the soft and spongy character of the lung is lo as it becomes consolidated by organization of the effus fibrine in the air-cells, and resembles the cut surface of t liver; this condition is called *Hepatization*. *Percuss* elicits great dulness over the whole of the affected pa During convalescence, as the air-cells open, *minute crepitati* may be again heard, and afterwards the natural vesicul murmur.

In the next, or third stage, purulent infiltration occu which consists of diffused suppuration of the lung-tiss In rare cases, a circumscribed abscess forms, and on applyi the ear to that part of the chest, a gurgling sound may heard; this condition is usually preceded by rigors; and hollow or cavernous sound follows when the abscess has be emptied by coughing and expectoration. The occurrence copious expectoration of whitish or yellowish mucus, gene perspiration, a sudden abundant discharge of urine, wi copious sediment, diarrhœa, or even bleeding of the no may be regarded as forming a crisis, encouraging the ho of a favourable termination.

Occasionally, in old or enfeebled constitutions, *gangre* of a portion *of the lung* may occur. This condition is easi recognised by a most intolerable odour of the patien breath, resembling that proceeding from mortification of t external parts. Unless the gangrenous portion is extreme limited, the case is almost certain to terminate fatally.

EPITOME OF TREATMENT.—

1. *At the onset.* Acon. in alternation with Phos. . healthy patients and in uncomplicated cases, these t medicines are sufficient.

2. *Pleuritic complication (pleuro-pneumonia).*—Bry. in alternation with Phos.

3. *Bronchial complication (broncho-pneumonia).*—Ant. Tart., in alternation with Phos.

4. *Other conditions.*—Cheled. Maj. *(liver complication)*; Ars. or Nit. Ac. *(aged persons or feeble constitutions)*; Iod. *(scrofulous patients)*; Sulph. *(tedious, or sub-acute)*; Rhus Tox., Ars., or Bapt. *(typhoid symptoms)*; Carbo Veg., Ars., or Lach. *(foul breath, gangrene, etc.)*

ACCESSORY MEANS.—A large, thick linseed-meal poultice, or *spongio-piline*, to fit the chest in front and back. A continuous poultice is one of the best methods of providing for the local loss of vitality in pneumonia and similar diseases. The patient must be kept very quiet, have mucilaginous drinks and farinaceous diet, and be treated generally as directed under *Typhoid Fever*, pages 119–124.

90.—Pleurisy *(Pleuritis)*.

DEFINITION.—Acute inflammation of the *pleura* (the serous membrane which invests the lungs and lines the thoracic cavity).

In health, the pleura has a smooth, lubricated surface, to permit the free motion of the viscera it encloses; inflammation destroys this polished surface, so that movement of the membranes, or of the lungs, is rendered difficult and painful.

PLEURODYNIA (false pleurisy) is pain in the *walls* of the chest, and does not belong to the pleura or lungs (see Section 53).

SYMPTOMS.—The disease comes on suddenly and violently, with rigors, fever, and *lancinating, stabbing pains*, often called "a stitch in the side," commonly felt below the nipple, and usually affecting only one side; the pains are acutely increased by coughing, by pressure, or by the least attempt at a deeper inspiration, which the patient soon refuses to take. There is tenderness at the intercostal spaces, and the breathing is diaphragmatic, the movements of the ribs being restrained, and the lungs only partially filled with air. There is also a short, frequent, dry cough; parched tongue; flushed face; hard, wiry, quick pulse (about 100 in the minute); scanty and high-coloured urine; and the patient constantly desires to lie on the affected side, or on the back. Should the lung also be involved, the expectoration will be very copious, and streaked with blood.

The inflammation, however, soon terminates in *resolution*, and the two surfaces of the pleura regain their smooth, moist character: or the roughened and inflamed surfaces become more or less *adherent*; or *effusion* takes place, and a dropsical fluid separates the surfaces, a condition known as *Hydrothorax*. In severe cases, the effusion may be so excessive as to compress the lungs and heart, and to suspend their functions. Sometimes there is a large collection of true pus, which fills the pleuritic cavity, when it is termed *Empyema*. This condition is likely to arise in bad constitutions, and also when the inflammation has resulted from injury, or the presence of foreign matter in the cavity. The quantity of effusion may be estimated by the dyspnœa with which the patient suffers, being greater in proportion as the lung is more completely compressed.

Physical Signs.—On applying the stethescope to the affected part of the chest at an early period, the dry inflamed surfaces may be heard rubbing against each other, and producing what is called a *friction-sound*; this rubbing may also be *felt* by placing the hand on the corresponding part of the chest; it is probably due to the pleura being preternaturally dry by exhalation, or to its being roughened by effusion of fibrine. This sound is only to be heard for a short time, because the opposite surfaces become glued together, or, more probably, separated by serous effusion; in this there is dulness on *percussion* at the lower part of the chest, as high as the level of the fluid. To the same extent, the respiratory murmur is also lost. *Ægophony* (a shrill, vibratory sound of the voice) may also be heard there. At the same time the patient, though at first he preferred to lie on the sound side, is compelled to turn to that which is affected, so that the movements of the healthy lung may not be impeded by the superincumbent weight of the dropsical pleura.

CAUSES.—Exposure to atmospheric vicissitudes, and sudden checking of the perspiration, are the most frequent causes, especially in persons of unhealthy constitutions; surgical operations and mechanical injuries are frequently exciting causes; thus the rough ends of a fractured rib may set up inflammation of the pleura. It may also be excited by extension of other diseases. The cause of the disease may materially alter the treatment.

TREATMENT.—*Aconitum.*—In the early stage of the disease. After administering two or three doses, its beneficial effects are often marked by the occurrence of perspiration, which contrasts most favourably with the hot, dry skin, urgent thirst, quick pulse, and general suspension of the secretory functions which existed before the exhibition of the remedy.

Bryonia.—This is a remedy of great power in pleurisy, even in its most violent forms. Its special indications are—laboured, short, anxious, and rapid respirations, performed almost entirely by the abdominal muscles; stinging, shooting, or burning pains in the side, aggravated by breathing or movement; painful, dry cough, or cough with expectoration of glairy sputa; weariness, disposition to retain the recumbent posture; irritability, restlessness, etc. A dose every one to three hours, alone, or in alternation with *Aconitum.*

Arsenicum.—Tedious cases; and when much effusion has

taken place, evidenced by painfully *oppressed breathing*, occasional attacks of suffocation, etc.; *coldness of the body*, and *general exhaustion*.

Iodium.—Scrofulous patients, in whom the disease is protracted. Even when effusion has occurred, *Iod.*, in alternation with *Acon.* or *Bry.*, will still be the best remedy in strumous constitutions.

Phosphorus.—If the lungs are affected *(pleuro-pneumonia)*; also in persons of weakly constitution, sensitive lungs, and predisposition to consumption. The expectoration is rusty-coloured, and there is much prostration.

Antimonium Tart.—Cough with rattling of mucous, oppressed breathing, sometimes nausea, *profuse expectoration*, violent throbbings of the heart, and a sense of suffocation.

Arnica.—Pleurisy supervening upon long-continued and laborious exercise, or from external injury; especially when pain and soreness remain, or when much fluid has been effused; in the latter case, *Arn.* tends to promote its absorption.

Sulphur.—When the lancinating pains in the chest have subsided, *Sulphur* every six or twelve hours, for several days, will often complete the cure. It is also advantageous as an intercurrent remedy when recovery proceeds very slowly, and when the breath and expectoration have a fœtid character.

Accessory Measures.—Applications of heat, in the form of poultices, flannel wrung out of hot water, etc., applied to the painful part, will often afford striking and immediate relief. Bleeding in every form should be avoided. The dietary should be the same as that prescribed in Section 9, p. 129.

CHAPTER IX.

DISEASES OF THE DIGESTIVE SYSTEM.

91.—Stomatitis *(Stomatitis)*—Inflammation of the Mouth.

SYMPTOMS.—Patches of redness on the lining of the mouth, which are sore, and from which an exudation occurs.

CAUSES.—Cold; gastric derangement; or the introduction of hot and acrid substances into the mouth. It usually occurs in children.

TREATMENT.—*Mercurius.*—When there is much salivation.

Kali Chloricum.—Fœtid breath, and great soreness. This remedy may also be used as a wash for the mouth: three grains of the *Chlorate of Potash* to four ounces of water.

ACCESSORY MEANS.—The cause should, if possible, be removed, and if stomachic, the diet corrected. As a rule, the patient's diet should be restricted to milk, or milk and soda-water in equal proportions, which is both nourishing and digestible, and may be taken without increasing the patient's sufferings.

92.—Thrush *(Aphthæ)*—Frog—Sore Mouth.

DEFINITION.—An inflammatory product, consisting of numerous minute vesicles terminating in white sloughs on the surface of the mouth, and sometimes extending to the whole of the gastro-intestinal mucous membrane.

SYMPTOMS.—Small vesicles or white specks appear upon all parts of the lining membrane of the mouth, and are sometimes so connected as to form a continuous covering over the tongue, gums, palate, and, in bad cases, through the intestinal canal. There is commonly feverishness, pain on swallowing, and the neighbouring glands are sometimes swollen and tender. Extension of the disease to the bowels, dark-coloured eruption and violent diarrhœa may arise in bad cases.

CAUSES.—A delicate or strumous constitution; insufficiency or unhealthy condition of the mother's milk; or, in infants who are fed by hand, an unsuitable quantity or quality of food; want of cleanliness; general disease. Thrush sometimes occurs during the course of measles, typhoid fever, consumption, and in the diseases attendant upon old age, and is then generally a sign of an early fatal termination.

TREATMENT.—*Borax* has a specific power over this affection, and will alone cure it if limited to the mouth. The mouth may also be washed with a weak solution of *Borax* (four grains to one ounce of water), by means of a soft brush.

Mercurius.—Dribbling saliva, diarrhœa, offensive breath, etc.; if administered when the white specks first appear, it is often alone sufficient. A dose every four or six hours, for several days.

Arsenicum.—Extension of the disease to the stomach and bowels; *dark-coloured eruption*, having an offensive odour; *exhausting diarrhœa.*

Sulphur may follow *Arsenicum* or any other remedy if that does no further good; also when the thrush has nearly subsided, to prevent a relapse; and when there are eruptions on the skin. A dose morning and night.

GENERAL TREATMENT.—Strict cleanliness, good ventilation, abundance of fresh, out-of-door air, and suitable diet. If the sore mouth be due to ill-health in the mother or nurse, the child should be at once weaned, and if under three months old, fed with *Sugar-of-Milk* (see Part IV), or if more than three months old, with *Neave's Farinaceous Food* (see Part IV). Emollient fluids—infusion of linseed, thin solution of borax and honey, etc., are grateful and useful. Vinegar, carbolic acid, sulphurous acid, etc., diluted with water, are also recommended as local applications or gargles, to cleanse the affected surfaces. Sulphurous acid is best applied by means of the *spray-producer*, in the proportion of one part of acid to twelve parts of water; it should be continued for two or three minutes, and repeated once or twice a day.

93.—Cancrum Oris *(Gangrena oris)*—Canker of the Mouth.

Definition.—A sloughing or gangrenous ulcer of the mouth, occasionally occurring in children who are ill-fed, or who live in low and damp situations.

Symptoms.—The inflammation generally begins at the edges of the gums opposite the incisors of the lower jaw; the gums appear white, become spongy, and separate from the teeth, as if *mercury* had produced its specific effects. Ulceration begins and extends along the gums until the jaws are implicated; and as the disease advances, the cheeks and lips swell and form a tense indurated tumefaction. The teeth are apt to fall out; and the parts assuming a gangrenous condition, the breath becomes intolerably fœtid. There is generally enlargement with tenderness of the submaxillary glands. In severe forms of the disease, the destructive process rapidly extends, so that in a few days the lips, cheeks, tonsils, palate, tongue, and even half the face, may become gangrenous, the teeth falling from their sockets, a horribly fœtid saliva and fluid flowing from the parts *(Aitken)*.

TREATMENT.—Merc. *(often specific in cases not caused by Mercury)*, Mur. Ac. *(canker associated with severe disease—measles, etc.)* Nit. Ac. *(from excessive doses of Mercury)*, Ars. *(extensive disorganizations of the mouth, and extreme prostration)*.

General treatment same as prescribed in the previous section.

94.—Teething *(Dentitio)*.

There are two sets of teeth; the first appears during the early period of life, and is called the milk-teeth; this set falls out in the seventh or eighth year, to be replaced by a permanent set, which is not completed till the commencement of adult life. The order in which the milk-teeth appear is generally as follows:—about the sixth month the two middle incisors of the lower jaw, followed in a few weeks by the corresponding incisors of the upper jaw; next appear the two outside incisors of the lower jaw, and soon after those of the upper; after another interval of perhaps about two months, the first four molars, then the eye teeth, and, lastly, four other molars, completing by about the second year the teeth of the first set. Should there be any little deviation from this order, or should dentition be a little prolonged, no great importance need be attached to it.

The changes occurring during the first dentition render the period an important one in the child's history. Concurrently with it, the whole organization appears to receive a new impulse. The face, hitherto without expression, receives distinctness of features; the eye acquires expression, the mind appearing to speak through it; the rounded facial outline becomes oval, the teeth separating the jaws further; the forehead becomes more expanded, and the general expression of the features are but signs of an evolution which ...ting the whole organism, of which the change in the ...ms but an inconsiderable part. Dentition being a natural process, should not certainly be regarded as in itself a disease, still less a dangerous one, but simply a natural period of the development of the child's organism. Notwithstanding, in many children, the process of teething is a trying one, and in some instances even dangerous.

Disorders of Teething.

The increased activity and excitement in the vascular system, combined with the nervous irritation which almost invariably attends dentition, may, in delicate or strumous children, give rise to a greater or less amount of local or constitutional disturbance. The period at which dentition occurs is important. In too early dentition, the constitution is rarely sufficiently strong to sustain the evolutions it has to undergo; while in late dentition, there is a languid condition, indicative of a scrofulous constitution. In either case, domestic treatment should scarcely be trusted to.

Symptoms.—Irritation in the mouth, swollen or tender gums, and increased flow of saliva; startings as if in fright, or interrupted sleep; sudden occurrence of febrile symptoms; various eruptions on the head or body; derangement of the digestive organs—diarrhœa, sickness, or constipation; and sometimes spasms and convulsions.

Causes.—Strumous constitution. The exciting causes are —*irregular* feeding; *excessive* feeding; *improper quality of food;* keeping the head too hot; too little out-of-door air. By such means, the stomach is disordered, the nervous system disturbed, and restlessness, crying, colic, and even convulsions follow. In nearly every case these causes may be avoided, and, though the child may have a strumous constitution and be otherwise predisposed to the disorders of teething, the sufferings may be reduced to a mininum.

Local affections of the gums, as inflammation; or disproportion between the jaw and the number and form of the teeth, are also causes of suffering which are often due to the conditions previously stated.

EPITOME OF TREATMENT.—

1. *Feverishness, etc.*—Acon., Cham. *(fretfulness; one cheek pale, the other flushed).*

2. *Diarrhœa.*—Cham. *(pinching-pains; slimy or yellow, sour-smelling motions)*; Merc. *(green or bloody)*; Coloc. *(much colic)*; Podoph. *(paroxysms of pain, with prolapsus ani)*; Bell. *(nervous irritability, flushed face, etc.)*; Calc. or Sulph. *(scrofulous children)*; Ars. *(emaciated constitutions).*

3. *Constipation.*—Bry., Nux Vom., Sulph., Acon.

4. *Sleeplessness, etc.*—Coff. *(nervous excitability)*: Bell. *(flushed face)*; Gels. *(simple wakefulness)*; Krea. *(agitation).*

5. *Convulsions.*—Bell., Cham., etc. See Section 49.

6. *Irregular dentition.*—Calc. Carb. *(too early or late)*; Phos. Ac. *(excessive weakness; rachitic constitution; see also* Section 35); Silic. *(perspirations about the head)*; Krea. *(thin, irritable children; teeth decay early).*

ACCESSORY TREATMENT.—*Regularity in the times of feeding and sleep*; correction of any habits in the mother which may affect the child unfavourably; restriction to *suitable quantities* of food at one time; *keeping the head cool* and the feet warm; washing the child daily in cold water, and allowing it to be much in the open air, tend to prevent determination of blood to the head. For children brought up by hand, we strongly recommend Neave's *Farinaceous Food.* If prepared strictly according to the directions supplied with the food, it is the ' st artificial diet we are acquainted with for infants. Purgives are to be strictly avoided. Costiveness in children is to errors in diet; if obstinate, or if worms are present, ctions of water may be used.

95.—Toothache* *(Odontalgia.)*

Causes.—Decay is the most common *predisposing* cause; sudden changes of temperature, derangements of the digestive organs, pregnancy, and general bad health, are the most frequent *exciting* causes. When the cavity of a tooth has been exposed by caries, the dental pulp is extremely liable to pain from contact with food, liquids, or atmospheric air; and if the health be much impaired, or the central pulp greatly irritated, acute inflammation, with extreme pain, may result.

Neuralgic Toothache occurs in paroxysms, which come and go suddenly (see Section 53).

Treatment.—If *Kreasote* or *Laudanum* have been used as a local application, the mouth should be thoroughly cleansed before taking any of the following remedies. After three or four doses of any medicine have been taken without mitigating the symptoms, another remedy should be selected.

Epitome of Treatment.—Acon. or Bell. (*congestive toothache*); Merc., Krea., or Staph. (*from decayed teeth*); Coff., Cham., Ign. (*nervous*); Cham. or Acon. (*in children*); Bell., Nux V., Coff., Cham. (*during pregnancy*); Ars., Krea., Merc. (*prophylactics*).

Leading Indications.—

Chamomilla.—Toothache from a draught, or sudden *suppression of perspiration*, and affecting the ear; the teeth feel too long and loose; the cheeks and gums are swollen, but the skin is not very red; and the pains are aggravated by eating or drinking, especially by warm drinks. It is particularly suited to children during teething, with watery, greenish, fœtid diarrhœa.

* "Toothache" does not occur in the "New Nomenclature," since it is not a disease *per se*, but only a symptom. Nevertheless, it is so common, that have inserted it amongst the diseases.

, throbbing pains, affecting several it is impossible to point out the exact bout, and are increased by contact or ions; determination of blood to the ve *sensitiveness to external impressions*, glands, dryness of the mouth and

eeth; violent scraping or lacerating , or pains aggravated by eating or ht in bed; pains affecting the entire ding to the temples, glands, and *livation* (not caused by *Mercury*); ich do not afford relief.

le jerking pains, coming on or 'his remedy may be continued for ion of pain, to prevent a recurrence

ent on extraction or other dental hould be rinsed with a mixture of trong tincture of *Arnica* to ten of

y of teeth, and easily-bleeding gums, *'eg.* and *Nit. Ac.* are also useful.

ging pain, or hard aching, relieved er; there is throbbing, heat of the lliness. There is not the mental s to noise, light, etc., which indicate ong tincture or of the first dilution, eans of a piece of lint, will promptly che.

r fifteen or twenty minutes till the ards, every four or six hours.

TOPPING CARIOUS TEETH.—If the ht, the decayed portions should be removed, and the cavity filled with a suitable material by a skilful dentist. If the patient be suffering from toothache, the pain should be removed before stopping. When it is not practicable to have a tooth stopped by a professional dentist, its cavity should be cleaned and filled with white wax, which, by excluding the atmospheric air and the irritation of food, retards the progress of decay. But a better and more durable stopping, for non-professional persons, is *gutta-percha*, which, if carefully introduced, after thoroughly cleaning out the affected tooth, may preserve it for years. *Gutta-percha* suitable for this purpose may be procured from chemists.

EXTRACTION OF TEETH.—In a very few cases the only remedy for toothache is *extraction*; this is especially the case if the decay has proceeded so far as to blacken the tooth, rendering it loose and useless for mastication, prejudicial to neighbouring teeth, and a cause of offensive breath. On the other hand, probably in ninety-eight cases out of a hundred, considerable experience justifies us in stating, that the most distressing cases of toothache are promptly cured by Homœopathic remedies. Our advice, therefore is, never extract a tooth merely because it aches, or has *begun* to decay; skilful treatment is usually sufficient to remove the pain; and, subsequently, local and general measures will prevent a recurrence of the trouble.

MEANS OF PRESERVATION.—The function of the teeth is so important, that their preservation is a matter of the highest moment. The teeth should be kept clean by rinsing the mouth with pure cold water, and brushing the teeth with a soft brush every morning; and, if possible, after every meal, especially when animal food has been used; and contact with any disorganizing agent avoided. Medicated tooth-powders—*Camphor*, *Kreasote*, *Laudanum*—are generally injurious; the unmedicated dentifrices, as prepared by homœopathic chemists, are the best. If drugs mitigate the [illegible] the gums can [illegible] The question of taking [illegible] be avoided, as [illegible] the counsel, and [illegible] On the other hand, the habit [illegible] of tempera- [illegible] avoided. Chewing [illegible] of strong drinks, [illegible] important means of [illegible] especially of the [illegible] the highest possible [illegible] food; cold [illegible] habits.

II.—[illegible]

[illegible] in the socket [illegible] through the gum or even through [illegible]

[illegible] from a decayed tooth. A [illegible] inflammation of the dental periosteum, the [illegible]

Symptoms.—Pain in a tooth, spreading over a portion of the jaw, with heat, throbbing, swelling, and the formation of a gum-boil. This may heal by resolution; or it may burst into the mouth, or even perforate the cheek. The sufferings are sometimes great, worse at night, and incessant till swelling has taken place, when it usually abates. There is frequently some febrile disturbance.

Treatment.—*Mercurius.*—Constant aching, much salivation, swelling of the gum, and throbbing. Persons who are subject to gum-boils should continue the use of this remedy as a preventive twice a day for *a week or two.*

Silicea.—May be alternated with the foregoing remedy

for feverishness. If prescribed very early, *Acon.* sometimes checks the disease at the onset.

Belladonna.—Two or three doses may be given if there be throbbing headache, flushed face, and sensitiveness to noise, light, etc.

Sulphur.—Gum-boils only partially cured by the above remedies; also when the tumour assumes a *chronic* form.

Accessory Treatment.—The application of a roasted fig, as hot as can be borne, to the inflamed gum, will speedily give relief. If the swelling be very extensive, and there are signs of the abscess coming through the cheek, a poultice of linseed-meal should be applied till suppuration is established, and continued for a short time afterwards. In some cases, prompt relief may be obtained by lancing the swelling as soon as its existence is ascertained. Sometimes extraction of the decayed tooth is necessary.

97.—Glossitis (*Glossitis*)—Inflammation of the Tongue.

Symptoms.—Heat and pain in the tongue, which rapidly swells, sometimes to an enormous size, so as to hang out of the mouth; there is profuse salivation; the patient may even become unable to eat, swallow, or speak; and suffocation seems imminent.

Causes.—Cold; wounds of the tongue; or, more frequently, mercurial salivation.

Treatment.—*Aconitum* and *Mercurius* in alternation every hour, for non-mercurial glossitis, till relief is obtained. If the disease be due to large doses of mercury, *Belladonna* should be alternated with *Hepar Sulph.* *Nit. Ac.* is also valuable in such a condition. If there be much swelling and *œdema*, *Apis* should be selected.

98.—Ulcer on the Tongue *(Ulcus Linguæ)*.

SYMPTOMS.—Soreness, slight swelling, and redness of the tongue; small ulcers form, and discharge pus.

FISSURES OR CRACKS sometimes appear upon the side of the tongue, generally opposite the molar teeth, from indigestion or the irritation of stumps.

TREATMENT.—*Mercurius* is generally the best remedy, except for patients who have been mistreated with large doses of that drug. *Nit. Ac.*, both internally and as a gargle, is useful for patients who have been overdosed with mercury. *Hydrastis Can.* is a most valuable remedy, and in many cases is alone sufficient; when used as a wash for the mouth, a few drops of the strong tincture may be added to a little water, and the mouth rinsed with the mixture several times a day.

99.—Sore Throat—*(Dolor faucium)*.

DEFINITION.—Simple soreness or swelling of the throat, uncomplicated by ulceration, quinsy, or syphilis.

CAUSE.—Catarrh; the sore throat being a simple extension of the catarrhal affection. This disease should not be neglected, as it is apt, in some persons, to degenerate into the troublesome form described in the next section.

TREATMENT.—*Belladonna.*—Red, raw throat, feeling as if scraped, with pain on swallowing.

Mercurius.—Sensation as of a lump in the throat, worse at night, sometimes accompanied by salivation.

Aconitum.—Dryness, roughness, and heat in the throat, with choky sensation, hoarseness, and febrile disturbance. If given early, *Acon.* alone will prove rapidly curative in catarrhal sore throat.

ACCESSORY MEANS.—Frequent draughts of cold water, and the application of the throat-compress (see Part IV).

Steaming the throat as directed under *inhalation* (Part IV) is a soothing and curative measure, but it should be done at bed-time, when the person has not to be again exposed.

100.—Relaxed Throat *(Resolutio Faucium)*; Ulcerated Throat *(Fauces Ulcerosæ)*; *and* Pharyngitis *(Pharyngitis)* — Clergyman's Sore Throat.*

The affections designated by the above names, being of a similar nature, and requiring similar treatment, are included in this section.

PATHOLOGY.—In the incipient state, there is irritation of the lining membrane of the fauces and pharynx; afterwards, congestion, inflammation, or relaxation of that membrane, enlargement of the tonsils, elongation of the uvula; and in its advanced stage, morbid deposit and ulceration of the mucous follicles.

SYMPTOMS.—The patient first complains of an uneasy sensation in the upper part of the throat, with a frequent disposition to swallow, as if something existed there which could thus be removed. If proper treatment be not adopted, the voice soon undergoes a change; it becomes feeble and hoarse, and sometimes, especially towards the evening, there is complete loss of voice. The patient complains of pain in the larynx, and makes frequent efforts to clear the throat of phlegm by coughing and spitting. On looking into the throat, the parts are found to have an unhealthy appearance, being raw and granular, and the mucous follicles filled with a yellowish substance; a viscid muco-purulent secretion may also be seen adhering to the palate and adjacent parts.

CAUSES.—This condition is probably most often induced by

* A paper on this affection, with cases of cure, is contained in *The Homœopathic World*, Vol. IV., p. 127, *et seq.*

the exercise of the organ of voice when in an inflamed state. An extension of the affection is almost certain to result from delivering an address or reading during an attack of sore throat or hoarseness, as the muscles of the larynx lose their nutrition through extension of the morbid materials from the inflamed mucous membrane. The disease may also result from an immoderate or irregular exercise of the voice, or it may follow inflammatory disease of the bronchial tubes or lungs, by much exercise of the voice before recovery has taken place.

EPITOME OF TREATMENT.—

1. *For the incipient and acute stages.*—Acon., Bell., Merc. (See the previous Section).

2. *For the chronic form.*—Bell., Merc. Iod., Kali Bich., Arg. Nit., Carbo Veg., Lach., Phyto.

3. *Occasional Remedies.*—Apis. *(much œdema)*; Ars. *(emaciated constitution)*; Phos. *(consumptive tendency)*; Sulph. *(as an intercurrent)*.

LEADING INDICATIONS.—

Belladonna.—Besides the symptoms mentioned in the previous section, *Bell.* is well adapted to ulcerated throat, with bright redness, and *much pain* on swallowing.

Mercurius Iod.—Less pain than for *Bell.*, and chronic cases in scrofulous constitutions. See under this remedy in the following section. It is one of the best medicines in Clergyman's Sore Throat.

Kali Bich.—Accumulation of tough and stringy phlegm, requiring considerable effort to eject it. Chronic ulceration.

Argentum Nitricum.—Ulcerated throat of a low type, with fœtid breath and foul mucus; and in cachectic individuals. A weak solution of the drug may be used as a gargle.

Carbo Veg.—Similar conditions, with hoarseness.

Lachesis.—Constant irritation in the throat, inducing much hawking, and a choking sensation; there is painful aching, but no deep-seated disorganization, the affection being more of a nervous character.

Hepar Sulph.—In scrofulous constitutions not requiring *Merc. Iod.* Also when the disease is consequent on the excessive use of *Mercury.*

Nit. Ac. is also useful under this condition.

Gargle.—To correct the foul breath arising in some stages of the disease, a gargle of *Condy's Fluid* should be used. See Part IV.

ACCESSORY AND PREVENTIVE MEANS. — 1st. PERFECT REST.—The first and most important is to exercise a sore and inflamed organ as little as possible. The treatment of an inflamed larynx, like that of an inflamed joint, should include a state of almost complete rest. As a preventive remedy in the case of clergymen, we would strongly urge the general adoption of Monday as a day of out-of-door recreation and cessation from all work, and thus compensate for the great mental and physical expenditure involved in the discharge of the duties of the earnest minister of the gospel on the Sunday.

2nd. THE THROAT COMPRESS (See Part IV).—When this is applied, the patient should retire to bed, and he will generally have the satisfaction of finding his throat-difficulty much relieved by the morning. In more obstinate cases, the compress should be worn in the day-time, re-wetting it as often as necessary. When discontinued, the throat and chest should be bathed with cold water, followed by vigorous friction with a coarse towel. However often repeated, the compress never relaxes the throat.

3rd. CULTIVATION OF THE BEARD.—The beard should be permitted to grow, as it affords an excellent protection to the throat, especially in the case of barristers, clergymen, public singers, and others subjected to the undue or irregular exercise of the organ of voice. After exercising the vocal organs, as in a public lecture, the throat becomes relaxed, and on entering the open air the unbroken force of the atmosphere is likely to induce an acute or chronic affection of the throat and bronchial tubes; while the natural respirator—the fine flowing beard—which our Maker intended to be one of the distinguishing features of the male sex, unshorn, would in many cases effectually protect these important parts. The hair on the human male face, planted there by the goodness and wisdom of our Creator, has its uses. Let the young man, therefore, never become a slave to the fashion which compels him to shave off his beard, since this natural appendage is found contributory to the health, if not to the improved personal appearance, of those who wear it. (See also under *Chronic Bronchitis.*)

These measures, faithfully and perseveringly carried out, would soon render obsolete the affection known as "Clergyman's sore throat."

101.—Quinsy (*Cynanche tonsillaris*).

Definition.—Acute inflammation of the tonsil or tonsils and subjacent mucous membrane, with general fever.

Symptoms.—It comes on quickly, with rapid swelling of one or both tonsils, severe throbbing pain, hoarseness, and difficult swallowing and expectoration, occasioning a painful and almost a constant effort to bring up and detach the viscid mucous which adheres to the inflamed surface; headache; pain in the back and limbs; foul tongue; offensive breath; and general febrile symptoms. The morbid action generally extends to the *uvula*, which, becoming swollen and elongated, rests on the base of the tongue, and gives rise to an unpleasant sense of titillation. If the disease be promptly and skilfully met, the inflammatory symptoms subside in a few days, leaving the tonsils enlarged; otherwise, suppuration ensues, indicated by rigors, and throbbing, darting pains in the throat, extending to the ears. When the abscess is fully mature, it ruptures, to the immediate relief of the patient. Often the abscess forms in one tonsil, and after its discharge another forms in the other.

CHRONIC ENLARGEMENT OF THE TONSILS.—Repeated attacks of acute inflammation, or attacks only partially cured, are followed by chronic enlargements and indurations, causing difficult swallowing, hoarse voice, noisy and laborious breathing, especially during sleep, affections of the ears arising from an extension of the disease along the mucous membrane, and extreme liability, from slight causes, to a frequent recurrence of acute inflammation.

CAUSES.—The *predisposing* are—scrofulous constitution, abuse of *mercury*, disorders of the digestive organs, and previous attacks of quinsy. The *exciting* are—cold, atmospheric changes, wet feet, etc. Quinsy is most frequent in young plethoric persons, between fourteen and twenty, and for several years is liable to occur frequently unless preventive means are adopted.

DANGERS.—Extension of the inflammation to the uvula, soft palate, the salivary glands, pharynx, and particularly to the root of the tongue, with difficult breathing, etc. But early and skilful treatment usually prevents the malady assuming such a serious form.

TREATMENT.—*Aconitum.*—Feverishness, headache, dizziness, and restlessness; a sensation of stinging, pricking, fulness, or even of choking in the throat, which on examination looks as if scorched.

Belladonna.—Bright redness and rawness of the affected parts; flushed face, glistening of the eye, headache, and pain and difficulty in swallowing. Useful either after, or in alternation with, *Aconitum.*

Mercurius Iod.—Swollen throat; copious accumulation of

etc., and gargling the mouth and throat every morning with cold water. After exposure to cold, and especially when symptoms of sore throat show themselves, the compress should be at once applied.

102.—Gastritis *(Inflammatio ventriculi)*—Inflammation of the Stomach.

Acute inflammation of the stomach, except as a result of poisoning by some irritant, is a rare disease.

SYMPTOMS.—Burning pain increased by pressure; constant thirst for cold drinks, with inability to retain either food or drink; constant nausea, coated tongue, and foul taste; dyspnœa; faintness, prostration, anxiety, etc.

CAUSES.—Indigestion; cold draughts, damp, wet, etc.; cold drinks when over-heated; mechanical injuries; poisons—arsenic, vegetable acids, caustic alkalies, etc.

EPITOME OF TREATMENT.—

Acon. *(usually sufficient in simple gastritis from cold)*; Ars. *(burning; agonizing distress; unquenchable thirst; wiry, quick pulse)*; Ant. Crud. *(thickly-coated tongue, nausea, eructations with taste of food)*; Merc., Bry., or Puls. *(chronic cases)*.

ACCESSORY TREATMENT.—In *acute* cases, small pieces of ice to suck, and during the severity of the symptoms the patient should be fed by nutritious enemata. Fomentations to the stomach give much relief. During convalescence the patient must only gradually return to solid kinds of food.

In *chronic* gastritis, the most important points are—attention to diet and general habits as recommended in the section on "Dyspepsia." Cold water and a spare wholesome diet are valuable adjuncts in the treatment.

103.—Chronic Ulcer of the Stomach
(Ulcus longum ventriculi).

This disease is more common than is generally supposed, owing to its non-acute character, its giving rise to some of the symptoms of chronic dyspepsia, and its tendency, in about fifty per cent. of cases, to disappear spontaneously. It occurs twice amongst women for once in men, chiefly during adult life, and is more frequent in the poor than the rich. There may be one, two, or more ulcers in the same stomach.

SYMPTOMS.—They are often not very clear; but there is generally pain over the middle of the back, and in the stomach, the latter felt just below the breast-bone, of a dull, sickening character, and worse after food. Sometimes there are violent pulsations accompanying the pain, or pyrosis, or nausea and vomiting; the patient loses flesh; and, in women, the monthly period is affected.

DANGERS.—The dangers to be apprehended are—*perforation*, when the contents of the stomach escape into the abdominal cavity, setting up *peritonitis* (see Section 123); *hæmorrhage*, which occurs in about four per cent. of cases, generally soon after a full meal; and *exhaustion*, consequent on want of nourishment from defective digestion.

TREATMENT.—*Ars.*, *Kali Bich.*, *Krea.*, or *Hydrastis Can.* are the chief remedies. *Ham.* or *Ipec.* for hæmorrhage. When ulcer of the stomach is suspected, it should always be under the care of a physician.

ACCESSORY MEANS.—Obstinate vomiting is benefited by sucking small pieces of ice; simple digestible food only should be taken,—*Neave's Farinaceous Food*, arrowroot, and beef-tea. In bad cases, complete rest for the stomach for some time, giving nutriment by enemata, is necessary.

104.—Hæmatemesis (*Hæmatemesis*)—Vomiting of Blood.

The following table will enable almost anyone to know whether a discharge of blood is from the lungs or stomach.

FROM THE STOMACH.	FROM THE LUNGS.
1. In hæmatemesis the blood is of a *dark* colour.	1. In hæmoptysis the blood is of a *bright-red* colour.
2. The blood is *vomited*.	2. The blood is generally *coughed* up.
3. The blood is often mixed with *food* and is *not* frothy.	3. The blood is *frothy* and mixed with *sputa*.
4. Is preceded by nausea and *stomach* distress.	4. Is preceded by pain in the *chest* and dyspnœa.
5. Blood is generally passed *with the evacuations* from the bowels.	5. Blood is not found in the *stools*.

TREATMENT.—*Aconitum.*—Hæmorrhage with flushed face, palpitation and anguish; also for the premonitory symptoms—shiverings, quick pulse, etc.

Hamamelis.—This is an excellent remedy for *venous* or dark hæmorrhage from any organ, and when the *state of the vessels* leads to the hæmorrhage rather than any change in the normal constituents of the blood. We have so often used it successfully that we now employ it probably more frequently for hæmorrhage than any other drug.

Ipecacuanha.—Bright-red hæmorrhage, with paleness of the face; inclination to vomit; frequent, short cough; salt taste in the mouth, expectoration streaked with blood. Often useful after, or in alternation with, *Acon.*

China.—*Debility* consequent on hæmorrhage, indicated by feeble pulse, cold hands or feet, fainting, etc.

[illegible] and to [illegible]

[illegible] necessary for the [illegible] The patient should [illegible] with the head and [illegible] lifting [illegible] should be [illegible] stimulants, and no talking, coughing, [illegible] permitted; at the same time the [illegible] and [illegible] about 35° Fahr. Food [illegible] time, a little cold water, or small [illegible] only being necessary. Should [illegible] be [illegible], because it is often nature's method [illegible] the bleeding. After the haemorrhage, the patient [illegible] be kept cool and quiet, and the diet be light [illegible]ing, while the position of the body should be [illegible] the return of blood from the bleeding organ.

105.—Dyspepsia (*Dyspepsia*)—Indigestion.

Physiology of Digestion.—Human life has been compared to a fire; for just as fire requires fuel for its consumption, life requires food its sustenance. Further, like fire, the processes of life are attended with the production of a certain amount of heat. The body, moreover, is in a condition of perpetual change, consequent on its various functions, and the wear and tear of life. This change continues even when a person lies at rest, for the heart continues to beat, respiration goes on, the blood circulates, the brain is in action, and numerous other functions uninterruptedly continue, from which a waste results which must be repaired.

Under ordinary circumstances, however, when both the mind and body are actively employed, the waste of human tissue is much more rapid, and a large amount of new material is required for its reparation. A man, for example, weighing from ten to twelve stones, loses in twenty-four hours, three to four pounds of matter in the performance of the various duties of life. Now the matter thus expended is replenished by *Digestion*, *Respiration*, and *Circulation*. The organs of digestion receive the food, and change it into a milky fluid, the *chyle*, which, being conveyed with the venous blood into the right side of the heart, is propelled by the contraction of that organ into the lungs; here it is intimately exposed to the atmospheric air, and thus the conversion into bright arterial blood is completed. It is now received into the left side of the heart, and thence into the general circulation, and in the *capillaries* (minute, hair-like vessels), it enters into the various tissues of which the body is composed. Again, the result of the functional activity of the body is, that it is maintained at a certain temperature. If a thermometer be placed under the tongue, the temperature will be found to be 98° Fahr., which is greater than that of the atmosphere, this heightened temperature being the result of the combustion of food in the system. The function of digestion, then, first repairs the waste of the body; and, secondly, it maintains it at a proper temperature.

Indigestion is a deviation from the healthy function just described, and is one of the most common affections the physician has to treat.

Symptoms of Indigestion.—These vary greatly, both in their character and intensity, but there is commonly one or more of the following:—Impaired appetite; flatulence; nausea, and eructations which often bring up bitter or acid fluids; furred tongue; foul taste or breath; heartburn; pain, sensation of weight, and inconvenience or fulness after a meal; irregular action of the bowels; headache; diminished mental energy and alertness; dejection of spirits; palpitation of the heart or great vessels; and various affections in other organs. Disturbances in remote parts may be due to *reflex action;* or to the effects of distension of the stomach, which, encroaching on the space occupied by the lungs, heart, or other organs, impede their healthy action.

Occasionally, one or two symptoms are so prominent as to exclusively concentrate the patient's attention, who regards them as diseases *per se.* *Loss of appetite, flatulence,* etc., are examples of the most commonly prominent symptoms, and to them we give a brief separate notice.

Loss of Appetite *(Anorexia).*—The natural requirements of the body might be neglected but for certain sensations—hunger and thirst—which, no doubt, depend upon some peculiar condition of the nerves. The receipt of alarming or startling intelligence often arrests, in an instant, the keenest appetite. Hunger is much influenced by habit, and returns with great regularity when meals are taken at a uniform hour. Many substances which are non-nutritious destroy or lower the susceptibility of the nervous filaments of the stomach, and thus blunt the natural sensations of hunger; such especially, are, tobacco, opium, and ardent spirits. *Too little out-of-door exercise, irregularity of meals, eating between*

late hours, are some of the most frequent causes.

Loss of appetite during acute disease or a weakened state of the system, should be respected; for if food be thrust into the stomach in spite of its dictates, it will generally give rise to more serious symptoms. Sometimes instead of loss of appetite there is *voracious* or *depraved* appetite; these symptoms are usually associated with nervous irritation from worms, chlorosis, etc.; they can only be removed by correcting the condition on which they depend. See Sections 40 and 112.

FLATULENCE *(Inflatio)*.—This is frequently a prominent and persistent symptom, and is caused by defective nerve-force, or general debility; food may be detained in the stomach and undergo fermentation, owing to imperfection or arrest of the vital and chemical processes characteristic of health. At other times it is apparently generated by the mucous membrane of the intestinal canal; for the symptoms are very apt to arise in dyspeptic persons when a meal is delayed beyond the accustomed hour, or when the stomach is empty. Flatulence is often associated with faintness, nausea, palpitation, and other disagreeable sensations.

HEARTBURN *(Cardialgia mordens)*.—An acrid or scalding sensation, commencing in the stomach and rising up the throat to the mouth, generally from excess of animal food, and is especially liable to occur in gouty constitutions. *Hiccough (singultus)* is a common accompaniment of heartburn, and consists of brief spasms of the œsophagus. In infants it is easily removed by administering a small quantity of milk or water.

NIGHTMARE *(Incubus)*.—In this condition the patient experiences confused and frightful dreams, with a sense of weight or pressure impeding breathing and producing great anguish; or he fancies himself in imminent danger or difficulty, from which he vainly strives to extricate himself, until at length he succeeds in uttering a cry, or moving, when the distressing condition terminates. It is caused by disorder of the digestive organs, and most frequently follows a late, especially a heavy supper. It may also be induced by fatigue, or an uneasy position in bed; sometimes the cause is very obscure, and requires professional examination and treatment.

Causes of Indigestion.—Irregularities in diet, such as indulgence in the luxuries of the table, partaking of rich, highly-seasoned, heavy, fat, sour, or bad food; *eating too quickly; imperfect mastication of food; eating too frequently*, or, on the other hand, too long abstinence from food; the use of warm and relaxing drinks, green tea, coffee, tobacco, wine, and alcoholic drinks; too little out-of-door exercise; excessive bodily or mental exertion; late hours; exposure to cold and damp; etc. Business and family anxieties are frequent causes of dyspepsia, and their operation is very general and extended, implicating not only the mucous coats of the stomach, but the liver, the bowels, and often the whole nervous system. "The battle of life" is too often fought, not only with much wear and tear, but with almost overwhelming anxieties and disappointments; and the digestive organs are often the first to suffer from depression of the mind. In this respect, the cause is often put for the effect, the common remark being that depression of spirits accompanies indigestion; but it is more true to say, that indigestion accompanies depressed spirits. When the mind is depressed by disappointment or anxiety, there is a corresponding depression of the energies of the nervous system, and so the stomach, in common with other organs (see Section 75), loses vital energy.

In the treatment of dyspepsia, the use of medicines and the observance of hygienic rules and habits, as suggested a little further on, must ever go hand-in-hand; for the former, however skilfully directed, will, alone, be unavailing in most

EPITOME OF TREATMENT.—

1. *Acute Dyspepsia.*—Nux Vom., Bismuth. (*severe pain towards night; spasm*); Puls. (*from rich or fatty food*); Ars., Coloc. (*sour fruits and vegetables*).

2. *Chronic.*—Nux Vom., Puls., Hepar Sulph., Bry., Carbo Veg., Calc., Sulph., Lyc., Ant. C., Kali Bich., Merc., Arn.

3. *From mental causes.*—Nux Vom. (*business anxiety*); Ign. (*grief*); Acon., China, or Nux Vom. (*night-watching, etc.*); Quin.

4. *Debilitating losses—Diarrhœa, Hæmorrhage, Suppuration, etc.*—China, Phos. Ac., Phos., Ferrum.

5. *From cold.*—Acon., Ars., Merc.

6. *Special symptoms:—Loss of appetite*—Calc., Ferr., or China; *Depraved appetite*—China or Cina; *Flatulence*—Lyco. (*with constipation*), Carbo Veg. (*with diarrhœa*); *Heartburn*—Puls., Caps., or Nux Vom.; *Hiccough*—Nux Vom., Ars., Sulph. Ac. (*with acidity*); *Water-brash*—Bry., Lyco., Nux Vom.; *Chronic acidity*—Calc., Sulph. Ac., Phos.; *Nightmare*—Nux Vom. (*from indigestion or abuse of spirits*), China (*with oppression*), Sulph. (*with palpitation*).

LEADING INDICATIONS.—

Nux Vomica.—Pain, tenderness, and fulness of the stomach after meals; heartburn; sour acid risings; flatulence; frequent vomiting of food and bile; sour or bitter taste in the mouth; the head is confused, the patient feels indolent and sleepy after a meal, and unfitted for mental or physical exertion; there is a sallow, yellowish complexion, and constipation, or *irregular* action of the bowels, with ineffectual urging. *Nux Vom.* is particularly indicated in persons of dark, bilious complexion, who take too little exercise in the open air, have much mental labour, eat too much, or drink alcoholic liquors. A tendency to piles is a further indication for *Nux Vom.* and also for *Sulphur*, which may often advantageously follow it.

Pulsatilla.—Indigestion from the use of fatty food or pastry, with much secretion of mucus; heartburn, with acid, bitter, or putrid taste; and frequent and loose evacuations. It is generally most suited to females with deranged period, and to individuals of a mild disposition.

Antimonium Crudum.—Aversion to food, or loss of appetite; sensation as if the stomach were overloaded; eructations, tasting of the food, nausea and inclination to vomit, or vomiting of mucus and bile; escape of flatulence, with an almost immediate reproduction of the symptoms; alternate diarrhœa and constipation. Pimply eruptions on the face, or sores on the lips or nostrils, are further indications.

Bryonia.—A sense of pressure or weight, as of a stone, after food; frequent *bitter or acrid eructations;* nausea, or bilious vomiting; stitch-like pain, extending from the pit of the stomach to the blade-bones; painful soreness at the pit of the stomach on coughing or taking a deep breath; confined bowels; obstinate and irritable disposition.

Lycopodium.—"It is in the thoroughly atonic dyspepsia of weakly subjects, where the digestion is delayed through deficient glandular secretion and muscular energy; where there is so little nervous force to spare for digestion, that during its process an irresistible drowsiness comes on, and the sleeper wakes exhausted; and where from like causes flatulence collects in abundance, and the bowels are utterly torpid, that *Lycopodium* displays its powers" *(Hughes).*

Hepar Sulphuris.—*Chronic* indigestion; nearly all kinds of food disagree; craving for stimulants; also if *Mercury* has been given too freely.

Sulphur.—Suitable in most cases of long standing, when only partial relief has followed the use of other remedies; and as an intercurrent remedy. It is particularly required in *strumous constitutions*, and for indigestion associated with or following acute or chronic *eruptions*, *piles*, *constipation*, irritability, glandular swellings, affection of the eyes, or other scrofulous affections.

Carbo Veg.—Chronic cases, with *flatulence*, heart-burn, headache, etc. Very useful in old persons.

Calc. Carb.—Well adapted to constitutions in which the digestion and assimilation of food does not lead to the formation of good blood and healthy tissues; there are—*obstinate acid eructations*; relaxed bowels; sensitiveness to cold and damp; fatigue after slight exertion; cough; gradual emaciation; and, in females, too frequent and profuse menstruation.

ACCESSORY MEASURES.—The following points in the treatment and prevention of indigestion should, as far as possible, be adopted.

1st. *Mastication.*—The reduction of food to a state of minute division in the mouth is a most essential step towards easy and perfect digestion. Digestion really means solution; and just as solid substances, intended by the chemist for solution, are first reduced in the laboratory by the pestle and mortar, so must the teeth perform a precisely similar process with the food. Not a particle capable of being further reduced by the teeth should be admitted into the stomach, as the appropriate work of the former can never be faithfully performed by the latter. A stomach, especially if weak, acts tardily and imperfectly upon food introduced into it in an incomplete state of comminution. Further, food requires to be well masticated that it may be duly mixed with saliva. In front of the ear we have the parotid gland; beneath the jaw at the sides, the submaxillary; and under the chin, the sublingual; all these secrete saliva, which pours into the mouth through minute openings during mastication. This salivary secretion is not only intended to moisten and lubricate the food, but is a most essential chemical aid in digestion, such as no other liquid can supply. We therefore warn the busy, the studious, the solitary, or on the other hand those persons who talk too much during meal-time, of the danger of neglecting the perfect mastication of their food. *The loss of teeth* is a frequent cause of indigestion, but now, happily, easily preventible; for when the natural teeth are lost, the skill of the dentist supplies us with useful substitutes.

2nd. *Overloading the Stomach.*—Too large a quantity of food interferes with digestion in two ways. (I) By so distending the stomach as to interfere with the churning motions which it undergoes during the process, and impairing its subsequent necessary contraction. (2) The secretion of gastric fluid is probably of a uniform quantity; therefore an inordinate amount of food would fail to be duly saturated with this indispensable fluid. The normal limits of the stomach are always exceeded when food has been taken in such a quantity as to produce an uneasy sense of distension. After long abstinence from food, as in the case of persons who dine late, there is great danger of eating too much, unless the meal be taken slowly, or finished before the sensations of hunger are completely appeased. The same danger is likely to arise from too many dishes, or too stimulating articles of food; a morbid craving is thus excited long after the natural appetite would have been satisfied. See Section 121.

3rd. *Suitable Food.*—As a rule, animal food is easier of digestion than vegetable, and it is well known that a weak stomach is much more liable to flatulence, and other symptoms of indigestion, after vegetable food than after animal. Indeed, the teeth of man partake of an intermediate character, as he is no doubt intended to subsist both on animal and vegetable food; so that a due admixture of both is probably more easily digested than a more or less exclusive use of either. It is important to remember that *starch* is not a nitrogenous or flesh-forming substance. Foods, therefore, the chief constituent of which is starch, as potatoes, rice, sago, etc., should be eaten only as additions to food containing a ge amount of nitrogenous materials. Further, it is espe-lly necessary that the dyspeptic should select *tender* animal d, and have it *cooked* so as to retain all its natural juices. e suggestions contained in the section on "Cooking," ges 31–3, are of great importance. Hard, dried, and cured ats—ham, tongue, sausages, and the like—are especially be avoided. In the same category we may place veal, rk, twice-cooked meats, salmon, lobsters, crabs, salads, umbers, raw vegetables, cheese, new-baked bread, coffee, d all substances known to disagree with the patient.

4th. *Beverages.*—As a general rule, patients suffering from ligestion are better without malt liquors, wines, or spirits; nigh standard of health being often best maintained alto-ther apart from the use of alcohol at all. Perhaps certain tients suffering from acute indigestion, or others in whom powers of life are much enfeebled, may be benefited by a *derate* and *temporary* use of stimulants. But if the use of se liquors be followed by excitement, flushing of the face, any other inconvenience, they should at once be given . Even when their use is at first attended by apparent nefit, *they should be discontinued when the circumstances which quired them no longer exist;* for in our practice we have ind that the most severe and obstinate forms of indigestion cur as the result of the excessive use of alcoholic beverages. addition to *Cocoa* for the morning, and tea for the evening al, the moderate use of *Pure water* is almost the only fluid quired. This liquid, so often despised, and even regarded many as prejudicial, is one of the most potent means for eventing or curing dyspepsia. Drinking water, however, ould be done in moderation. Two or three glasses a day is ough for most people. It is best to avoid drinking cold ter at meals, except very sparingly; not, as is generally pposed, because it dilutes the salivary secretion or the stric juice, but because it lowers the temperature of th *mach, and checks its* action. (See *Beaumont* on Digestion

5th. *Disposition in which to eat.*—A cheerful and tranquil frame of mind, especially during meals, is a most essential point in the treatment and cure of indigestion. Cheerful conversation and ease of mind favour digestion by increasing the secretion of gastric juice. At meal times, the mind should be disburdened, the conscience untroubled, and study, straining the head, business anxieties, and everything that occupies the mind either too intently, or disagreeably, should be avoided. None of the other functions of the body are more completely under the influence of the emotions than those of digestion. The sight and smell of food make the "mouth water" in anticipation of the sweet morsel to "roll under the tongue," and the pleasant excitement of agreeable associations enhance the enjoyment of eating. On the other hand, distress, fear, or any sudden unfavourable intelligence, exercise an influence directly the reverse. Let meals, then, be taken with pleasant and cheerful companions; or if compelled to eat alone, let the thoughts from some pleasant book relieve the tedium of solitude. The aliment received under such pleasurable circumstances, may be expected to furnish in abundance, and in the highest state of perfection, those secretions which are necessary to good digestion.

6th. *General Habits.*—Mental or bodily occupations should not be resumed immediately after a full meal; nor should food be taken without a few minutes' pause after exhaustive fatigue. Violent muscular exertions arrest digestion by engaging the nervous energies in other directions. The weary man, whether weary from the sweat of the brow or the sweat of the brain, should rest before he eats. We particularly recommend the "Plan of General Dietary," as sketched in the introductory chapter, pages 25–8, for general adoption. *Regularity* in the habits of life, such as taking food, sleep, exercise, etc., is an important condition in the treatment of dyspepsia. Feather beds, and too much sleep should be avoided; the patient should retire early and rise early, bathe or sponge the body every morning with cold water, and take moderate exercise daily in the open air. An occasional *change of air* and scenery exercises a wonderful influence in removing or preventing an attack of indigestion, divesting the mind of its ordinary train of thought, business and family anxieties, or gloomy pondering over personal ailments. Fortunately, our railway system is now so perfect, and widespread, and withal so economical, that few, by the exercise of a little foresight, need be deprived of so potent an aid to good health.

106.—Gastrodynia *(Gastrodynia)*—Pain or Spasms in the Stomach.

Pain in the stomach may be spasmodic or neuralgic. The latter has been already treated of in Section 53.

SYMPTOMS.—Severe pinching, gnawing, or contractive pains in the stomach, generally occurring after taking food.

CAUSES.—Highly-seasoned or indigestible food; stimulants, coffee, and tobacco; long fasting; exposure to cold or damp; etc. Gastrodynia is usually but a symptom of indigestion.

TREATMENT.—Nux Vom. *(severe spasm)*; Bry. *(in rheumatic patients)*; Arn. *(soreness)*; Bisthmuth. *(dull, pressing pain, with frontal headache)*; Ars. *(pain and vomiting after food; it is often the best remedy)*.

ACCESSORY TREATMENT.—In severe cases two or three folds of flannel, wrung out of hot water, and applied as hot as can be borne; in mild cases, warmed dry flannels. Attention to the "Accessory Measures" suggested in the previous section is often alone sufficient to cure gastrodynia.

107.—Pyrosis (*Pyrosis*)—Water-brash.

Symptoms.—Eructations of an acid or tasteless watery fluid, sometimes in considerable quantities. It seems to arise from closure of the œsophagus by muscular spasm, so that the trickling saliva is prevented from passing into the stomach, and rises into the mouth without any effort. It is often accompanied with pain, and is sometimes a symptom of organic disease of the stomach (see Section 103) or liver.

When arising from indigestion it is generally due to the too exclusive use of a vegetable diet, or to other indigestible food; it is of common occurrence amongst the poorly-fed.

Treatment.—*Carbo Veg.*—Acid or acrid eructations, with flatulence, and, usually, constipation, sometimes diarrhœa; *Lycopodium* in chronic cases; *Nux Vom.* other gastric symptoms (see Section 105). *Sulph. Ac.*, *Bry.*, *Puls.*, and *Acet. Ac.*, are also recommended.

108.—Vomiting (*Vomitus*)—Sickness.

Causes.—Too large a quantity of, or improper, food; a disordered condition of the digestive functions; pregnancy;* disease or irritation in other organs, as the brain, kidneys, uterus, etc.; cancer of the stomach; mechanical obstruction of any part of the intestinal canal; morbid states of the blood; it also occurs in most of the eruptive fevers. See also the following Section.

Prognosis.—Nausea and vomiting occurring in diseases of the brain, as in epilepsy, are unfavourable indications; on the contrary, in pregnancy or hysteria, no alarm need be felt, as they are merely symptomatic of irritation conveyed by the nervous system to the stomach. We may learn much

* For the treatment of "Morning Sickness" in pregnancy, see the "Lady's Homœopathic Manual."

by observing the time of the occurrence of vomiting, the nature of the matters ejected, and the extent and urgency of the symptoms. If vomiting afford relief, and the nausea, oppression of the chest and stomach, and headache cease, the case may be considered favourable; if, on the other hand, the symptoms preceding vomiting are not relieved by it, but increase, the disease must be regarded as having taken an alarming form.

TREATMENT.—Should vomiting arise from overloading the stomach, or from the use of indigestible food, it is truly a conservative act, and should be encouraged, within proper limits, by drinking warm water, or tickling the throat with a feather, until the offending material is expelled. If sympathetic of organic disease in any organ, the treatment should be directed to the primary cause, while temporary relief from the vomiting may be obtained by the use of one of the following remedies. Under other circumstances, a remedy may be selected according to the causes which give rise to the vomiting, and the symptoms which exist.

Kreasotum.—Chronic *persistent* vomiting. When the affection does not depend on simple indigestion, *Kreas.* is its best remedy; also for *persistent retching*, without vomiting.

Ipecacuanha.—*Simple copious vomiting*, with a disagreeable sickly feeling; also when it is attended with diarrhœa.

Secale.—Chronic vomiting of sour mucus, with offensive eructations.

Arsenicum.—Vomiting, purging, great prostration, with a burning sensation in the stomach and throat, and cold hands and feet. When caused by cancer or malignant disease of the stomach, this remedy often relieves.

Zincum.—The food is *suddenly ejected*, without retching; and the patient becomes emaciated.

Ant. Crud.—Nausea, heaviness of the stomach, foul tongue, and dislike to food, which continue unabated after free *vomiting.*

ACCESSORY MEANS.—Small pieces of ice placed on the tongue are very grateful and tend to allay the sickness. The diet must be simple, nourishing, and free from any irritating principle. Beef-tea is, probably, the most suitable form of nourishment, and may be given every one to three hours in small quantities, till other food can be borne. The stomach will often retain a small quantity of bland liquid diet, when it would reject a larger quantity.

109.—Sea-Sickness* (*Nausea Marina*).

This affection, though very distressing, is not serious; it is caused by the motion of the vessel. The seat of the affection is in the brain, and the sickness probably arises from a deficient amount of blood supplied to that organ. The retching and vomiting frequently recur, with intervals of extreme physical prostration, a sinking sensation at the pit of the stomach, vertigo, headache, etc. The symptoms, especially the vertigo, are most severe in the upright posture, and are at once relieved by a strictly horizontal posture.

Persons of delicate and sensitive organization, with a weak heart, a quick pulse, and a tendency to palpitation, are most liable to be affected, and are sometimes subject to similar derangement from the oscillations of a carriage or swing.

The best remedies are *Petroleum*, *Cocculus*, and *Nux Vomica*, as preventives; and *Kreas.*, *Tabac.*, or *Petrol.*, during the sickness. *Petroleum* should be taken on going on board, a drop on a small piece of sugar, repeated every two or three hours. When actual sickness comes on, *Tabacum* is the best remedy, and may be taken every ten or twenty minutes.

ACCESSORY MEANS.—If the previous statement be correct—that sea-sickness is caused by an insufficient supply of blood to the brain—our first effort should be an attempt to facilitate

* *Sea-Sickness* is not mentioned in the "New Nomenclature."

the afflux of blood to that organ, by a favourable position, and by imparting strength to the heart's action. The *horizontal posture*, therefore, should be enjoined; and small quantities of arrow-root, good beef-tea, or such light diet as best agrees with the patient. Champagne—iced if possible—is the best beverage, if it suit the stomach. Soda-water and a small quantity of brandy often suits well. When the symptoms are subsiding and the appetite is returning, a cup of good coffee without milk or sugar, with a plain biscuit or a small slice of toast, is often grateful.

PREVENTION.—For several days before embarking, indigestible food, overloading the stomach, or any irregularity in diet should be avoided. At the same time one or more of the preventive remedies should be taken. Dr. Marsden informs the author that he has found those medicines most efficacious which, taken a day or two before going on board, improve the digestion, and act downwards. During the early part of the voyage, unless the weather be very fine, the patient should remain in his berth, in a horizontal posture, and take chiefly liquid food—beef-tea, chicken-broth, etc. A girdle, moderately tight, round the waist and abdomen, or a stomach-compress, without mackintosh, has also been recommended. Warmth to the stomach and feet tends very much to prevent sea-sickness. Anything to amuse, and divert the attention from the waving position, is useful.*

* POWER OF THE MIND OVER SEA-SICKNESS.—The powerful effect of mental emotion in bracing us up against sea-sickness is very remarkable, and associates its pathology closely with that of other functional paralysis. This is said to be observed in a striking manner in shipwrecks, when fright renders every soul alert, though before there was any danger they had been exclaiming that they recked not what became of them. Of that I have no experience; but I remember once lying prostrate with nausea in a Peninsular steamer, when the captain, knowing I was a doctor, begged me to come and attend to an engineer who had got rolled into the machinery. Only one finger was crushed, but the binding up that and the encouragement of the frightened man quite cured me (*Dr. T. K. Chambers*).

110.—Dysentery (*Dysenteria*)—Bloody-Flux.

DEFINITION.—A febrile disease, consisting of inflammation and ulceration of the minute lenticular and tubular glands of the mucous membrane of the large intestine, attended with *tormina* (severe griping pains), followed by *tenesmus* (straining), and scanty *mucous* or *bloody* stools.

HISTORY.—Dysentery being an attendant upon war—a practice both old and universal—it was well known to the the most ancient writers on medicine. It has been the scourge of all the great armies which have traversed Europe during the last two hundred years, being particularly fatal in all unsanitary camps and garrisons. "It is the disease of famished garrisons, besieged towns, barren encampments, and fleets navigating tropical seas, where fruits and vegetables cannot be procured. During the Peninsular war, the first Burmese war, and the war with Russia, *dysentery* was one of the most prevalent and fatal diseases which reduced the strength of the armies."

Even in England, before the sweeping changes which have followed in the wake of the sanitary reformer, it was as frequent and fatal as it still is in unsanitary tropical countries. To the higher degree of civilization we enjoy, including in its train well-constructed, well-ventilated, and well-lighted dwelling-houses and streets, a more general and perfect system of drainage, with an abundant supply of good water, temperate and cleanly habits of the population, and enlarged general information on the laws of health, we may in truth ascribe our present comparative exemption from dysentery and analagous diseases.

SYMPTOMS.—These vary considerably with the type of the disease. Simple cases occur, and run their course, with little constitutional disturbance; but an acute attack comes with a chill or rigor, and is soon followed by quick pulse, hot skin, flushed face, and often, pain in the head, thirst, furred tongue, nausea and vomiting. Griping, irregular pains in the abdomen, called *tormina*, are experienced, and the patient is often tormented by a sensation as if there were some excrementitious matter in the bowel ready to be evacuated, and he is irresistibly impelled to strain violently to remove the irritation. This, the most marked symptom of dysentery, is called *tenesmus*, and although the desire to go to stool is frequent and urgent, the patient is unable to pass anything except a little mucous and blood, shreds of fibrine which the patient often thinks to be the coats of his own bowels, and, sometimes, balls of hardened fæces, called *scybala*. In hot climates the attacks are acute and violent, the pain being very severe around the navel and at the bottom of the back-bone. The bladder often sympathises with the rectum, exciting frequent efforts to pass water. In unfavourable cases, loss of strength and flesh follow, small and rapid pulse, anxious and depressed countenance, the abdomen becomes increasingly tympanitic, with bearing-down of the lower bowel, burning heat, hiccough, sudden cessation of pain, cold sweats, sharpened features, delirium and death. In favourable cases, the strength is not much reduced, while warmth and moisture of the skin, and a more natural character of the evacuations, indicate a tendency to recovery.

Causes.—"I believe dysentery to be caused by the action of a poison in the blood having a peculiar affinity for the glandular structures of the large intestine. This poison I believe to be a malaria generated in the soil by the decomposition of organic matter" *(Maclean)*. The effluvia from dysenteric stools are infectious, and consequently, are a cause of the disease. It is probable that the following are efficient agents in the *propagation*, rather than in the *causation* of dysentery:—Exposure to extreme and sudden changes of temperature, as from heat of day to the cold and damp of night; impure water; insufficient protection from cold and wet, as sleeping on the ground with the abdomen insufficiently covered; intemperance; a poor or irregular diet, etc. It is therefore often epidemic among people reduced by privation.

TREATMENT.*—*Aconitum.*—If febrile symptoms are well marked, the early use of this remedy often arrests the disease at its onset. It should be administered several times, at intervals of an hour. Afterwards, if required, one of the following:

Mercurius Corrosivus.—Bloody evacuations, or mucus mixed with blood; severe pain and straining before, and especially after, a discharge.

Colocynth.—This remedy is often required after *Mercurius*, especially when the *colicky* pains are very severe, when the abdomen is distended, the tongue coated white, and the discharges are slimy and bloody.

Arsenicum.—Burning pain with the evacuations; excessive *weakness;* coldness of the extremities; cold breath; putrid and offensive fæces and urine, often passed involuntarily. It is especially indicated in constitutions enfeebled by previous disease.

Ipecacuanha.—Autumnal dysentery, with nausea and vomiting, great uneasiness, straining, and colic; the evacuations are frothy, fœtid, and afterwards bloody. This remedy is often administered advantageously in alternation with *Bryonia.*

China.—Dysentery in marshy districts; putrid and intermittent dysentery.

Rhus Tox.—Involuntary nocturnal discharges; cutting pains in the abdomen; almost constant urging to stool.

Sulphur.—Obstinate cases, where ordinary remedies fail in

* Dr. Teste recommends *Ipecacuanha* and *Petroleum*, in alternation, as curative of dysentery under all circumstances. In case of intense fever, one or two doses of *Acon.* to be first administered.

affording relief, especially where there is constitutional taint, or hæmorrhoidal disease; also as an intercurrent remedy.

Administration.—In urgent cases, a dose every twenty minutes, half-hour, or hour; in less severe cases, every three or four hours.

Chronic Dysentery.—*Phos.*, *Nit. Acid.*, *Sulph.*, *China*, *Calc. C.*, *Verat.*, and *Phos. Ac.*, are our chief remedies.

Accessory Means.—The patient should maintain a reclining posture in bed, in a well-ventilated apartment, and in severe cases use the bed-pan instead of getting up. Local applications afford great relief, the best of which is the *cold abdominal compress* (see Part IV). If the pains are very severe, flannels wrung out of *hot water* should be applied over the abdomen, a second hot flannel being ready when the first is removed. Great benefit often results from injections, if there be not too much inflammation to admit of the introduction of the enema-tube. They may be administered after each evacuation if they prove beneficial. The first two or three injections may consist of from half-a-pint to a pint of tepid water, the temperature being afterwards gradually reduced. Mucilaginous injections are also frequently of service. The drink should consist of cold water, toast-water, gum-water, barley-water, etc.; the diet must be restricted to cold milk, arrowroot, cocoa, broths, ripe grapes, and other liquid forms of food. Animal food and stimulants should be avoided; when recovery has considerably advanced, and in chronic cases unattended by fever, beef-tea and other animal broths may be taken.

Preventive Measures.—Besides avoidance of the conditions pointed out under "Causes," it is absolutely necessary promptly to remove, disinfect, and bury the evacuations from a dysenteric patient, and to adopt the "Accessory" and "Precautionary Measures" pointed out under "Typhoid Fever," page 124.

111.—Hernia (*Hernia*)—Rupture.

Nature.—Hernia is a protrusion of some portion of the intestines through the walls of the abdomen, causing a swelling.

Varieties.—The following are the most common:—*Umbilical* hernia makes its appearance at the navel, usually in infantile life; *inguinal*, in the groin; *femoral*, also in the groin, but a little lower than the inguinal region; and *scrotal*, in the scrotum. *Reducible* hernia is one that can be returned into the abdomen; *irreducible*, cannot be returned; *strangulated*, is so constricted that the contents of the bowel cannot pass onwards, and the circulation of blood is impeded.

Symptoms of Strangulated Hernia.—A painful, tense, and incompressible swelling; flatulence, and colicky pains; obstruction; desire to go to stool, and inability to pass anything, unless there be fæcal matter in the bowel *below* the seat of rupture. If relief be not obtained, inflammation sets in, with vomiting, extreme pain, small wiry pulse, etc.; and, finally, mortification, with cessation of pain, and death.

Causes of Hernia.—*Weakness* of the abdominal walls from disease, injury, or congenital deficiency; *violent exertion*, as in lifting; *immoderate straining*, as in passing urine through a stricture, or in relieving the bowels.

Treatment.—No time should be lost in trying to push the tumour back into the abdomen, force being exerted chiefly upwards and outwards as the patient lies with the hips raised, and the thigh on the ruptured side flexed. If not quickly successful, lay the patient on *a board*, so placed as to form *a steep inclined plane*, so that the patient's feet and hips are very much higher than his head; he should be firmly held in this posture by an assistant, when, by pressure on the swelling, and often without any, the bowels will fall towards the chest, drawing with them the constricted portion. After returning the hernia, a truss should be employed to exert a sufficient amount of pressure to prevent subsequent protrusion. *Salmon* and *Ody's* self-adjusting truss is the one we generally use. A truss should be worn constantly during the day-time, and applied *before* rising from the horizontal posture. The skin of the part on which it presses should be washed daily, and for the first few weeks bathed with *Eau de Cologne* or spirit-and-water to prevent excoriation and the formation of boils.

If the rupture resist the measures just recommended, the best surgeon within reach should be *immediately* sent for, as an operation may be necessary to save the life of the patient. In the mean time *Acon.* and *Nux Vom.* should be administered every fifteen or twenty minutes in alternation.

112.—Parasitic Disease of the Intestines *(Morbus parasiticus intestinorum)*—Worms.

It is a curious fact, and a humiliating one, that the human body should furnish both a dwelling-place and food for a host of animal and vegetable parasites, not only after death, but also during life. Indeed, additions are constantly being made to the list of verminous creatures who get within, and subsist upon, the human body. It has been well remarked, "The wisdom of creative design is not easily fathomed when we see the higher orders of animals, and man himself, perishing in order to afford food and a means of propagation to the marvels of organization which appear to us always obnoxious and destructive—born for evil, and not calculated to play in this world's *rôle* any other than an offensive part."

There are *fifty-five* well-marked parasites which infest the human body. Of these thirty-five live *within*, hence are called *Entozoa;* and eight live *upon* or *outside* the body, and are called *Ectozoa* (see the Section "Parasitic Diseases of the Skin"). There are twelve other parasites which are of *vegetable* growth, and are called *Entophyta*, or *Epiphyta*, according as they live within or upon the body. There are many others which have been reported, but their characters or existence are still the subject of enquiry. Even the parasites themselves are infested with parasites—"an observation embodied," says Dr. Aitken, "in the Hudibrasian couplet:—

'These fleas have other fleas to bite 'em,
And these fleas, fleas, *ad infinitum*.'"

The parasites of man are divided into three classes:— A. *Cœlelmintha*—hollow worms—worms with an abdominal cavity; B. *Sterelmintha*—solid worms; and C. *Accidental Parasitics*—internal parasites, having the habits, but not referable to the class, of entozoa. The round-worm and thread-worm are examples of the first class; the tape-worm, of the second; and the larva of the gad-fly belongs to the third class. There is scarcely a tissue or organ of the body that has not been invaded by parasites: by far the greater number of the *entozoa* dwell in the intestines; but many are found elsewhere—the *Guinea-worm* in the skin and subcutaneous tissues, the *Trichina Spiralis* in the muscles, and others in the eye, kidney, liver, brain, heart, etc., etc., and even in the blood.

The three parasites which are most common, and to which we refer in the following remarks, are—the *Round-worm*, the *Thread-worm*, and the *Tape-worm*.

1. The *Ascaris lumbricoides*—the long or round-worm—inhabits the intestines of children, where it feeds on the *chyle*, attains a length of six to sixteen inches, and in appearance is similar to the earth worm. It sometimes travels upwards into the stomach, and is vomited; or downwards into the colon, and is passed with the stools.

2. The *Oxyuris vermicularis*—the thread- or maw-worm—has the rectum for its *habitat*, and is most common in children,

though of frequent occurrence in adults. It is very small, from a quarter to half-an-inch long, and multiplies rapidly. It may often be seen in the stools of those affected, or crawling about the anus, especially after the patient gets warm in bed.

3. The *Tænia solium*—the common tape-worm—is found both in children and adults, its *habitat* being the intestines. It is nearly white, flattened, and of a jointed structure; it attains a great length, even upwards of eleven yards, by repetition of the joints, which are sometimes one thousand in number. There is seldom more than one worm at a time, yet as each joint or segment possesses an ovary, its eggs are millions, but are discharged with the fæces, and are frequently eaten by unclean animals—swine, ducks, and rats in these creatures they become developed, but not always into tape-worms, for they appear to go through several generations before returning to the jointed form. They are probably introduced into the human body by means of unwholesome animal food, especially tripe, sausages, and sausage-skins. The *ova* sometimes reach the circulation, and in the liver or other organs are developed into *encysted entozoa*, commonly called *Hydatids*; when in the heart they are sometimes a cause of sudden death.

Production of Worms.—Intestinal worms spring from germs introduced from without, and which find in the interior of other living bodies the only conditions compatible with their development and growth. To suppose the *spontaneous* origin of intestinal worms would be contrary to the evidence of facts; there is no instance of a living structure being developed from apparently inanimate matter, except through the instrumentality of a previously-existing principle.

Most of the parasites affecting man are furnished with digestive organs, instruments of locomotion, and with male and female organs of generation. This last fact is conclusive that they proceed from ova or germs, which quicken whenever they are introduced into their proper element. Some of the entozoa are peculiar to certain localities, and strangers visiting such places contract them. The tape-worm invades the intestines of persons travelling in the country to which it belongs; thus the tape-worm of England is the *Tænia solium*, that of Switzerland is the *Tænia lata;* but an Englishman visiting Switzerland is liable to the *Tænia lata*, and, on the other hand, a Swiss in England is liable to that variety common to our country. The following curious story was related by Mr. Abernethy:—"A shepherd had to drive a flock of healthy sheep to a distant part of the country. The journey occupied two or three days. On the road one of the animals broke its leg, and was carried the rest of the way on horseback. All the flock, except this hurt individual, were turned for one night into a marshy pasture. The broken limb was set, and the patient got well, and was the only one of the flock that did not subsequently become affected with the rot, the only one that escaped having flukes in its liver. Is it not almost certain that the germs of these parasites were swallowed with the herbage cropped by the sheep in the damp meadow?" *(Watson).*

INTRODUCTION OF WORMS INTO THE HUMAN BODY.—The following are some of the most common vehicles and modes of introduction:—Imperfectly-washed *water-cresses*, in which condition aquatic animalcules which adhere to them are swallowed; *market-garden vegetables*, especially those in the production of which filthy water or liquid manure has been used to increase the fertility of the crop; *drinking-water*, containing the ova of entozoa which, having escaped from the alimentary canal of dogs, have been transported, in easily-understood ways, into ditches, ponds, lakes, or rivers; or food which has been immersed or washed in water polluted as above; raw or underdone meat, etc. People who live in places where dogs abound are very liable to the hydatid-forming tape-worm which is derived from dogs;* hence this disease is very prevalent in Iceland, where every peasant owns, on an average, half-a-dozen dogs. Even the *Ascaris mystax*, which infests every domestic cat, must now be regarded as a human parasite *(Aitken)*.

The dissemination of tape-worms from man to animals, and *vice versâ*, is easily explained. The pork tape-worm is said to contain at least 45,000 eggs, and these, escaping from the joints either before the latter leave the body, or subsequently, are distributed by water, sewage, or other means, reaching the stomach of pigs or even man, where the shell of the egg is dissolved and the embryo liberated. Parasitic maladies in the pig chiefly abound in districts where swine live most among human beings. Enclosed in farm yards, or in piggeries at a proper distance from human habitations, these animals are generally free from worms which are likely to exist in the body of man. The Irish pig, allowed the free range of house and road, where every kind of filth is devoured, charged with the ova of parasites expelled by man or some of the lower animals, is most commonly injured by entozoa. "The observations of helminthologists prove that it is not unattended with danger for human beings to sleep together when one is affected with tape-worm or trichina. How much more dangerous, then, for animals to live with people who disregard all habits of cleanliness! Though we refuse to believe that filth breeds parasites, we must not forget that dirt protects the ova and favours their transmission from one nest to another. The terrible hydatid disease, which is the direct cause of one-fifth of the human mortality of Iceland, is due to negligence and dirt. The

* In the British Islands the pig holds the same position in propagating entozoa that the dog does in Iceland.

Icelanders slaughter their animals, and leave the offal to decompose. Dogs devour the entrails, which abound in entozoa, and, breeding tapeworms within them, disseminate eggs over the whole country" *(Gamgee)*.

GENERAL SYMPTOMS.—The symptoms indicating the presence of *tape-worm* are generally masked, its presence being unsuspected until portions are passed in the motions; and almost every case has special symptoms of its own, either local, reflex, or general. Irritation at the mucous orifices (mouth, nose, and anus), and an indescribable distressed feeling in the abdomen, are common evidences of the presence of tape-worm.

The *thread-* and *round-worm* have many symptoms in common:—there are, usually, frequent changes in the colour of the face; dark semi-circles under the eyes; copious flow of saliva; nausea; insipid, acid, or fœtid odour of the breath; voracious, alternating with poor, appetite; a frequent feeling of malaise; itching of the anus; talking and grinding the teeth during sleep; thick and whitish urine; tightness and swelling of the lower part of the abdomen; and, if much irritation be occasioned by the presence of worms, the nervous system may become implicated, and convulsions, epilepsy, chorea, or delirium, ensue. Perhaps the only *irrefragable* sign is the presence of worms in the stools, or in the matter vomited.

When a discharge of worms occurs, whether spontaneously or by means of purgatives, it is, in itself, no evidence that the patient is more clear of the disease than he was before.

EPITOME OF TREATMENT.—

1. *As Anthelmintics.*—Cin., Cupr., Filix Mas., Teuc.

2. *For constitutional conditions commonly associated with worms.*—Ars., Calc. Carb., Sulph., Sil., Merc.

3. *Occasional remedies.*—Acon. *(feverishness and restlessness)*; Bell. *(flushed face and nervous irritability)*; Nux Vom. *or* Puls. *(indigestion)*; Ign. *(nervous depression)*.

LEADING INDICATIONS.—

Cina.—A valuable remedy for all parasites of the intestines, with the following symptoms:—boring at the nose; livid circles round the eyes; tossing about, or calling out suddenly during sleep; voracious appetite, even after a full meal; nausea and vomiting; griping; itching at the anus, and crawling out of thread worms when the patient is warm in bed; white and thick urine, sometimes passed involuntarily; wetting the bed; lassitude; occasional convulsive movements in the limbs, or even epilepsy; etc.

Mercurius.—This is an invaluable remedy in worm affections, but is more indicated by the nature of the evacuations than by the presence of worms. The motions are whitish or greenish, pappy, and sometimes bloody, with straining; there may be also distension of the abdomen, restlessness at night, fœtid breath, augmented secretion of saliva, etc.

Teucrium.—Thread-worms with much irritation in the rectum, irritability of the nervous system, sleeplessness, vertigo, etc. It is especially efficacious in adults.

Filix Mas.—This remedy is chiefly employed against the tape-worm, and if continued for some time, twice a day, often effects a cure.

China.—Suitable for the treatment of children with thread-worms and tendency to diarrhœa, irritation at the anus, pallor of the face and livid appearance under the eyes.

ACCESSORY MEANS.—The diet should be simple, easy of digestion, and include wholesome, properly-cooked animal food, especially mutton, beef, fowl, and rabbit; pastry, sweetmeats, sweet-made dishes, pork, and veal, should be avoided. Salt, as a condiment, may be advantageously taken with the food. A draught of spring-water should be swallowed every morning on rising; and the whole body, the stomach, and abdomen in particular, bathed with cold water, and afterwards rubbed till the whole surface is in a glow; daily exercise taken in the open air; also injections as recommended in the next paragraph.

Injections are useful for expelling the worms; half-a-pint to a pint of water, in which a spoonful of common salt has been dissolved, once or twice repeated, will often suffice to relieve a patient of these troublesome parasites. An effort should be made to retain the salt injection for some hours, or even during the night. Afterwards, a simple cold or tepid injection should be used regularly about three times a week, for two or three months, to wash away the slime in which the ova exist. But the general and medicinal treatment can alone be relied upon for improving the health and preventing the re-formation of worms.

PREVENTION OF WORMS.—1.—Avoid open waters, either for drink, or for use in the preparation of food, into which the carcases of dogs are sometimes thrown, or into which worm-eggs may be washed by rain, or other agencies, or to which even dogs or other animals have access. All suspected water should be previously boiled, distilled, or well filtered. 2.—Doubtful pieces of meat should be destroyed by *fire*; if thrown to dogs, or allowed to accumulate on the ground, or even buried, worms are propagated, and human health and life endangered. 3.—Raw or underdone meat, especially ham, bacon, sausages, etc., should be carefully avoided. Cooks, butchers, etc., are more liable to be infested with *tænia* than other persons; and in countries where uncooked flesh, fowl, or fish, is consumed, worms abound. Good cooking ranks next in importance to the attempt to exterminate parasites from the animals we eat, or the water we drink. 4.—Vegetables and salads, eaten raw, should be first most scrupulously washed, as it is through such media that the ova of parasites often find their way into our bodies.

113.—Diarrhœa (*Alvus soluta*)—Purging.

Definition.—Frequent, *excessive*, fluid evacuations from the bowels, without *tormina* or straining, from functional or structural changes in the small intestines, of a local or constitutional origin.

Simple frequency of evacuation may exist while there may be no increase in the quantity of fæcal matter discharged, or it may even be deficient. True diarrhœa depends upon defective absorption of the intestines, so that an excess of matter passes through them, and less is taken up for the nourishment of the body.

Forms.—The following are the chief: *Irritative diarrhœa*, from excessive, stimulating, irritating, or impure food or drink; *Congestive or inflammatory diarrhœa*, from cold, cold drinks or ices when the body is overheated, checked perspiration, or suppressed accustomed discharges; *Diarrhœa lienterica*, or discharges of unaltered food from arrest of the digestive and assimilative functions; and *Summer-diarrhœa.*

Symptoms.—Nausea, flatulence, griping pain in the bowels; followed by loose motions, which may vary as regards *consistence*—being fluid or watery; in their *nature*—slimy, bilious, or bloody; and in their *odour* and *colour*. A furred tongue, foul breath, and acrid eructations, are generally superadded. The circulation, breathing, and other functions are usually unaffected. In Summer-diarrhœa, or English cholera, the discharges are chiefly bilious, and there are often violent pains in the abdomen, cramps in the legs, and great prostration.

Causes.—1. *Excess in the Pleasures of the Table.*—Overrepletion of the stomach may occasion irritation and diarrhœa by the mere quantity of the aliment introduced, but these results much more frequently follow the *mixture* of various kinds of food and drink in one meal.

2. *Indigestible kinds of Food.*—Such are, especially—sour, unripe, or decaying fruits or vegetables; badly-cooked food; various kinds of shell-fish; *putrid* or *diseased* animal food; Numerous proofs are furnished in the public journals that the flesh of animals slaughtered in a state of disease is extensively sold for human food.*

3. *Impure Water.*—This is a fruitful cause of diarrhœa. Water contaminated with sewage or sewage gases, or with decomposing animal matter, is almost certain to occasion diarrhœa, especially in recent visitors to a neighbourhood supplied with such water.

4. *Atmospheric Influences.*—The heat of summer, the hot days but chilly nights and mornings of autumn, are frequent exciting causes of diarrhœa; so is the application of cold to

* The following will suggest great caution as to the selection and purchase of animal food, and may serve as an explanation of frequent attacks of diarrhœa.

Mr. Gamgee, appointed by the Lords of the Privy Council to institute a full inquiry into the subject of diseased animal meat as used for human food, finds that "Disease prevails very extensively in the United Kingdom amongst horned cattle, sheep, and swine; that the diseased state of an animal not only does not lead the owner to withhold it from being slaughtered for consumption as human food, but, on the contrary, in large classes of cases, where the disease is of an acute kind, leads him to take immediate measures with a view to this application of his diseased animal; and that, consequently, a very large proportion, perhaps a fifth part, of the common meat of this country—beef, veal, lamb, mutton, and pork—is derived from animals considerably diseased. . . . . . The presence of parasites in the flesh of an animal never prevents the owner from selling it as food. Carcases, too obviously ill-conditioned for exposure in the butcher's shop, are sent in abundance to the sausage-makers, and are also 'pickled' and 'dried;' and though specially diseased organs are generally thrown aside by most sausage-makers, some will even utilize the most diseased parts that they can obtain. Finally, in connection with some slaughtering establishments, pigs—destined themselves to become human food—are habitually fed on the offal and refuse of the shambles, and consume, with other abominable filth, such diseased organs as are below the more conscientious sausage-makers' standard of proper condition!"

the perspiring body, or the sudden checking of perspiration. Hot weather is a frequent exciting cause of diarrhœa, termed, on this account, Summer or English cholera. Dr. Farr says that diarrhœa "is as constantly in English towns when the temperature rises above 60°, as bronchitis and catarrh when the temperature falls below 32°." Probably, to the influence of the change of temperature—from the excessive heat of the day to the cool of the evening in the autumnal months—may be added bad drainage, and the impurities of our rivers and springs which then exist.

5. *Mental Emotions.*—The depressing influences of fear or anxiety, or the violent excitement of anger, are frequent exciting causes. A sudden fright excites in many persons the action of the bowels as certainly as, and much more quickly than, a *black-draught.*

6. *Functional or organic disease.*—Diarrhœa is often a symptom of other diseases arising from local or constitutional causes, as in typhoid fever; and in hectic fever, and phthisis, when it is called *colliquative* diarrhœa, because it appears to *melt down* the substance of the body; *cachectic* diarrhœa, as from chronic malarious diseases; bilious diarrhœa, from excessive flow of bile, as in hot weather or after passing a gall-stone. Looseness of the bowels is also a very common precursor of cholera, when that disease is epidemic.

Treatment.—The attempt to arrest diarrhœa by the astringent measures of the old school has, in many ways, a most prejudicial effect; for should one symptom be relieved, it is too frequently followed by aggravation of others. When loose evacuations afford relief to a patient they should not be interfered with, for in such cases they are Nature's mode of curing disease. The evacuations following the too free indulgence of the table, or those of children during teething, are of this class.

6. *From mental causes.*—Ign., Verat., Cham., China.

7. *During dentition.*—See Section 94.

8. *In weak and aged persons.*—Phos., Phos. Ac., Ant. C., Nit. Ac.

9. *Chronic diarrhœa.*—Ars., Phos., Calc. Carb., Phos. Ac., China, Sulph., Ferr. Iod. See also Section 34.

10. *Other conditions.*—Ipec. *(with vomiting)*; Ferr., China, or Ars. *(undigested food in the stools)*; Merc. Cor., Caps., or Ipec. *(bloody discharges: see also Section 110)*; Podoph., Merc., China, or Iris *(bilious diarrhœa)*.

Leading Indications.—

Camphor.—In *sudden* and *recent* cases, with chilliness, shivering, cold creeping of the skin, severe pain in the stomach and bowels, cold face and hands. Two drops on a small piece of loaf sugar, repeated every twenty or thirty minutes, for three or four times.

Dulcamara.—Diarrhœa traceable to cold, particularly in the summer or autumn; when the evacuations take place at night, and are slimy or bilious; and attended with impaired appetite and dejection of spirits.

Pulsatilla.—Purging from fatty or rich food, bitter taste in the mouth, nausea, eructations, and colicky pains, especially ·ight.

Ant. Crud.—Watery diarrhœa, with disordered stomach, loss of appetite, white-coated tongue, eructations, and nausea. It is more especially adapted to aged persons.

China.—*Simple summer-diarrhœa;* also after eating, or in the night, and containing undigested food, with colic; or painless diarrhœa, with debility, thirst, and loss of appetite.

Apis.—Painless, greenish-yellow diarrhœa *recurring every morning.*

Iris Versicolor.—English cholera or summer diarrhœa; bilious evacuations, with vomiting and headache.

Arsenicum.—Diarrhœa accompanied or ushered in by vomiting, with heat in the stomach, and a *burning sensation* attending the effort of expelling the motions, with griping or tearing pains in the abdomen. It is well indicated in cases marked by extreme weakness, emaciation, coldness of the extremities, paleness of the face, sunken cheeks, etc. It is therefore more suited to diarrhœa associated with deep-seated disease than to mere functional disorder.

Mercurius Cor.—Bilious or bloody stools, preceded by colic and griping, and followed by painful *straining.*

Bryonia.—Diarrhœa during the heat of summer, especially if caused by cold drinks, or by sudden change from heat to cold wind.

Podophyllum.—Dysenteric and bilious diarrhœa, with prolapse of the bowel.

Veratrum.—Thin, *watery* evacuations, with *cramps, vomiting, coldness of the body,* and *rapid sinking.*

Phosphoric Acid.—Chronic, *exhausting,* painless diarrhœa, particularly when there is involuntary action of the bowels.

Phosphorus.—Weakly, nervous patients, especially young persons with a tendency to phthisis.

Ferrum.—*Anæmic* patients; chronic diarrhœa, with undigested food.

Calcarea Carb.—Chronic diarrhœa, with weakness, emaciation, pale face, and sometimes variable appetite. It is especially useful in scrofulous persons.

DIET.—In recent cases of diarrhœa, food should be given sparingly, consisting of light, non-irritating articles—gruel, rice, arrowroot, *Neave's Food* prepared with an extra quantity of milk, and other farinaceous substances, which should be taken *cool.* In chronic diarrhœa, the diet should be nutritious, but restricted to the most digestible kinds of food—mutton, chicken, pigeon, game, and white fish are generally suitable, if not overcooked. Beef, pork, and veal, and all tough portions of meat should be avoided. Starchy foods—arrow-root, sago, etc., are insufficient for prolonged cases of diarrhœa, but are improved by admixture with good milk. *Old* rice, well cooked, with milk, taken directly it is prepared, is excellent nourishment. Raw or half-cooked eggs, and wholesome ripe fruit in moderation, may generally be taken. Mucilaginous drinks—barley-water, gum-water, nitric lemonade, linseed tea, etc., are the most suitable: see Part IV. Probably, however, the best diet is *milk and lime-water*, as recommended by Dr. T. K. Chambers; it may be iced in feverish conditions, and soda-water occasionally substituted for lime-water. Restricting a patient entirely to this diet is often alone sufficient to cure all kinds of diarrhœa not depending on a permanent chronic cause. Even in the latter case much temporary benefit is gained. The alkaline milk diet may be taken frequently and in small quantities.

ACCESSORY MEANS.—The extremities should be kept warm, and exposure to cold or wet avoided. Rest, in the recumbent position, is desirable in acute cases. Severe griping pains may be relieved by warmed flannel, dry, or wrung out of hot water, and applied to the abdomen. Persons liable to diarrhœa should wear flannel abdominal-belts. Night air and late hours predispose to attacks. Except in severe cases, moderate out-door exercise should be taken daily. On recovery from diarrhœa, relapses should be guarded against by shunning all exciting causes in food, clothing, etc.; mental excitement, and excessive or prolonged exertion should also be avoided.

114.—Colic *(Colum)*—Spasms of the Bowels.

The seat of this affection is the large intestine; the pain being due to violent contraction (*spasm*) of the muscular fibres of that portion of the intestinal canal.

Symptoms.—Severe twisting, griping pain in the abdomen, chiefly around the navel, relieved by pressure, so that the patient doubles himself up, lies on his belly, or rolls on the floor, writhing in agony. The bowels are generally constipated, but there is a frequent desire to relieve them, although little passes but flatus; there is no fever, nor is the pulse even quickened, unless after a time it become so from anxiety. The paroxysms of pain are owing to the efforts of the bowel above to force downwards the mass of accumulated gas or fæces, or while the lower portion is contracted.

Diagnosis.—Colic is sometimes mistaken for *Enteritis* (inflammation of the bowels), and for *Hernia* (rupture); but it may be distinguished as follows:—In colic, there is no fever, no acceleration of the pulse, no serious apprehensive anxiety, the pain is relieved by pressure, and there are intervals of almost complete relief. *Enteritis*, on the other hand, is attended with fever and extreme tenderness of the abdomen, causing the patient to avoid any movement which would bring into action the abdominal muscles, so that he breathes by the chest alone; and, although there are *paroxysms* of severe pain, there are no complete intermissions. Colic may be distinguished from *Hernia* by the tumour which exists in the latter disease, but which is absent in the former.

Causes.—Errors of diet, such as eating a mass of heterogeneous, acrid, indigestible food, or acid fruits; cold, from wet feet or suppressed perspiration; worms; constipation; etc. It may also arise from stricture of the intestines (*intussusception*).

TREATMENT.—*Colocynth.*—*Cutting* or *griping* pains, extremely severe, with flatulence or diarrhœa.

Chamomilla.—In women and children; the pain is pinching and twisting, the bowels feel sore, and there is nausea.

Nux Vomica.—Spasmodic flatulent colic, with pain as if the bowels and bladder were pressed upon with a cutting instrument; irregularity in the action of the bowels. *Nux Vom.* will also correct the tendency to recurrence of the affection.

Iris Versicolor.—*Severe flatulent colic.* We are indebted to Dr. Dalzell for the special recommendation of this remedy, who informs us that colic which used to last three to five days, in spite of *Nux Vom.*, *Coloc.*, *Cham.*, *Puls.*, etc., he has been able to cut short by a few doses of this remedy.

Belladonna.—Paroxysmal colic, griping, and sensation as if a ball or lump were forming; there may be distension of some part of the abdomen.

Plumbum.—Violent constrictive shooting or pinching pains in the region of the navel; constant desire to eructate and expel flatus; torpor, numbness, stiffness, and weakness in the limbs; pressure and cramps in the stomach; *flatulence* and *obstinate constipation;* face and skin pale, bluish, or yellow; cold extremities; melancholy; etc.

Veratrum.—Severe *crampy pains*, with coldness of the whole body; flatulent colic, especially in the night; colic affecting the whole abdomen, with swelling, or loud rumbling.

Bryonia.—In less severe forms of the disease, when in addition to fulness and distension of the bowels, there are sharp stitching-pains in the sides or in the bowels, and irritability of temper.

Other remedies sometimes required are—*Coce.*, (menstrual

colic); *Merc.* or *Podoph.* (bilious colic); *Puls.*, *Dioscorea Villosa*, etc. For *Lead-Colic*, see the Index.

ACCESSORY MEANS.—Hot flannels over the abdomen; or a copious enema of warm water, is often followed by immediate relief. Food of a flatulent character, and every kind that has been found to disagree with the patient, must be avoided. Persons subject to colic may be benefited by wearing a piece of flannel around the abdomen, and having the feet well protected from damp.

115.—Constipation *(Alvus adstricta)*—Confined Bowels.

DEFINITION.—A collection or impaction of excrementitious substance in the rectum—the residuum of the various processes concerned in the nourishment of the body—occasioning irregularity in the evacuations from the bowel, increase in their consistence, and often a sensation of fulness and tension in the bowel and surrounding parts.

CONSTIPATION AND PURGATIVES.—Now, while we admit that constipation is not desirable, and may almost invariably be avoided by such measures as are pointed out further on, yet a tendency thereto is not so prejudicial as many persons suppose; indeed, people thus predisposed are generally long-lived, unless they injure themselves by purgative medicines;* while those who are subject to frequent attacks of diarrhœa are soon debilitated, and seldom attain old age. The importance of a daily evacuation from the bowels, as nearly as possible about the same hour, is generally admitted; while the fact is by no means so generally known that more than one evacuation a day is as unfavourable as the former is favourable. But the most erroneous and dangerous idea on

* See illustrative cases in *The Homœopathic World*, Jan., 1869.

this subject is that extremely popular one,—that aperient medicines contribute to health, not only during sickness, but also occasionally in health, inasmuch as impurities are thereby expelled from the body.

The fallacy of this may be easily demonstrated: Let purgatives be taken for a week, and however good may have been the health previously, at the termination of this period very much impurity will be discharged, especially after taking *jalap* and *calomel*. As this is an invariable result, even in the case of those who have never been ill, it seems to prove that *impurities are produced by the drugs*.

Aperients during sickness are also most injurious.

"Temporary relief is afforded by powerful purgatives, but the delicate mucous membrane of the intestinal tract is weakened, a sort of chronic catarrh is induced, and the very condition sought to be removed is aggravated tenfold" *(Habershon)*.

The unphilosophical practice of resorting to purgatives is well put by Dr. Yeldham, who argues that as disease weakens the whole system, so

"The bowels, in common with the legs, the arms, the stomach, the brain, and every other organ, partake of the general debility, and become deprived of that power by which, in a state of health, they are enabled to discharge their proper functions. Why, then, should they, more than the other organs, be impelled to the performance of a duty to which, at the time, they are totally unequal?

"Again, under the process of disease, the whole vital power is devoted to the struggle which is going on in the affected part. The attention of the system is, as it were, drawn off as well from the bowels as from every other organ not immediately engaged in the contest. On this account also they remain quiescent; and any interference with that quietude, by diverting the vital energy, weakens that force which nature requires to be undivided, to enable her to conduct her combat with disease to a successful issue—an additional reason why purgatives should be avoided. Constipation is an *effect*, not a *disease*. If it were, there might be some show of reason in the use of aperients. But being merely a temporary loss of power, we can no more restore that power by *forcing* the action of the bowels, than we can impart strength to a weakened leg by *compelling* it to walk. In the latter instance, we should instinctively rest the part, until, by the removal of the disease, motion might be resumed. The same reasoning applies with equal force to the removal of constipation. The exercise of a little patience, and the employment of judicious means for the eradication of that disordered condition on which the inaction depends, will as infallibly restore the bowels to their duty, as in every other instance the effect must cease when the cause is removed.

Purgation produced by drugs is an *unnatural condition*, and although relief often follows the use of aperients, they tend to disorganize the parts on which their force is chiefly expended. The intestinal canal is not a smooth, hard tube, through which can be forced whatever it contains without injury; it is part of a *living organism*, and needs no force to propel its contents on their way; nor can such force be applied with impunity. Not only does the frequent use of purgatives over-stimulate the liver and pancreas, but also especially the numerous secretory glands which cover the extensive surface of the intestinal canal, forcing them to pour out their contents in such excessive quantities as permanently to weaken and impair their functions, and so produce a state of general debility. The normal action of the stomach and intestinal canal being thus suspended, nausea, vomiting, griping, and even fainting are produced. The brain and vital energies are disturbed, occasioning lowness of spirits with melancholy, alternating with mental excitement and peculiar irritability of temper. But the most serious result of purgatives is the damage inflicted on the mucous lining of the whole intestinal canal, leading to impairment of the functions of digestion, and resulting sooner or later in ulceration of its surface, with a long train of evils.

An important end will be gained when we can lead persons to regard constipation as a mere result of other causes—a want of balance in the general system; and when our general and remedial measures shall be directed to the correcting of this condition as the only adequate means of curing constipation.

Constipation in Old Age.—Daily evacuation, which is the rule in youth and middle life, is often an excess in advanced life, when three or four times a week is sufficient. It is desirable that this physiological fact should be known, as old persons often trouble themselves needlessly on this point. If constipation give rise to any inconvenience in the aged, it is best met by oleaginous articles of diet—butter, bacon, etc., which should be taken as largely as can be digested.

SYMPTOMS ASSOCIATED WITH, OR FOLLOWING, CONSTIPATION.—Headache; feverishness; pressure or distension in the stomach and bowels; urging, and repeated but fruitless efforts to evacuate the contents of the bowel, or complete torpor without desire; pulsation or pain in the abdomen; piles and varicose veins; uneasy breathing; disturbed sleep; depression of mind; etc. If constipation be persistent, it may be attended with vomiting.

CAUSES.—*Sedentary habits;* anxiety; dissipation; an improper quality or quantity of food; the use of *superfine flour;* neglect in attending to the call of nature to relieve the bowels; disease of the liver; derangement of the digestive organs, inducing diminished contractile power in the coats of the rectum; mechanical obstruction preventing the progressive motion of the contents of the tube; inflammatory disease of the intestines, brain, or spinal cord, or their membranes. But a frequent cause of constipation, as shown above, is the loss of tone of the mucous lining of the bowels produced by the habitual use of purgatives.

TREATMENT.—The following remedies, it should be distinctly borne in mind, are not intended merely to *act upon* the bowels but to correct the derangement upon which the constipation depends.

Epitome of Treatment.—

Chronic Constipation.—Sulph.; Plumb. *(with colic);* Opi. *(with drowsiness);* Nux Vom. *(with headache, and ineffectual urging);* Bry. *(with throbbing headache and torpor of the bowels);* Lyco. *(with flatulence);* Hydras. Can. *(simple cases);* Alumina *(dry and pale motions);* Æsculus Hippo., Aloes, *or* Collinsonia (*with piles:* see Section 117); Nat. Mur., Podoph.; Sep., Carbo Veg., Verat.

Leading Indications.—

Nux Vomica.—Constipation occurring in connexion with other affections; habitual constipation, *with frequent ineffectual efforts* to stool; also with nausea, *congestive headache*, ill-humour, and uneasy sleep. It is especially useful when the affection is consequent on indigestion, the use of intoxicating drinks, tobacco, or coffee; and for persons who take little out-of-door exercise.

Bryonia.—Chilliness, *throbbing headache*, pain in the region of the liver; also in persons having a tendency to rheumatism; and when there is no inclination to stool.

Opium.—Constipation, with complete *torpor* of the bowels, especially after unsuccessful remedies; it is particularly indicated when there are hard, lumpy motions, headache, drowsiness, dizziness, congested face, and retention of urine. *Opium* is well adapted to the aged, and to persons of a torpid or plethoric temperament, who do not readily respond to other remedies.

Lycopodium.—Constipation with rumbling *and flatulence;* fulness and distension of the abdomen; heartburn; water-brash; difficult evacuations.

Plumbum.—Obstinate cases, as from palsy of the intestines, either painless or with severe colic; unsuccessful efforts to evacuate, with a painful, constricted feeling about the anus; the motions are dark, and passed in small balls. For persons of a paralytic diathesis, and particularly in such as have had attacks of palsy, it is strongly indicated.

Ignatia.—Confined bowels, with *prolapsus* of the rectum on slight efforts to evacuate; creeping, itching sensation in the rectum, as of thread worms.

Sulphur.—Habitual costiveness, with flatulent distension of the abdomen, piles, etc. As an intercurrent remedy it acts like *Opium*, but having a wider sphere of action, and being useful in numerous forms of disease, it is an agent of far greater value.

Aconitum.—Constipation during acute disease.

Diet and Accessory Measures.—Meals should be taken with regularity, animal food eaten sparingly, but vegetables and ripe fruit freely. Coarse oatmeal porridge, with treacle, may be taken for breakfast; and *brown bread should always be preferred to white.* If brown bread be not eaten exclusively, a little should be taken with nearly every meal; its effects will thus be more uniformly exerted through the alimentary canal than if only taken occasionally. Water is an extremely valuable adjunct, both as a beverage and for external use. Strong or green tea, spirituous liquors, highly-seasoned food, and late suppers, should be strictly avoided. Sections 1 and 2, in Part I, pp. 25–31, should be read.

Walking-exercise in the country, with the mind unencumbered with care, is useful, particularly in the morning; but it should not be carried to the point of inducing fatigue or much perspiration.

Frictions over the abdomen are frequently of great utility; they tend to rouse the paralyzed action of the bowels, and to dispel accumulations of flatulence. The frictions may be performed by towels, horse-hair gloves, or the hands.

The Abdominal Compress (see Part IV) is extremely valuable in correcting constipation, and in obstinate cases may be worn day and night; it is only contra-indicated in aged and weakly persons, in whom there does not exist vital energy sufficient to excite reaction, and the wet linen continues to feel cold long after it has been applied. In other cases the chill produced by the sudden application of the wet cloth rapidly disappears, and in from five to ten minutes a comfortable warmth results, proving its suitability to the patient.

REGULAR HOUR.—Regularity in attending to the calls of nature should be observed, as there is probably no function of the animal economy more completely under the influence of habit, than the one in question; nor is there any that may be more effectually deranged through the influence which the will can oppose to it. By fixing the mind on this operation for a short time, the bowels will at length respond, and a habit become established which will tend to procure both comfort and health.

INJECTIONS.—In obstinate and protracted constipation attended with feverishness, and hardness or fulness of the bowels, and when it is ascertained that the lower bowel is obstructed with fæcal matter, too large, or too hard and dry for discharge, and the means before suggested have not proved at once effectual, the enema may be used as an almost certain means of obtaining temporary relief. The injection should consist of about half-a-pint to a pint of cold or tepid water, which should be carefully injected up the rectum by means of the enema syringe. The temperature of the water on commencing the use of injections should not be lower that 72° Fahr., and gradually reduced to 64°. Unirritating in its operation, and acting directly on the seat of obstruction, an injection is far preferable to deranging the whole alimentary tract with strong drugs, which excite violent action only to settle hack into a state of greater debility and torpor than before.

116.—Fistula in ano (*Fistula in ano*).

DEFINITION.—A fistula in ano is a narrow pipe-like track, lined by an imperfect mucous membrane, secreting pus, having a narrow callous opening, situate within a short distance of the verge of the anus, and with no disposition to heal.

SYMPTOMS.—There first appears on one side of the rectum a small hard lump, which, as it continues to enlarge, occasions considerable pain, and not unfrequently much constitutional disturbance. The surrounding parts soon become much swollen, the skin red, and suppuration quickly follows. During the formation of the abscess, the patient complains of pain in passing his motions, which are sometimes slightly tinged with blood. Great relief follows the discharge of the abscess, which is generally of a most offensive character, and the swelling subsides; but there still remains a small opening near the anus, and upon pressure a hardened track may be felt, leading towards the bowel. This is the fistula. The external orifice of the fistula is often very small; is frequently difficult to find in the folds of the thin skin near the anus, and is sometimes concealed by a papilla.

VARIETIES.—(1) The *complete* fistula communicates at one extremity with the interior of the rectum, and at the other opens through the skin, and is most common. (2) The *blind external* only opens through the skin, and a probe does not penetrate into the interior of the bowel. (3) The *blind internal* is not so readily detected, but is indicated by pain at stool, and discharge of blood and pus with the fæces; it may also be detected by a finger or probe, or seen by a speculum, about an inch to an inch-and-a-half within the rectum.

CAUSES.—These fistulæ originate in abscesses, which are prevented from healing by the movement of the *sphincter ani* and the bowel itself; or by the ulceration of the mucous membrane of the rectum, and generation of feculent fluids and gases, which gradually excite progressive ulceration towards the surface. The disease is frequent in consumptive patients, probably from deposit of tubercle under the mucous membrane of the rectum, or the areolar tissue about the rectum losing its fat, and falling into a watery, unhealthy condition.

TREATMENT.—The administration of one or more remedies will aid the cure of fistula, and in many cases, as we have found in practice, render unnecessary any operative measures. Several bad cases, previously under the care of allopathic surgeons, by whom operations were said to be absolutely necessary, have been completely cured by such remedies and measures as we have prescribed. In one case it was arranged for a London surgeon to operate, but it being inconvenient for the patient to leave his engagements for a few weeks, we were requested to undertake the case in the mean time, and when the period for the operation arrived it was no longer necessary.

The following are the chief medicines, the choice from which must be made according to the general symptoms and condition of the patient:—*Silic.*, *Calc. Phos.*, *Lyc.*, *Caust.*, *Nux Vom.*, and *Sulph.* At the same time, *local* applications of *Hydrastis* or *Calendula* are useful to assist the curative process.

ACCESSORY MEANS.—An occasional poultice; frequent washings with cold or tepid water; the sitz-bath; daily injections as directed in the following Section, combined with the local applications previously recommended, afford comfort to the patient, prevent the extension of the disease, and favour a radical cure. Nourishing, digestible diet, abundance of fresh air, and general good hygienic conditions are necessary to increase the reparative powers of the system.

Operative measures may be required in a few cases. They should, however, never be undertaken indiscriminately, if the patient be decidedly phthisical, or if there be disease of the kidneys or liver, no operation would be justifiable, the artificial wound would probably never heal, and the patient's weakness would be aggravated by an additional discharge.

117.—Hæmorrhoids (*Hæmorrhoïdes*)—Piles.

DEFINITION.—Small tumours, consisting of folds of mucous and sub-mucous tissue, in different stages of congestion, inflammation, or permanent enlargement, situated within or just outside the anal aperture, and originating from dilatation of the hæmorrhoidal veins.

Piles are of a pink or purplish hue, forming one or more distinct pendulous tumours, varying from the size of a pea to that of a damson or walnut, are often intensely painful, and constitute the most frequent disease of the anus.

VARIETIES.—Piles are classified as (*a*) *internal* and (*b*) *external* according as they are situated within the rectum or at the verge of the anus. The *external* are covered by skin; they vary in number from one to several clustering together like a bunch of grapes. The *internal* are covered by mucous membrane, and are always within the bowel; they are very liable to bleed, especially during the passage of fæces. The blood thus lost is of a bright-red colour, being arterial, proceeds from the capillaries of the vascular surface of the tumours, and varies in quantity from a few drops to such a profuse discharge as is truly alarming; if hæmorrhage be long continued, an anæmic condition is induced that is highly prejudicial to the constitution. The piles are seated in the vertical folds of the mucous membrane which lines the bowel; that portion of membrane which invests them being extremely vascular, numerous minute vessels of brighter colour than the body of the piles may be seen ramifying on the surface.

Piles that do not bleed are called *blind;* this variety is prone to inflammation, when they become tense, appear ready to burst, and are so excessively sensitive, that the patient can scarcely sit, walk, or lie.

Symptoms.—These vary considerably according to the amount of inflammation present. When indolent, the chief inconvenience arises from their bulk and situation; or from their getting within the *sphincter* muscle, occasioning more or less pain when the bowel is acting, prolapse, and often a sense of weight and discomfort which quite unfits the mind for deep thought. But when inflamed, or, in common language, "during a fit of the piles," there are pricking, itching, shooting, or burning pains about the anus, increased on going to stool, and a feeling as if there were a foreign substance in the rectum. After emptying the bowel, there is often painful straining, as if it were not emptied, occasioned by the piles or the elongated mucous membrane to which they are attached, being protruded during the expulsion of fæces, and not replaced sufficiently quick, and so grasped and constricted by the *sphincter ani*, the function of which is to close the aperture of the bowel after defecation. This condition is greatly aggravated if the patient stand or walk much after going to stool, or if the bowels are constipated, so that the rectum is much distended or the fæces become hard. If proper remedial measures be not adopted, the inconveniences and suffering become seriously augmented, the general health implicated, the patient loses flesh and strength, and the countenance wears an anxious and care-worn expression.

Causes.—The *predisposing causes* are—a general plethoric condition of the system, or any circumstances which determine blood to, or impede its return from, the rectum; such are *sedentary habits*; *luxurious living*, especially the use of highly-seasoned food, wines, and spirits; tight-lacing; pregnancy; confined bowels; and diseases of the liver. Residence in moist, warm, and relaxing climates; soft, warm beds or cushions, and over-excitement of the sexual organs may also be classed among predisposing causes. The *exciting causes* include anything which irritate the lower bowel, such as straining at stool, hard riding, and the use of drastic purgatives, especially *aloes* and *rhubarb*.

Probably the most potent causes of this disease are the indolent and luxurious habits of the wealthy classes, which, by diminishing tone, occasion plethora and a tendency to abdominal congestion, and so exercise a considerable influence in producing the malady. Accordingly we find piles much more prevalent among the wealthy than among the industrial and frugal classes.

Age and sex appear to exercise considerable influence on this disease. In early life, it is probably much more frequent in young men than in young women. The comparative exemption of young women is readily accounted for by the regular action of the catamenial function which probably obviates congestion that might otherwise occur. At a later period, after the cessation of the menses, or during the pressure of the gravid uterus in pregnancy, congestion is apt to occur in certain neighbouring organs, and so give rise to piles (see the "Lady's Manual").

Epitome of Treatment.—

1. *From luxurious or sedentary habits.*—Nux Vom., Sulph., Podoph.

2. *From constipation.*—Sulph., Æsculus Hippo., Nux Vom., Collinsonia, Carbo Veg. See also Section 115.

3. *During pregnancy.*—Aloes, Collinsonia Can., Nux Vom.

4. *Bleeding-piles.*—Ham., internally and externally; Sulph. *(dark blood)*; Acon. *(excessive bleeding)*; China *(after losses of blood)*.

5. *Blind-piles.*—Nux Vom., in alternation with Sulph.; Acon., internally and externally *(great pain)*; Caps. *(burning and itching)*.

6. *White-piles—discharges of mucus.*—Merc. *(with excoriation)*; Acon. *(frequent discharge of white mucus)*.

7. *Chronic.*—Ars. *(in emaciated persons)*; Ferr. *(cachectic constitutions)*; Nit Ac., Sulph., Hep. Sulph.

8. *Suppressed.*—Acon., Puls., Sulph.

LEADING INDICATIONS.—

Nux Vomica.—Piles associated with sedentary habits; luxurious living; indulgence in stimulating beverages; depressing mental emotions; confined bowels, or ineffectual urging to stool; prolapsus, or loss of power of the muscular structure of the bowel. *Sulphur* may advantageously follow this remedy, a dose being given night and morning for four or five days; or *Sulphur* and *Nux Vomica* may be given in alternation, the former in the morning and the latter at night.

Hamamelis.—Very valuable in bleeding-piles; or even when there is only a varicose condition of the hæmorrhoidal veins, particularly if the patient be also troubled with a varicose state of the veins of the lower extremities. For cases in which there is considerable loss of blood, it should be used both internally and externally, a lotion being made by adding thirty drops of the strong tincture to four ounces of water, and applied by means of two or three folds of linen, covered with oiled-silk, and renewed several times daily.

Æsculus Hippo.—*Bleeding*-piles, with much *pain in the rectum*, and also in the *back and loins*.

Collinsonia.—Piles associated with constipation.

Aconitum.—Piles in an inflamed condition, with feverish restlessness, a sensation of heat, and discharge of mucus or blood. For the *excessive pain* often associated with piles, besides its internal use, *Acon.* may be used as a *lotion*.

Arsenicum.—Burning sensation, and sometimes a feeling compared to passing red-hot needles through the piles, with intolerable pain in the back, protrusion of the tumours, and *prostration of strength.*

Sulphur.—This remedy is regarded as one of the most valuable in every variety of piles, especially in chronic cases, occurring in scrofulous individuals, and associated with constipation, or thin evacuations mixed with blood.

DIET AND ACCESSORY MEANS.—Patients should avoid coffee, peppers, spices, stimulating or highly-seasoned food, the habitual use of beer, wine, spirits, and all kinds of indigestible food. Light animal food, a liberal quantity of well-cooked vegetables, and ripe and wholesome fruits, form the most suitable diet. During an attack of piles, animal food should be sparingly used.

Sedentary habits and much standing, on the one hand, and extreme fatigue on the other, are prejudicial; as also is the use of cushions and feather-beds. The pain attending *blind-piles* may be relieved by ablution in cold water, or in tepid water if that is found more agreeable. *Bleeding-piles* may be relieved by drinking half a tumbler of cold water, and then lying down for an hour. The horizontal position should be maintained as much as possible, that being most favourable to recovery. When piles protrude, the use of *petroleum soap* will be found of great utility.

INJECTIONS.—Great relief and permanent benefit will also follow an occasional injection of from half-a-pint to a pint of cold or tepid water up the lower bowel. This acts beneficially, by constricting the blood-vessels and softening the fæces before evacuation, and by giving tone to the relaxed structures. Injections of cold water are also of service after each evacuation, when any feculent matter remains; at the same time the application of water exercises a most favourable influence on the blood-vessels and nerves of the bowels. As a rule, tepid injections are most suitable for patients of a full habit of body, and cold ones for those of relaxed constitutions.

When piles are excessively sensitive or painful, the patient should sit over the steam of hot water, or keep his bed, or recline during a great part of the day on a couch. Strict cleanliness is also essential. The parts should be frequently washed with soap and cold water; or when the tumours are inflamed and painful, with tepid water. A warm- or vapour-bath (see Part IV) may be occasionally used at night, when the liver is inactive and the skin dry and harsh. It should be followed in the morning with a cold bath, or the body should be rapidly rubbed, first with a wet cold towel, and then with a dry one.

The Abdominal Compress (see Part IV), is strongly recommended as *preventive* of piles, and should be adopted directly the first symptoms are felt; also as a *curative* means in connexion with others pointed out.

Another most important point for patients troubled with piles is, that the habit should be acquired of going to stool at night, immediately before retiring to bed, instead of morning, so that the horizontal position may favour the early subsidence of the tumour, instead of its remaining in an inflamed and prolapsed condition, to the great annoyance and distress of the patient, and to the permanent injury of the parts.

Surgical measures are sometimes necessary; bût, happily, these are rarely required under Homœopathic treatment, the most inveterate cases generally yielding to our prescriptions without the use of the knife, the ligature, or nitric acid.

118.—Pruritus Ani *(Pruritus ani)*—Itching of the Anus.

Definition.—A peculiar itching of the anus, at first of a voluptuous character, but afterwards violent and almost unbearable.

SYMPTOMS.—Crawling, tingling, irritating sensations about the anus, often most troublesome at night, as the patient gets warm in bed, and preventing sleep. It is frequently complicated with an excoriated or fissured condition of the anus.

CAUSES.—Irritation of piles; worms; lodgment of fæces; suppressed period, or any suddenly-suppressed discharge or cutaneous eruption. Frequently, itching of the anus is only a symptom of disease of the liver, of some portion of the digestive apparatus, especially the rectum, or of some part in immediate proximity thereto.

TREATMENT.—*Sulph.*, *Nit. Ac.*, *Lyc.*, *Ant. Crud.*, *Ars.* The selection of the remedy must be guided by the cause of the affection and by the symptoms present. See Section 135.

If connected with piles, worms, or indigestion, the Sections on those subjects should be referred to.

119.—Prolapsus ani *(Prolapsio ani)*—Falling of the Bowel.

DEFINITION.—A protrusion of the mucous lining of the rectum through the anal aperture; occasionally, in complicated cases, a portion of the muscular structures of the rectum is protruded with the mucous membrane.

In slight cases the protrusion only takes place after the action of the bowel, and goes back of itself, or is easily returned; in other instances, however, it may protrude from riding, walking, or even standing, and be replaced with difficulty.

CAUSES.—The disease may be due to constitutional laxity and delicacy of structure, but more frequently to immoderate straining at stool, or when urinating; also to long-continued diarrhœa, constipation, piles, stone in the bladder, or stricture of the urethra. Although not confined to them, it is most frequent in children.

TREATMENT.—*Ignatia.*—This remedy is often specific, and is generally the first to be used, especially for infants and children. The indications are—frequent ineffectual urging to stool, straining, difficult passage of fæces, itching, and prolapse of the bowel.

Nux Vomica.—For males and adults of either sex of a vigorous constitution, this remedy should be substituted for *Ignatia.*

Mercurius.—Prolapsus with itching, diarrhœa, discharge of a yellowish mucus, and hard, swollen abdomen.

Lycopodium.—Obstinate cases, after other remedies have only effected a partial cure; also *Sulphur.*

Podophyllum.—Prolapsus accompanying diarrhœa, with straining and offensive stools; irritation from teething, etc.

ADDITIONAL REMEDIES.—*Calc.*, *Sep.*, *Ars.*, *Bry.*

ACCESSORY MEANS.—These must include—(1.) *The return of the protruded part*, which should be carefully washed and replaced with the forefinger, well oiled, pushing it up into the anus, and carrying the protruded part before it. If the prolapsus be large, the aid of a surgeon should be secured. (2.) *Removal, if possible, of the cause.* If, as is most frequently the case, indigestion, constipation, or piles, be the cause, the suggestions contained in the sections devoted to those subjects should be observed. The diet should be plain, nourishing, and include such kinds of food as favour the healthy action of the bowels. Bathing the parts and loins every morning with cold water, and occasional injections of cold water, give tone to the relaxed structures. As long as the prolapsus continues, the patient should lie down for a short time after the action of the bowels, or acquire the habit of going to stool in the evening, just before retiring to bed, as recommended in the Section on "Piles," page 417.

120.—Hepatitis (*Hepatitis*)—Inflammation of the Liver.

Acute inflammation of this organ is not frequent in this country, although it is very common in tropical climates.

SYMPTOMS.—The disease is usually ushered in by rigors, which are quickly followed by hot skin, thirst, and scanty urine; sometimes nausea and vomiting; white- or yellow-furred tongue; bitter taste; pain more or less severe in the region of the liver, aggravated by pressure, deep breathing, or coughing, and extending to the top of the right shoulder; fulness, from enlargement of the organ; a yellow tinge of the conjunctivæ, and often a general jaundiced state of the skin; the breathing is short and thoracic, being performed almost entirely by the intercostal muscles; sympathetic cough and vomiting. The fever sometimes assumes a typhoid character.

The symptoms vary, however, according to the portion of the gland implicated in the inflammatory process. When the disease is in the convex side of the liver, it is accompanied by a burning, stitching pain in the right side, which extends into the chest, under the collar-bone, between the shoulder-blades, to the top of the right shoulder, and sometimes down the arm, and is aggravated by external pressure. If the inflammation be in the inner portion of the liver, there will be the symptoms already indicated,—saffron-coloured urine, yellow colour of the eyes and skin, etc. If the substance of the gland be involved, the pain is of a dull, tensive character; if the thin serous covering which invests the organ, the pain is sharp and lancinating. Whatever part of the liver is diseased, increased secretion of bile, some degree of jaundice, dyspnœa, cough, etc., are present.

TERMINATIONS.—1. *Resolution.*—This is indicated by an amelioration of the febrile symptoms, copious perspiration, and an abundant deposit in the urine. 2. *Abscess.*—Matter forms, sometimes enclosed in a cyst, at other times diffused, the patient experiencing throbbing, pulsating sensations in the part, with the general symptoms of hectic fever, the abscess discharging itself into the stomach, duodenum, or colon, or externally by perforation of the chest or abdominal wall. 3. *Enlargement.*

CAUSES.—In India the disease is most frequent, from the climate and diet not suiting European constitutions, and is seated in the substance of the liver: in this country it arises from cold, nervous depression, pregnancy, drunkenness, and other causes, and is then usually seated in the peritoneal covering, resembles pleuritis, and ends in adhesion to the diaphragm or other adjacent parts.

EPITOME OF TREATMENT.—

Acon. *(fever)*; Bry. in alternation with Merc. *(after the fever is abated)*; Hep. S. *(if abscess form or be threatened)*. For *Simple enlargement* see next Section.

ACCESSORY MEANS.—When there is severe pain, the whole of the affected part should be covered with two or three thicknesses of linen, squeezed out after immersion in a lotion of half-a-drachm of the strong tincture of the root of *Aconitum* to half-a-pint of *hot* water, and covered with oiled-silk and flannel, or spongio-piline.

See also "Accessory and Preventive Means" in next Section.

121.—Simple Enlargement of the Liver *(Amplificatio simplex jecinoris)*—Congestion of the Liver—Liver-Complaint—Biliousness.

SYMPTOMS.—Fulness on the right side in the region of the false ribs; sense of weight on assuming the upright posture; uneasy sensation when the part is pressed upon; the complexion may be pale, sallow, or dusky; the tongue coated; the bowels constipated; the appetite faulty; and there may be nausea, vomiting, headache, languor, lassitude, and depression of spirits. The pulse is usually slow and irregular.

CAUSES.—Sudden chills; *too abundant, highly-seasoned, stimulating diet; the habitual use of alcoholic or malt drinks*; anger, or other mental influences; excessive bodily exercise in the heat of the sun. As before intimated, Hepatitis is also an occasional cause. It is a very common disease, and Dr. Budd thus accounts for its frequency: "Amid the continual excesses at table of persons in the middle and upper classes of society, an immense variety of noxious matters find their way into the portal blood that should never be present in it, and the mischief which this is calculated to produce is enhanced by indolent or sedentary habits. The consequence often is, that the liver becomes habitually gorged. The same, or even worse effects, result in the lower classes of our larger towns from their inordinate consumption of gin and porter."

Functional derangement, with suppressed secretion, sometimes accompanies congestion of the gland. Dram-drinking often leads to a hard, contracted condition of the liver, called *Cirrhosis* or *hob-nailed liver*, which leads to dropsy.

EPITOME OF TREATMENT.—

1. *Enlargement of the liver.*—Phos., Merc., Nit. Ac., Agar. Mus., Ars., China *(after fever and ague: see Section 11)*.

2. *Hepatalgia (pain in the liver).*—Acon. *(hard-aching; or shooting-pains after exposure)*; Bry. *(tensive and burning, or stinging-pains; and in rheumatic persons)*; Merc. *(dull pain)*; Sabadilla *(dull scraping sensation)*.

3. *Biliousness.*—Bry. *(vomiting of bile and mucus)*; Nux Vom. *(from stimulants and over-feeding; also when associated with piles)*; Sulph. *(constipation)*; Merc. *(white, costive stools, and depression)*; Acon. *(bilious attack from cold)*; Cham. *(from anger)*; Iris *(sick-headache)*; Lyco., Hep. S., Puls., h., Cheled. Maj., Tarax.

4. *Bilious diarrhœa.*—Podoph. *(with bitter taste and dark urine)*; Iris. *(in hot weather, with vomiting)*; China *(simple cases; and in summer)*; Cham. *(in children and females; and when caused by passion)*.

5. *Dropsy of the abdomen from liver-disease.*—Ars. See Section 41.

LEADING INDICATIONS.—

Bryonia.—Enlargement and hardness of the liver, with shooting, stinging, or tensive burning pains, increased on pressure, and accompanied by constipation, without inclination for stool. *Bry.* often acts better in such cases when alternated with *Merc.*

Mercurius.—Dull, pressive pain, which prevents the patient from lying long on the right side; yellow tinge of the "white" of the eyes; sallow skin; shivering, followed by profuse clammy perspiration; loss of appetite; foul taste in the mouth; constipation of the bowels, with white stools; or relaxation, with bilious motions. *Merc.* is one of the best hepatic medicines in simple cases. See also *Bry.* But patients who have been dosed largely with *Mercury* should select *Hep. S.*, especially when the stools are clay-coloured.

Nux Vomica.—Liver-derangement from the use of intoxicating drinks, excessive or stimulating food, or sedentary habits; with constipation, deep-red urine, etc. Also, when associated with piles: in this case, *Sulph.* should be alternated with *Nux Vom.*

Lycopodium.—Sometimes required instead of, or after, *Nux Vom.*, when the latter is insufficient; constipation with flatulence; and continual pain in the right side and back.

Chamomilla.—Bilious attacks in females and children, from exposure to cold, or from anger; with nausea or vomiting of bile, yellow-coated tongue, and sometimes bilious diarrhœa.

Aconitum.—Sudden, acute bilious attacks, following chills, with febrile disturbance.

Podophyllum.—Bilious vomiting, and diarrhœa, with prolapsus ani; bitter taste in the mouth; dark urine; sallow complexion.

Arsenicum.—Extreme, also chronic cases, with great weakness, intense burning pain, vomiting of bile, and exhausting diarrhœa.

Chelidonium Majus.—Chronic liver-complaint; thick and yellow-coated tongue; nausea; dull headache; urine deep-yellow and thick; pain and fulness; constipated bowels.

Nitric. Ac. or *Phos.* are required in long-continued, obstinate cases, with jaundice, more especially if there be reason to fear organic disease of the liver; the former if there be dropsy; the latter if there be fatty degeneration, cirrhosis, etc.

Accessory and Preventive Means.—The patient should strictly avoid everything mentioned as "Causes" in a foregoing paragraph, for wrong habits will render a cure impossible; on the other hand, self-denial, abstinence, and correct habits, in conjunction with the medicinal treatment pointed out, will generally ensure the most gratifying results.

To residents in India and other tropical climates, the foregoing remarks are especially appropriate. The food should be properly cooked, and the quantity taken should be proportioned to the amount of physical work and exercise.

The food supplied to soldiers not in action in India errs in two ways: it is too much in quantity; and, in addition, there is a very large amount of condiments (spices and peppers) with it—articles which may be fitted for the rice and vegetable diet of the Hindu, but particularly objectionable for Europeans.

The *abdominal compress* (see Part IV) is a most valuable adjunct in all liver-affections; a cold salt-bath also should be used daily.

In some parts of India, entozoic influence may be at work in the production of hydatid disease of the liver, or other diseases of the same class, more generally than is supposed *(Parkes)*.

122.—Jaundice *(Morbus regius)*—The Yellows.

The above terms are used to express conditions in which many of the tissues and fluids of the body become yellow, especially the whites of the eyes and the connective tissue of the body. Jaundice is often a symptom of some acute or chronic affection of the liver, rather than a disease *per se*.

Symptoms.—Yellow tinge, first of the whites of the eyes, then of the roots of the nails, and next the face and neck, and finally the trunk and extremities. The urine becomes yellow-coloured or deep-brown, and stains the linen; the fæces whitish or drab-coloured; there is constipation; lassitude; anxiety; pain in the stomach; bitter taste in the mouth; and, generally, febrile symptoms. Sometimes, especially in children, the bowels are relaxed from the food not being properly digested and occasioning irritation. There are also, usually, depression of spirits, prostration of strength, and slowness of the pulse. The presence of the yellow tint in the conjunctivæ and urine is very conclusive that the patient is suffering from jaundice, and not merely from the sallowness of anæmia. If nitric acid be added to the urine, it changes it to a deep green colour. When there is obstruction from a gall-stone, the most acute suffering is induced; the pains come on in paroxysms, and are often accompanied by vomiting and hiccough.

Causes.—Jaundice, as pointed out by Dr. Budd, may be produced in two ways:—(1st) By some impediment to the flow of bile into the duodenum, and the consequent absorption of the retained bile; and (2nd) by defective secretion on the part of the liver, so that the constituents of the bile are not separated from the blood.

Derangement in the functions of the liver connected with the secretion of bile, consequent on atmospheric changes, dietetic errors, dissipation, fits of passion, etc., are frequent causes. A not uncommon impediment to the flow of bile is the impaction of a *gall-stone* in the natural channels of the bile. A gall-stone consists of bile in a crystalline form, the solvent properties having been released. The excessive use of quinine, rhubarb, or calomel in some fevers, may also be stated as a cause, as these drugs obstruct the bile-duct. Pressure of the enlarged womb in pregnancy, or the growth of tumours, causing obstruction of the gall-ducts, are also occasional causes of jaundice. But *sedentary occupations* and *high-living* are probably the most frequent causes.

Epitome of Treatment.—

1. *Acute jaundice.*—Acon., Merc., Nux V.

2. *Chronic.*—Cheled. Maj., Podoph., China, Dig., Ars., Phos., Nit Ac. See also the previous Section.

3. *From impacted gall-stones*—Acon., and the application of a large hot compress over the seat of pain. Drs. Bayes and Hughes recommend Calc. 30, as the best remedy for the relief of pain attendant on their passage along the biliary ducts.

Leading Indications.—

Aconitum.—Jaundice, with symptoms of inflammation, and great pain in the region of the liver.

Mercurius.—This is one of the most valuable remedies, and will often effect a speedy cure; it is especially useful after the use of *Acon.*

China.—Jaundice from marsh miasmatic influences; or with bilious diarrhœa; or if the disease have an intermittent character.

Nux Vomica.—Jaundice with costiveness, sensitiveness in

the region of the liver, or from sedentary habits, or indulgence in stimulants.

Chelidonium Maj.—Jaundice, with pain or tenderness in the liver and right shoulder, deep-red, clean tongue, bitter taste; light-coloured, formed, stools, etc.

Phosphorus.—Brownish-yellow colour of the skin and conjunctivæ; frequent, copious, whitish-gray evacuations; blackish-brown urine; dejection and despondency; sometimes loss of voice, cough, and other symptoms of malignant jaundice.

Arsenicum.—Malignant cases, with typhoid symptoms; great emaciation. *Ars.* is also useful for the dyspepsia sometimes following an acute attack; for jaundice arising from the free use of *Mercury;* and for obstinate cases resulting from fever and ague.

Jaundice during pregnancy, or from cancer or other tumour of the liver, requires professional treatment.

Diet.—Light and digestible—chicken-broth; beef-tea; *toasted* bread, scalded with hot water, with a little sugar; roasted apples; and as much cold water as the patient desires.

Accessory Means.—Flannel squeezed after immersion in *hot* water, or a hot hip-bath, relieves pain. Jaundice from inactivity and chronic congestion of the liver requires change of air and scene, travelling, *daily walking- or horse-exercise*, regular and temperate habits, and the use of the abdominal compress, as described in Part IV. See also the previous Section.

123.—Peritonitis *(Peritonitis)*—Inflammation of the Peritonæum.

Definition.—Inflammation of the serous membrane which lines the interior of the abdomen, and invests and supports the viscera contained therein.

among this class of patients (see "Lady's Manual").

Symptoms.—Shivering and febrile disorder frequently, but not invariably, usher in the disease. There is a stitching, burning, and more or less constant pain, generally first felt below the navel, and soon extending over the entire abdomen; there is great sensitiveness, so that pressure even of the bed-clothes becomes unendurable; the pulse is quick and small, and nausea, vomiting, and, generally, constipation and tympanites are present. The patient lies on his back with his legs flexed so as to relax as much as possible the muscles of the abdomen. When peritonitis arises from perforation of the stomach or intestine, the pain is *sudden* and *intense*, the abdomen becomes excessively sensitive, and the patient is liable to succumb suddenly.

Causes.—Mechanical violence, as a kick, operations, etc.; sudden and excessive changes of temperature; errors of diet; frequent intoxication, the disease termed *gin-colic* being but a chronic peritionitis. Inflammation of the peritoneum is often secondary to enteritis, hepatitis, perforation of the intestine, stomach, etc.

Treatment.—In uncomplicated peritonitis the following treatment, if commenced early, will be rapidly curative. Owing to the complications which frequently arise, the disease should always be under professional care.

Aconitum.—Peritonitis from cold, with predominance of febrile symptoms. A dose every hour till relief is experienced. It is also required in alternation with any other remedy selected early in the disease. A low dilution should be used.

Bryonia.—Stinging and burning pains, greatly increased on movement; constipation, general uneasiness, etc.

Mercurius Cor.—Sallow skin, yellow-coated tongue, and when tympanites and abscesses occur. It is especially useful in scrofulous patients.

Belladonna.—Brain disturbance—headache, flushed face, throbbing, etc. A few doses usually suffice.

Accessory Means.—Hot fomentations to the abdomen to relieve pain; perfect quiet; frequent sips of cold water. When the acuteness of the attack is passed, mild, unstimulating diet, and the use of the abdominal compress (see Part IV).

CHAPTER X.

Diseases of the Urinary System.

124.—Bright's Disease (*Morbus Brightii*)—**Albuminuria.**

Definition.—"A generic term, including several forms of acute and chronic disease of the kidney, usually associated with albumen in the urine, and frequently with dropsy, and with various secondary diseases resulting from deterioration of the blood."

1. Acute Bright's Disease (*Morbus Brightii acutus*)—acute renal dropsy.

Symptoms.—Anasarca of the upper as well as the lower parts of the body—the hands and feet as well as the face being puffy and swollen; there are febrile symptoms—a dry, harsh skin; quick, hard pulse; and, often, sickness from sympathy of the stomach with the kidneys. The skin is tense and does not pit; the urine is scanty, high-coloured, and albuminous, coagulating with heat and nitric acid; and by the microscope there may be seen in it the blood-corpuscles, and also granular casts of the minute tubes of the kidneys, owing their granular appearance to numerous spheroidal tubes of epithelium, the kidneys being in an active stage of congestion if not of inflammation. This condition has been called *desquamative nephritis*, owing to the rapid separation of epithelium which goes on.

As may be inferred from what has been stated, both a ical and microscopical examination of the urine is ssary, and should be made frequently, to determine the ress or otherwise of the disease.

CAUSES.—The effects of fever, especially *Scarlatina* (see page 100), exposure to cold, the action of irritating drugs, etc. The digestive and secretory functions being impaired, the blood and nervous system become deteriorated, and the balance in the circulation and the secretion of the kidneys becomes destroyed.

2. CHRONIC BRIGHT'S DISEASE (*Morbus Brightii longus*).

SYMPTOMS.—Debility, general impairment of the health, and pallor of the surface, coming on insidiously, with pain in the loins, and frequent desire to pass water, particularly at night, the urinary secretion being at first increased in quantity. The patient's face becomes pallid, pasty, and œdematous, so that his features are flattened, and there is loss of appetite, acid eructations, nausea, and frequent sickness, which nothing in his diet can account for. His urine is found to be of less specific gravity than natural, as shown by the depth to which the urinometer sinks below its surface; it is also albuminous and coagulable by heat and nitric acid. There is most albumen at the beginning of the disease, because the kidneys are more congested; but it is of lowest specific gravity at the end, when the urinometer may go down to 1004, and then the quantity of urine is very small. At first the urine may be of a very dark or smoky colour, from containing blood-corpuscles; but afterwards it becomes paler.

The disease progresses slowly; but sooner or later there is *anæmia*, in consequence of the tenuity of the blood from loss of its albumen, so that it is incapable of producing or maintaining the floating cells characteristic of healthy blood. Œdema of the feet and ankles is present, and, in advanced stages, there may be ascites, or general dropsy. But dropsy is not invariably a very marked symptom of the disease; it is sometimes scarcely observed, death arising from *uremiæ*—accumulation of urea in the blood from inability of the kidneys to excrete it; the urea acts as a poison on the brain, producing delirium, convulsions, and coma; and of coma the patient dies. Sometimes, from the poisoned state of the blood, inflammation of a serous membrane arises, especially pericarditis or endocarditis, setting up valvular disease of the heart, and then the patient becomes extremely dropsical, and is carried off by asphyxia, from a complication of heart and kidney disease. At this advanced stage the kidneys are found to be nearly white, anæmic, of the colour of a parsnip, sometimes enlarged, and sometimes diminished in size.

CAUSES.—Chronic Bright's Disease often follows acute desquamative nephritis; sometimes it is a result of bad living, intemperance, constant exposure to wet; struma, gout, etc. It is a constitutional disease; both kidneys are equally affected, probably from some defect in assimilative or other minute changes in nutrition.

TREATMENT.—In detail this must be strictly adapted to the peculiarities of individual cases. The results of the remedies and means employed must be tested at regular intervals by an examination of the urine. Patience is necessary; after carefully deciding as to the line of treatment, it must be steadily persevered in, as marked improvement can only be seen after considerable time.

Leading Remedies.—Ars., Phos., Canth., Krea., Nux Vom., Phos. Ac., Opi.

SPECIAL INDICATIONS.—Acon. *(from cold, with dry skin, thirst, and febrile heat).*

Tereb. *(scanty, dark, bloody urine, and general œdema).*

Canth. *(drop-by-drop and painful micturition, with head-symptoms—delirium, coma, etc.)*

Ars. *(chronic kidney-disease, and post-scarlatinal dropsy, and when there is dropsy of the chest and abdomen, and general anasarca).*

Ferr. *(when the acute symptoms have yielded, to restore the healthy constituents of the blood).*

Krea. *(excessive vomiting).*

Nux V. *or* Ars. *(from alcoholic drinks).*

Opi. *(symptoms of uremic poisoning).*

Phos. Ac. *(from suppuration or other cachectic conditions).*

ACCESSORY MEANS.—In the acute disease, warm-baths, or vapour-baths, should be had recourse to early, to promote the functions of the skin, lessen the dropsy, and to carry off from the blood deleterious matters which may be retained in it by inaction of the kidneys. Vapour-baths are preferable to warm-baths, because they can be used at a higher temperature. If there be much anæmia, warm-baths should be employed with discretion. Further, to favour the free action of the skin, warm clothing—flannel and woollen garments—should be added, and chills and draughts guarded against. In chronic or convalescent cases, a healthy residence is necessary, including a sandy or chalky soil, and mild, dry air, so that out-of-door exercise may be taken. Patients with symptoms of Bright's disease should be encouraged to take abundance of open-air exercise as long as possible, chills and fatigue being guarded against. Bathing or cold sponging, and frictions with a sheet or bath-towel, tend to arrest the disease and invigorate the health. By such means, and the administration of appropriate remedies, patients suffering from chronic disease of the kidney may live for years, enjoying the pleasures, and fulfilling the duties of life.

125.—Cystitis *(Cystitis)*—Inflammation or Catarrh of the Bladder.

a. ACUTE CYSTITIS is a disease of rare occurrence, except when arising from gonorrhœa, or from wounds, calculi, the introduction of instruments, or other mechanical causes. Occasionally, cold or damp may induce inflammation of the bladder. There is usually pain, sense of weight, tenderness on pressure, and extreme irritability in the region of the bladder, with considerable constitutional irritation. The urine is ejected by a sort of spasmodic action as soon as it collects, with straining and, often, much suffering; and there may be discharge of mucous or pus, tinged with blood.

b. Chronic Cystitis is more common; it may be the sequel to an acute attack; but is more generally caused by calculi, disease of the prostate gland, stricture, etc. The symptoms are the same as above described, though in a modified form: but while the pain is less, the discharge is often greater.

From *inflammation of the kidneys*, cystitis may be thus diagnosed—in the latter the pain travels *upwards*, towards the loins; while in the former the pain extends from the loins *down* to the bladder.

Treatment.—The treatment of cystitis must be regulated by its causes and associations. When simple, and resulting from cold, *Aconitum* in alternation with *Cantharis*; if from exposure to damp, *Dulcamara*; if there be much nervous irritability, *Belladonna*. For the chronic form of the disease, *Canth.*, *Cannabis Sat.*, *Apis*, *Kali Iod.*, *Puls.*, and *Chimaphila Umbellata*, are the best remedies.

Accessory Measures.—For the relief of pain, hot fomentations; and in acute cases, rest in the horizontal posture. The warm hip-bath; the abdominal compress; and mucilaginous drinks, favour recovery.

126.—Calculus *(Calculus)*—Stone—Gravel.

In the urine are washed away the refuse matters resulting from digestion, assimilation, and the wear and tear of the body. Any deviation, therefore, from a healthy state of digestion and nutrition is sure to be followed by a deviation from the healthy properties of the urine. A deposit may exist occasionally in small quantity unnoticed; it is the constant or abundant presence which is the important evidence of disease.

When a precipitate is let fall from the urine after it has been voided, it is called a *sediment;* when precipitated in the bladder or kidneys, it is called *gravel*, being muddy as it passes; and when gravel, lodging in any of the urinary passages, becomes concrete, it is called *stone* (*Druitt*). When the urine of a person habitually presents any one kind of deposit, he is generally said to have a corresponding *diathesis;* as the lithic diathesis, etc.

There are several varieties of calculus; but the most common are, the uric or lithic, the phosphatic, and the oxalic.

The *lithic* deposits are observed in fever, chronic liver-disease, etc., forming pink or brick-dust colouring-matter in the urine. When this is abundant it is commonly called *red-gravel.* The lithates chiefly occur in robust persons of florid appearance, who live high and suffer from irritable gastric dyspepsia; and are often associated with gout, rheumatism, and chronic skin disease.

The *phosphatic*, unless arising from changes in the bladder, usually depend on low dyspepsia, an anæmic or broken-down state of the constitution, and occur chiefly in aged persons.

The *oxalic*, are evidences of feeble powers of assimilation, and exhaustion of the nervous system, arising from over-work, mental anxiety, or venereal excesses. The patient is usually pale and hypochondriacal, suffers from disturbed sleep, acid dyspepsia, etc. There is no gravel or sediment, properly speaking; the particles of oxalate float as crystals in the urine, or subside if the urine be allowed to stand, but are not in large quantity.

Various tests are employed by physicians to determine the character of urinary deposits; but to these we cannot further refer.

TREATMENT.—First and foremost, all avoidable causes must be removed—high living, the use of alcoholic liquors, and insufficient exercise, on the one hand; and over-work, anxiety, and excesses of all kinds, on the other. Dyspeptic symptoms must be treated according to the instructions given in the 105th Section; and any other concurrent affection suitably met.

Among the medicines found useful in the treatment of calculus, the following are probably the most successful:—*Phos. Ac.*, *Oxalic. Ac.*, *Lyco.*, *Cann.*, *Canth.*, and *Natrum Carb.*

When a stone becomes dislodged, and is passing from the kidney down the ureter towards the bladder, or from the bladder through the urethra, the pain is extreme; the membrane of the canals is liable to be lacerated, and inflammation and suppuration may supervene; or irritability, spasm, or incontinence, may trouble the patient for a long time.

All cases in which there is even room for suspicion of calculus, should be at once placed under the care of a Homœopathic physician or surgeon.

127.—Irritability of the Bladder (*Vesica Irritabilis*): *and* Spasm of the Bladder (*Spasmus Vesica*) —Stranguary—Difficulty in Passing Water.

These conditions are usually consequent on some diseases of the urinary organs—cystitis, calculus, gonorrhœa, etc.; or are associated with gout, hysteria, or other conditions.

SYMPTOMS.—Frequent desire to urinate; the fluid is forcibly or spasmodically ejected in small quantities; and its passage is attended by burning, aching, or spasmodic pain (*stranguary*); the pain is confined to the bladder, or extends to the end of the penis, round the pelvis, or down the thighs. The urine may or may not be unnatural; but if the disease have become chronic, mucous or pus is passed with it *(catarrh of the bladder)*. In children, irritability of the bladder is sometimes caused by worms (see Section 112).

EPITOME OF TREATMENT.—Nux Vom. *(spasm)*; Ferr. *(simple irritability during the day)*; Bell. *(irritability in children and hysteric females)*; Apis *(stranguary)*; Acon. *(stranguary from cold)*; Dulc. *(from damp)*; Camph. *(in urgent painful cases)*; Canth. *(with or after inflammation of the parts)*; Lyco. *(with much red sediment or gravel)*.

ACCESSORY MEANS.—Mucilaginous drinks, the tepid hip-bath, etc.; see Section 125. It is important to recollect that stranguary is not a substantive disease, but a symptom resulting from various causes, the removal of which is necessary before the bladder can regain its healthy sensibility and tone.

128.—Incontinence of Urine *(Incontinentia urinæ)*—Wetting the Bed.

In this disease there may be partial or entire loss of power to retain the urine in the bladder. The patient has almost constantly an urgent inclination to pass water, which, if not immediately responded to, results in an involuntary discharge, but there is no pain or spasm as in stranguary. If the patient be troubled with a cough, the inconvenience is much increased, as during each paroxysm the urine escapes. When the loss of voluntary power is more complete, the urine continues to dribble away as fast as secreted. The constant discharge excoriates the parts, so that there is much soreness felt when the patient moves about; at the same time, an offensive urinous odour is exhaled from the person, thus rendering the condition one of a most distressing character.

In children the trouble is not uncommon, and occurs chiefly at night.

CAUSES.—Paralysis of the muscular fibres which surround the neck *(sphincter)* of the bladder, and are designed to open or close that organ; this may result from injuries, the pressure of tumours, calculous deposits, syphilitic disease, or from constitutional causes. The most frequent causes of this disease in children are—*irritation of the bladder from worms*; strumous constitution; too large a quantity of fluids, especially warm, or if taken towards evening; improper food or drink, giving rise to acid urine, which *irritates* the mucous coats of the bladder, etc. An examination of the urine of children who wet their beds an hour or two after falling asleep will find it loaded with lithic acid crystals.

TREATMENT.—It is often an obstinate complaint, requiring professional treatment.

The chief remedies are, Bell., Caust., Canth., Nux Vom., Phos. Ac., Podoph., Calc. Carb., Nit. Ac., Gels. *(in the aged)*; Opi., Lyc., Benzoic. Ac. *(high-coloured and strong-smelling urine)*; Cina *or* Spig. *(from worms;* see Section 112); Ferr. *(diurnal)*; Scilla *(profuse discharge)*; Acon., Canth., or Cham. *(in children, with uneasiness in micturating)*.

ACCESSORY MEANS.—As incontinence of urine is generally the result of disease, punishing children cannot remove the annoyance, but only suitable medicinal and general treatment, which must be entirely regulated by the cause. All salt, sharp, and sour articles of food, malt liquors, spirits, tea, and coffee, should be avoided. Meat may be eaten in moderate quantities, but only a small quantity of fruit, and no flatulent food. Nothing hot should be taken in the afterpart of the day. Simple water, milk-and-water, and cocoa, are the most suitable beverages. Cold water or mucilaginous drinks tend to diminish the acrid properties of the urine, when used in moderation. Children who wet their beds ought to sleep on hard mattresses, with light clothing at night take much exercise in the open air, and have shower-baths or daily ablutions with *cold* water. The whole process of ablution, including drying with a rough towel, should not occupy more than five minutes.

Patients troubled with nocturnal incontinence should be prevented from falling into a morbidly profound sleep, as it is then that the discharge of urine usually occurs. Heavy sleep may be obviated by waking up the patient about the second hour of sleep, or in the case of adults, by an alarum set so as to rouse him at the proper time.

129.—Retention of Urine (*Retentio urinæ*).

Definition.—Obstruction to the discharge of the urine contained in the bladder.

Diagnosis.—Retention is liable to be confounded with *suppression* of urine; but in the latter condition, the kidneys are the seat of the disease, and do not secrete the urine; in retention, the urine is secreted, but the fault is in the bladder, its sphincter, or in the course of the urethra, in which there is some cause of obstruction, as stricture, diseased prostate, etc. Suppression may be easily distinguished from retention, for in the latter disease the bladder is distended with urine, and may be felt at the bottom of the abdomen; while, in suppression, the bladder is empty and can scarcely be felt. If it be deemed necessary to introduce the catheter, the diagnosis will be confirmed; in retention the bladder will be found full, but in suppression, empty; the latter condition, however—except in temporary cases, when *Tereb.* will be rapidly curative—is attended with extreme peril, as the urea and other elements of urine accumulate in the blood when the kidneys have fallen into disease, and no longer secrete the urine; the patient becomes uneasy, then drowsy, and soon coma and effusion upon the brain supervene.

Causes of Retention.—Acute febrile disease; fibrinous

exposure to cold, etc. Spasmodic stricture is not likely to occur except in persons already suffering from a slight degree of permanent stricture, or gleety discharge, or an abnormal condition of the urine.

TREATMENT.—*Aconitum.*—Inflammatory symptoms, often in alternation with some other remedy, especially *Cantharis.*

Camphor.—Spasm at the neck of the bladder, especially if caused by *Cantharides* (a drop on a piece of loaf-sugar every fifteen minutes for three or four times).

Cantharis.—Urging to pass water, with cutting and tearing pains.

Clematis.—Difficult passage of urine; heat or slight burning, with occasional stitches in the course of the urethra while passing water; stricture of the urethra after repeated attacks of gonorrhœa, and in cases temporarily relieved by the introduction of bougies. Dr. Hirsch has administered this remedy in such cases with complete success.

Nux Vomica.—Painful, ineffectual efforts to urinate, caused by abuse of wines or spirits; spasmodic stricture.

Sulphur.—In alternation with the last remedy, if the patient be troubled with piles.

In addition to the above remedies, the following are often useful:—*Cann.*, *Tereb.*, *Uva U.*, *Phos. Ac.*, *Bell.*, *Iod.*, *Ars.*

ACCESSORY MEANS.—The introduction of the catheter, so

frequently resorted to under the old treatment, is often superseded by the more efficient remedies we employ; still it may be necessary in some cases; but this requires professional skill. External applications—warm baths, hot fomentations—bland drinks, and injections by the rectum, will greatly aid the medicines in restoring the functions of the parts, if there be not incurable organic disease. The diet must be sparing, and, in some severe cases, restricted to demulcent drinks—barley-water, gum-water, etc.

130.—Gonorrhœa (*Gonorrhœa*)—Venereal Disease.

Definition.—A specific disease characterized by inflammation of, and a muco-purulent discharge from, the mucous membrane of the urethra, and other portions of the genitals. It may exist in both sexes.

Cause.—Gonorrhœa is produced by contact of the genital organs with a specific and highly-contagious animal poison during impure or indiscriminate sexual connexion. At the same time it is well known that the urethra may become inflamed and pour out a purulent discharge, from connection with a woman not suffering from disease of a specific venereal character. On the part of the female—the menstrual fluid, acrid leucorrhœa, want of cleanliness, etc.; or, on the part of the male—an acid state of the urine, a gouty or rheumatic diathesis, the irritation of stricture, etc., may give rise to a discharge having many of the characteristics and even the obstinacy of a specific gonorrhœal disease. The poison of gonorrhœa, then, though by far the most frequent, is but one among several causes capable of exciting inflammation of, and purulent discharge from, the urethra.

The special cause, however, it is scarcely necessary to add, is generally avoidable, and *ought* to be avoided. See the remarks under "Preventive Measures," in next Section.

SYMPTOMS.—These have been divided into three stages, the *initiatory*, the *inflammatory*, and the *chronic*. There is first experienced a tingling or itching sensation, with some degree of heat, at the orifice of the urethra, especially when urinating. The orifice of the urethra soon becomes red and swollen, and then muco-pus exudes. As the inflammatory stage sets in, there are burning or scalding pains on passing water, with increased secretion from the affected part, at first thin, but soon becoming thick, milky, yellow, green, or even bloody; during this stage, broken rest at night, a good deal of constitutional disturbance, and complications, such as are afterwards mentioned, are prone to arise.

After the disease has continued for about seven to fourteen days, the inflammatory symptoms begin to subside, and the chronic stage sets in: there is more or less irritation in passing water, and a yellow discharge, which, under unfavourable circumstances, may persist for a long time, and then terminate in an obstinate, thin, transparent, painless discharge *(Gleet)*; this is especially likely to occur in strumous, phlegmatic, or gouty constitutions, and in patients subject to chronic cutaneous diseases.

COMPLICATIONS OF GONORRHŒA.—(1.) *Irritation, congestion*, or even true *inflammation of the urinary organs*, causing a frequent desire to pass water, but extreme difficulty in doing so; or there may be complete retention of urine. (2.) In the male, frequent and involuntary erections, crooked and painful, occurring chiefly during the night *(Chordee)*. (3.) A thickened and constricted condition of the glans penis, and effusion under it, so that the foreskin cannot be retracted *(Phimosis)*. (4.) Inflammation of the lymphatic glands of the groin *(Sympathetic bubo)*. (5.) *Inflammation of the testicles (Orchitis)*, coming on at a later stage of the disease, when the discharge has nearly ceased, and is probably an extension of the inflammation from the urethra; it is marked by pain, greatly increased by allowing the organs to hang unsupported, excessive tenderness, great swelling, fever, and, often, vomiting.

TREATMENT.—In the treatment of this disease homœopathy offers the following advantages over the old system: her medicines are safe, pleasant, and effective, sometimes rapidly so; they generally steer the patient clear of all or most of the usual sequelæ; and they do not interfere with the comfort, occupation, or health of the patient.

The treatment may be preventive or curative. The *preventive period*, which intervenes between the exposure to the infection and the occurrence of any symptom, averages about three days.

The *forming stage*, when the symptoms of disease first occur—slight redness and tingling at the end of the penis, and an augmentation of the natural secretion of the parts. This stage lasts from twelve to forty-eight hours. The treatment in these stages, *before* any acute symptoms have set in, is an astringent lotion, prepared according to one of the following formulæ:—

Argenti nitras, gr. ij; aquæ des. ℥viij;
or, Zinci sulph., gr. viij; aquæ des. ℥viij.

The selection of the lotion, and the frequency of its use, must be determined by the circumstances of the case. A glass syringe, of a suitable size and form—the nozzle of the instrument being well lubricated—is necessary for the application of the lotion to the diseased surface; also tact and care in the mode of injecting, upon which much of the efficiency of the lotion depends. This proceeding is strictly homœopathic, and if employed early will almost certainly arrest the disease. If, however, *acute* symptoms have set in, astringent injections are improper. Avoidance of intoxicating beverages and stimulating food, with quiet, rest in the *horizontal posture*, and frequent washing the parts with soap and water, will greatly facilitate the cure.

The *acute* inflammatory stage usually continues from eight to fourteen days, but may be shorter or longer, according to the treatment adopted, and the constitution of the patient. The most useful remedies are:—*Acon.*, *Cann.*, *Canth.*, *Apis*, *Mer. Cor.*, *Copaibæ*. The remedies should be administered in low dilutions, those indicated in the list, page 72, being, in our experience, inefficient. In addition to the administration of one or more of the above, the treatment must embrace a moderate diet, with linseed-tea, gum-water, barley-water, or similar demulcent drinks, taken *ad libitum*, and the exclusion of fermented liquors. Also frequent ablutions with warm or cold water, and keeping the parts as free as possible from the irritating discharge. It is, probably, the infectious nature of this matter which renders the disease so obstinate, for it operates as a continual exciting cause.

The *chronic stage* is that form of the disease termed *Gleet*. Besides the local measures pointed out below, the administration of one or more of the annexed medicines is necessary:—*Ferr.*, *Merc.*, *Lyc.*, *Nux V.*, *Thuja*, *Petro.*, and *Sulph.*

Injections are often useful. We mainly depend upon those recommended by Dr. Yeldham. Liq. *Plumbi Diacet* (ʒss ad aquæ dest. ℥j), and an infusion of *Hydrastis* (℥j ad aquæ dest. O). In addition to these, *Nitrate of Silver*, *Tannin*, *Lime-water*, and *Cold-water*, are often prescribed.

Combined with these remedies, cold baths, or if practicable, sea-bathing, regular and early hours, and good temperate living, are necessary to ensure successful results.

We have entered only very superficially into the management of this disease: its difficult nature, its numerous and annoying complications, and the risk of exposing another to contagion, if the best curative measures be not adopted, are circumstances which render professional treatment necessary.

In certain constitutions the disease is sometimes tedious.

131.—Spermatorrhœa (*Spermatorrhœa*)—Involuntary Emissions.

Definition.—Involuntary seminal discharges, occurring either during sleep, or under various conditions during the day, and associated with irritability and debility of the generative organs.

Causes.—Spermatorrhœa generally occurs as the result of a bad habit—*self-abuse*—either accidentally acquired, or learned from somewhat older associates, especially in schools, and continued under the influence of a morbid imagination, or from the excitement occasioned by "sensationals," divorce-court trial reports, impure conversation, etc., often in ignorance of the consequences of the vicious practice. Public schools, especially boarding-schools and colleges, are the most fruitful sources of instruction and irritation into this vice. Other causes may be—morbid conditions of the urethra, or of the rectum; sexual excesses; frequent excitation of the sexual passion; irritation from worms, piles, horseback-exercise, etc.; disease of the brain or spinal marrow; etc. Under such conditions, the organs become extremely debilitated, and liable to excitation, with secretion and discharge of seminal fluid, from slight emotional causes,—a thought, a glance, a word,—or by trivial and common physical agents,—the oscillations of a carriage, the efforts of straining at stool, etc.

Effects.—The effects of spermatorrhœa are—depression of spirits, often to an extreme degree; loss or weakness of memory and other senses; indigestion with oppression after food, flatulence, palpitation, headache, etc.; impotence;

sunken eyes, and loss of the healthy tints of the lips and face, the patient looking older than his years. If indulgence in the habit were commenced early, and have been frequent and long-continued, the effects on the physical and mental state of the patient are more serious and general. Happily, a course of judicious treatment is sufficient in nearly every case to effect a cure, and to restore the patient to a life of usefulness and happiness.

EXTENT AND EVILS OF THE HABITUAL CAUSE.—In the previous editions of this book, and elsewhere, the subject of this section has been more or less distinctly mentioned, and, as a consequence, we have been consulted by many hundred persons, in various and remote places, suffering from different degrees of weakness, or morbid, irregular action of the generative organs. Our correspondence and practice prove to us that the evils of this affection are wide-spread, beyond the credibility of those who have not thoroughly investigated the subject. The notion that boys are ignorant of the subject, and that we ought not to remove that ignorance, is wholly incorrect. Self-abuse is of such extreme frequency that it is a question whether even a majority of the youth of all classes of the community do not practise it. The consequences of the habit, if not serious as involving immediately fatal results, occasion the deepest mental distress, and too often disqualify the patient for the discharge of the ordinary duties of life.

Notwithstanding the magnitude of the evil, our experience forces us to the conclusion that the subject has been much overlooked or under-rated by medical men generally. Probably in many cases we have been consulted from an insuperable dislike of the patient to confront a medical man in his own neighbourhood on a subject of such extreme delicacy. The whole question, however, demands far more attention from the profession that it has yet received, both on account of the physical and mental sufferings involved, and the charlatanism and imposture which professional neglect involves. In untold instances, shattered health, and exhausted resourses, have resulted from falling into the hands of any of the numerous advertising quacks who in all large towns prey on the sufferers from this disease.

TREATMENT.—The treatment, both medical and hygienic, should include all available methods for establishing the constitutional strength, soothing local excitement and irritability, and forming healthy habits both of mind and body.

The *medical* treatment involves the administration of Homœopathic remedies, only a few of which are described in this work —*China*, *Canth.*, *Phos.*, *Phos. Ac.*, *Staph.*, *Nux Vom.*, *Sulph.*, etc.), the selection and the doses of which can only be determined by the local and general symptoms of individual cases. Amplitude of resources, beyond those possessed by amateur practitioners, are necessary in the management of this affection.

An important feature in the medical treatment should be the correction of any concurrent affection from which the patient may suffer.

The *hygienic* treatment includes many points, and should extend to the commercial, social, and moral relationships of the patient—occupation, recreation, literature, and mental and moral discipline; diet, sleep, bathing, etc. The management of these several points must be regulated according to the exigences of each case.

PREVENTIVE MEASURES.—The sexual instinct in man is strong, and has been rendered so by Providence for the important purpose of perpetuating the race. But the precocious development of this passion may be prevented; and when, on account of youth and other circumstances, its gratification would be imprudent, it may be kept in abeyance by proper measures and correct discipline—the discipline contributing to manliness of character, and at the same time better fitting him for the duties and enjoyments of mature manhood.

The following suggestions are intended to aid in effecting this important object, and in guarding youth against sexual vice.

1. *Good physical and mental training.*—The systematic adoption of muscular and mental exercises expend the nervous energy, diverting it from the sexual organs, so that amorous thoughts and propensities become less prominent. Mental occupations also exercise a like tendency, though, perhaps, to a less degree. Constant and congenial occupation and recreation, bodily and mental, is a *sine quâ non.*

Fashionable and idle habits are the great cause of solitary vice on the one hand, or of venereal excesses and diseases on the other. The establishment of systematic exercises at home and in schools—athletic sports, gymnasia, etc.; libraries, literary and scientific institutions, including the instructive and interesting experiments in chemistry, electricity, mechanics, and other sciences; all these are highly useful by pre-occupying the mind, and so preventing loose thoughts and habits.

2. *Chaste thoughts and conversation.*—The cultivation of pure thoughts and conversation among the young would remove occasions of great temptation to sin. Parents, guardians, and teachers, should exercise a strict supervision over the books that are read. Much of the literature of the present day is of a character that tends to emasculate the mind of the reader, to crowd it with fancies and follies, inciting it to passions, and paving the way directly to the evils under consideration.

3. *Avoidance of stimulants and luxurious habits.*—The free use of meat and highly-seasoned dishes, coffee, wine, late suppers, etc., strongly tend to excite animal propensities,

which directly predisposes to the evil. Soft beds and too much sleep, are also to be avoided. Strict temperance, both in eating and drinking, is a great preventive.

4. *Direct instruction and caution.*—Young persons who, there is reason to believe, are ignorant of the practice of self-abuse, should be kept so, but watched, and it may soon be observed if he or she be addicted to this vice. Self-pollution may generally be detected by such signs as the following—bashfulness; paleness of the face, sunken eyes, and dull, heavy expression, especially in one previously healthy, with beaming eyes, and intelligent appearance and manner; weakness, with more or less pain, in the back; inability or indisposition to look frankly into the eyes of another, especially of the same sex; irritability, sadness, fearfulness, with indecision. These are strong evidences that the person is addicted to the habit. "The first sentiment that this species of sensuality awakens in young persons is a sort of bashfulness, incompatible with the innocence of their age" *(Teste).*

When such symptoms exist, a careful examination should be made, and the actions closely but unobtrusively watched. An examination of the linen generally affords conclusive evidence in the case of boys; the genital organs of these patients it may be noticed, too, receive an undue share of their attention. If the practice be found to exist, its discontinuance must be made imperative, and the dangers pointed out that will inevitably follow a persistence in the habit. The delicacy of the subject must never be allowed to operate as a barrier to an important duty. The patient should be constantly watched during the day till he falls asleep at night, and be required to arise directly he awakes in the morning. In confirmed cases, the night-dress should be so arranged that the hands cannot touch the genital organs.

Nurses should never be permitted to take any liberties with the genitals of children; and children should be early taught that *it is immodest,* and even wrong, to handle the parts.

If the habit have been acquired, and any of the effects already stated developed, a proper course of homœopathic treatment will suffice to restore the health, *providing the habit be relinquished.* The best Homœopathic doctor within reach should be consulted; or if there be none near, one should be consulted by letter. Under any circumstances, all advertising quacks, and all advertised quack medicines, should be avoided.

We have aimed to say as little as is consistent with our desire to arouse parents and teachers to a sense of their duty to the young in this matter. It may be deemed by some an offence against decency to write of such things in a work like this; but so wide-spread an evil, affecting the health and happiness of future generations and even the welfare of the nation itself, demands that false delicacy and modesty be cast aside, that the sin may be known, and its progress stayed. As guardians of health, we must deal with things *as they are.*

CHAPTER XII.

DISEASES OF THE CUTANEOUS SYSTEM.

132.—Erythema (*Erythema*)—Inflammatory Redness of the Skin.

DEFINITION.—A morbid redness of the skin, of a superficial character, sometimes called "inflammatory blush."

VARIETIES.—The varieties are named according to their characteristics When it occurs on the surface of an œdematous swelling it is called *Erythema læve*. *E. fugax* is simply a fleeting, patchy-redness. *E. marginatum* designates a redness with a well-defined circumference. *E. papulatum* consists of small red spots varying in size from a pin's head to a split-pea,—raised after a time into a papular form, of a vivid colour, becoming pale on pressure, and dying away in a few days with slight desquamation. The spots may be aggregated or distinct, and are seen especially on the back of the hand, the arm, neck, and breast. The disease lasts about three weeks, and seems to be associated with rheumatic symptoms. It occurs mainly in young people. *E. tuberculatum* is the same disease, in which the erythema becomes somewhat tuberculated: it is often seen in servants who make a change of residence from country to town. *E. nodosum* is a more marked stage of the last; the spots are sometimes as large as a walnut or even much larger, oval in shape, the long diameter being in a majority of cases parallel to that of the limb: they are

EPITOME OF TREATMENT.—Bell. *(simple redness, and E. papulatum)*; Acon. *(febrile disturbance, and flushing of the face from excitement)*; Apis *(E. læve, and E. nodosum)*; Kali Bich. *(E. papulatum, if* Bell. *be not sufficient)*; Nux Vom. *(flushing after food)*; Bry., Mang., Ferr., Ars.

ACCESSORY MEASURES.—Regular open-air exercise; sufficient time for, and freedom of the mind during, meals; simple food; and the free use of cold water internally and externally.

133.—Intertrigo *(Intertrigo)* Chafing—Soreness of Infants.

DEFINITION.—Redness and chafing produced by the friction of two folds of skin, especially in fat children and adults: it is seen in the groin, axilla, and neck; sometimes a fluid is exuded, the acridity of which increases the local mischief, and presently an offensive raw surface is produced.

Intertrigo differs from eczema in its acute course, and in the character of the secretion, which is clear, and does not stiffen linen.

EPITOME OF TREATMENT.—Cham. *(in infants)*; Calc. Carb. *(scrofulous children)*; Lyco. *(obstinate cases)*; Merc. *(rawness and great soreness)*; Sulph. The parts should be *well washed with cold or tepid water, and carefully dried* two or three times

be laid between the opposed surfaces; or in bad cases, a lotion composed of one part of tincture of *Hydrastis* to ten of *Glycerine* may be applied in the same manner.

134.—Roseola (*Roseola*)—Rose-rash—False Measles.

Definition.—A simple rash, of a *rose-red* or *pink* colour, occurring in patches, about half-an-inch in diameter; it is associated with more or less febrile disturbance; and is non-contagious. There is also slight itching, sense of heat, and sometimes redness of the mucous surfaces of the palate and fauces.

Roseola may at first be mistaken for *measles* or *scarlet-fever*; otherwise the disease is of little importance.

Its varieties are:—*Roseola æstiva*—appearing in summer-time only; *R. autumnalis*—in autumn; *R. symptomatica*—occurring during the course of other diseases; and *R. annulata*—distinct rings of redness, with an unaffected centre.

The disease is apt to occur in infants, when it comes and goes perhaps for several days, accompanied by local heat and itching, especially at night.

There are no "wheals," as in *urticaria;* no catarrhal symptoms, as in *measles;* and no grave symptoms, as in *scarlatina.*

Treatment.—*Acon.* is usually sufficient. A dose may be given every three or four hours several times. If the itching be very troublesome, the parts may be moistened with a lotion of one part of *Acon.* tincture to twenty of water. *Rhus Tox.* or *Bell.* are sometimes required.

135.—Urticaria (*Urticaria*)—Nettle-Rash.

Definition.—A transient, non-contagious, cutaneous affection, characterised by an eruption of prominent patches or wheals, either redder or whiter than the natural skin, of

the great number, and frequent coalescence, of the "wheals." *Chronic* urticaria may be *U. evanida*—evanescent, without febrile symptoms, and with trifling redness; *U. perstans*—persistent nettle-rash; *U. subcutanea*—"subcutaneous nettle-rash, a nervous affection of the limbs, accompanied at intervals with an eruption of nettle-rash;" and *U. tuberculata*—characterized by the production of elevations of considerable size, extending deeply into the subcutaneous cellular tissue.

SYMPTOMS.—Similar, or more intense than those produced by nettle-stings, *urtica* being the Latin for a nettle. The eruption consists of elevations, occurring in streaks or wheals of an irregular shape, on a red ground; the character of the rash becomes much more marked after scratching or rubbing, "so that it is possible, by using the nail of the finger, to write one's name on the skin;" it is generally worse in the evening, and when the body is exposed to cold air. There is much tingling and burning, and often the eruption, after disappearing suddenly from one part, shows itself in another. The spots contain no fluid, and end in desquamation of the skin. It is most common in spring and early summer, is not contagious, may occur at any age, and in the same person repeatedly.

CAUSES.—Derangements of the digestive organs, following the use of some particular kinds of food, among which we may specify bitter almonds, cucumbers, mushrooms, oatmeal; shell-fish are a common cause of nettle-rash, especially mussels; and certain kinds of medicines, such as cubebs,

The skin being extremely sensitive, it is easily excited by external irritants—such as the wearing of flannel next the skin (see pp. 47–8), the bites of fleas, etc.

Chronic and intermittent urticaria is frequently associated with uterine or other diseases, and is often very obstinate. Cold, rapid changes of temperature, and, in children, teething, favour its development in patients predisposed.

Epitome of Treatment.—

1. *Simple Urticaria.*—Apis, Urtica Urens, Acon.

2. *From Gastric disorder.*—Ant. Crud., Nux Vom., Puls.

3. *From cold.*—Acon. *(from draughts and cold winds)*; Dulc. *(from damp)*.

4. *Associated with other affections).*—Bry., Cimic., *or* Rhus Tox *(rheumatic patients)*; Colch. *(gouty subjects)*; Ars. *or* Ipec. *(asthma)*; Puls. *(uterine irregularities)*.

5. *Chronic cases.*—Ars. *or* Quinine *(intermittent)*; Apis., Sulph.

6. *Special symptoms.*—Acon. *(febrile disturbance)*; Bry. *(sudden retrocession of eruption)*; Ign. *or* Anacardium *(mental depression and confusion)*; Coff. *(sleeplessness and nervous irritability)*.

Accessory Measures.—A general *warm bath* is invaluable; it soothes the skin and promotes the cure. When the eruption is thoroughly out, the heat and irritation may be materially alleviated by smearing the whole surface of the body with fresh-cured bacon, prepared as directed on page 84.

The patient should enjoy a dry, uniform, and moderate temperature; have plain food; take plenty of exercise in the open air; and observe great cleanliness. Draughts, changes of temperature, indigestible food, and all exciting causes, must be removed and avoided. If flannel be worn, it should be over a linen garment.

136.—Prurigo (*Prurigo*)—Itching of the Skin.

DEFINITION.—"A chronic affection of the skin, characterized by a thickened and *discoloured state* of that membrane, attended by *excessive itching*, and, generally, an eruption of *papulæ* (*pimples*).

SYMPTOMS.—*Intense itching*, and creeping sensation; patients scratch and tear themselves till the blood flows; their sleep is frequently disturbed, and their existence is often almost unendurable; or the impulse to incessant scratching is so powerful as to induce the patient to seek seclusion. Sometimes the itching is diffused irregularly over the surface; at other times it affects the extremities; frequently it occurs round the anus, or on the scrotum, or on the female genitals. It is often a horrible and most obstinate disease.

CAUSES.—The *predisposing* are—constitutional taint, senile decay, chronic disease, etc. It is generally a symptom of lowered vitality, or of decay of the skin; the skin loses its elasticity, firmness, and fat, and its secretion is disordered. It has been thought that the disease was caused by *pediculi*; but it is not so: pediculi are only present in prurigo in uncleanly persons. *Exciting* causes are—rich, indigestible food, stimulating drinks, extreme heat or cold, etc. In summer-time a mild form sometimes attacks young persons.

TREATMENT.—*Aconitum*.—Furious itching all over the skin, *with febrile symptoms*.

Sulphur.—Severe itching, attended with thirst and dryness of the skin, worse in the evening and in bed. This is generally a prominent remedy, and it is frequently specific, especially in recent cases.

Arsenicum.—Itching with burning; or an eruption emitting watery-fluid like sweat, and attended with much constitutional weakness. It is most suitable in chronic cases.

digestible food generally, must not be indulged in. The se of ointments is generally injurious. In severe cases, mporary relief may be obtained by bathing the parts with cohol and water in equal proportions; or with *Mezereum tion* (one part to ten of water); or by sponging the skin, on tiring to bed, with a warm infusion made by pouring oiling-water on bran.

The Wet Compress.—Prurigo, if confined to one or two laces, is much benefited by the constant use of a wet mpress over the affected part; for although it often increases e irritation at first, it finally assists nature in expelling the orbid matter.

SCRATCHING.—Notwithstanding the incentive to scratching prurigo and other skin affections, the practice greatly aids keeping up the irritation and increasing the disease. On is point the following remarks by Dr. Tilbury Fox well xpress a condition we have often observed:

"When the disease is *non-contagious*, secretion, if present, may be ansferred (by scratching), and, when acrid, sets up local inflammation; d when *contagious*, scratching is the surest method of inoculation, as in e case of the contagious impetigo or porrigo. Children in this way ansplant the disease from the head to various other parts of the body. others, beyond a doubt, get it about their hands from children. As an stance of the effect of scratching, I may mention the case of a gentle-an I have recently seen in consultation, who has tried every remedy and

and thickened. When disappearing, very fine, dry, greyish scales are formed.

The disease appears on different parts of the body, but generally on the back of the fore-arms and hands, the sides of the neck, and the face.

VARIETIES.—The disease may be *Lichen simplex*—occurring in summer; *L. pilaris*—the follicles of the hair being the seat of the affection; *L. circumspectus*—the pimples being grouped in small circular patches, with a well-defined border, sometimes with a clear centre; *L. agrius*—which is the most serious form of the disease, is seen in grocers, bakers, brick-layers, and washerwomen, sometimes called "baker's itch;" the pimples are very close, red, inflamed, and have a secretion, with intense itching and burning, febrile symptoms, pains in the limbs, gastric derangements, etc., and lasting, in the acute stage, ten or fifteen days; or, *L. tropicus*—"prickly heat," which occurs chiefly in hot climates, attacking the parts covered by the clothes, accompanied by a peculiar tingling and pricking; the papillæ are of a vivid-red colour, about the size of a pin's head, but there is no redness of the skin generally: the disease sometimes occurs in this country.

Causes.—Constitutional predisposition; irregularities in habits or diet; certain occupations, as those of cooks, bakers, grocers, etc.; hot weather or climate.

Epitome of Treatment.—Sulph. (*simple cases*); Ant. Crud. (*associated with derangements of the digestive organs*); Apis *or* Ledum Pal. ("*prickly heat*"); Ars. (*L. agrius; and chronic cases*); Nux Juglans.

Accessory Treatment.—Simple, unstimulating food and drink; proper attention to the general health. See "Causes," and also "Accessory Measures," in the two previous Sections.

Strophulus (*Strophulus*)—Red-gum—Tooth-rash—is supposed by some to be to children what lichen is to adults; but though there is a similarity, yet the seat of the former is probably in the sweat-glands; it occurs chiefly in children who are kept in heated rooms, or are muffled up from the fresh-air; and shows itself mostly on the exposed parts of the body—the face, neck, or limbs. It is generally seen during changes of season, teething, etc.

Its *Treatment* includes an abundant supply of fresh-air, the use of clothing which, while sufficient to protect the body from cold, permits the access of air to the skin, the daily cold or tepid bath, and the administration of *Cham.* thrice daily for several days; or, should there be derangement of the digestive system associated with the affection, *Ant. Crud.*; *Puls.*, or *Calc. Carb.*—the latter if there be *chronic acidity.*

138.—Pityriasis (*Pityriasis*)—Branny Tetter—Dandriff.

Definition.—A superficial cutaneous affection, in which there is desquamation—the skin falling off in whitish scales or bran-like powder. There may be more or less redness, *itching, and heat.*

The disease may occur on the head *(dandriff)*, eye-lids, or other parts of the body. The scales are continually shed and reproduced, but there is no discharge.

TREATMENT.—*Arsenicum* is generally the most Homœopathic remedy. A dose may be given thrice daily. *Graph.* or *Lyco.* may be given if *Ars.* be not sufficient.

ACCESSORY MEANS.—Strict attention to cleanliness; and well drying the parts after washing.

139.—Psoriasis *(Psoriasis)*—Lepra—Dry Tetter.

DEFINITION.—A non-contagious cutaneous affection, characterised by well-formed, dry, and whitish scales, without vesiculation or pustulation, accompanied by cracking of the skin, and having a disposition to recur.

The general health is not appreciably affected, there being few if any symptoms beyond slight itching, which is worst at the commencement.

The cutaneous eruption which has long been known as *Lepra* is now allowed to be merely a variety or a declining stage of Psoriasis, and not a separate affection *(Tanner)*.

VARIETIES.—In the common form of Psoriasis there are whitish, minute spots, made up of dry, silvery-looking scales, heaped together on tawny-red patches of skin about the elbows and knees *(P. vulgaris)*; when the spots are larger, they resemble drops of mortar, and are found on the breast, back, and limbs *(P. guttata)*; then the eruption may be more developed, and extend over a larger surface, sometimes covering an entire limb *(P. diffusa)*; when the eruption runs together in a serpentine form, the scales are thin, and quickly reproduced *(L. gyrata)*; when the scales are large, dry, and adherent, and the patches thickened and cracked, a slight discharge may occur, causing scabs,—this is the chronic form *(L. inveterata)*.

Psoriasis progresses by an increase in the size and number of the patches, and their extension along the extremities to the trunk. On the other hand, the cure of the disease is marked by diminution of the scales, and more full exposure of the surface beneath, until gradually the eruption disappears, leaving little or no trace of its former existence. It is sometimes, however, a most obstinate disease.

CAUSES.—Psoriasis occurs in persons apparently in good health, but who are probably suffering from some form of defective nutrition. Too rapid growth, bad living, overstudy, anxiety, too prolonged lactation, etc., are likely to excite an attack, where a predisposition, often hereditary, exists.

TREATMENT.—Merc., Iodine, Nit. Ac., Sulph.; Arsen. *(chronic and inveterate cases)*.

ACCESSORY MEANS.—*Local.*—Warm-baths; preparations of *Glycerine* (see Part IV, art. "Glycerine"), if the skin be much cracked, or occasional poultices if it be very hard. *General.*—Simple, nourishing diet, and, in growing persons, Cod-liver-oil (Möller's: see Part IV, art. "Cod-liver-oil"). Any defect in the functions of digestion and assimilation should be corrected. Patients who have been overtaxed in mind or body should have rest and change.

140.—Herpes *(Herpes)*—Shingles—Tetter.

DEFINITION.—*Large vesicles* or small blebs, occurring distinct from each other, in patches on different parts of the body, having an inflamed base, containing a fluid—at first clear, then milky, afterwards quickly disappearing—and ultimately shrivelling, leaving scabs; or, becoming ruptured, they dry up into light-brownish scabs.

VARIETIES.—There are four varieties of Herpes—*H. phlyctenodes*, sometimes called nirles—commences with a sense of local heat and inflammation; upon this ground arise round grouped vesicles, from ten to twenty, in patches varying from the size of a six-penny to that of a five-shilling piece, of which there are several, surrounded by a red areola, and mostly occurring about the face, neck, and upper limbs. *H. circinatus*, *vesicular* (not the common) ring-worm—disposes of itself in rings; and *H. iris*—in the form of rainbows. *H. zoster* or *zona*, commonly called *shingles*—has the nature of the first variety, but derives its name from its manner of encircling one half of the body. It is an acute disease, lasting about fourteen to twenty days, and follows the course of one or more of the cutaneous nerves, generally stopping short in the middle, though it may extend across to the other side, and has the appearance of a line of patches, like a belt, half round the body. It generally affects the trunk, chiefly of the right side, but occasionally the face, shoulder, abdomen, or upper part of the thigh. It is most common in the young, particularly during change of weather, and is often preceded by neuralgic pains, the eruption following in the same locality. In some rare cases, ulceration may supervene; there may be much pain, smarting, or burning; and the scars may remain for some time. There is a remarkable connection between *Herpes zoster* and the nervous system: the latter always determines the seat of the former. Zona is much dreaded, and uninstructed nurses foolishly state that if the patches extend round the body death is certain to result. There, however, is no danger, unless the patient be very old and feeble.

General Symptoms.—In addition to what is stated above, there is often a feeling of *malaise*, feverishness—headache, shivering—and, perhaps, neuralgic pain in the side *(pleurodynia)*, which may be very acute, especially in shingles (see pp. 264–7). The disease is mostly accompanied by sensations of heat, tension, and burning, felt even before the appearance of the eruption; and is followed by weakness and depression. When the disease occurs in the aged, or in persons of feeble constitution, there is much debility, and ulceration may arise, further debilitating the patient. It sometimes occurs during the course of other diseases.

CAUSE.—*Irritation of the nerves*—as when catarrh affects the air-passages, and herpes is developed on the nose or lips.

EPITOME OF TREATMENT.—

1. *Earliest symptoms.*—Acon. *(and when there is neuralgia consequent on anxiety, etc.)*

2. DEVELOPED HERPES.—Rhus Tox. *(in all simple cases)*; Sulph. *(to follow* Rhus *if necessary)*; Ars. *(neuralgia, and in debilitated constitutions)*; Phyto. *or* Graph. *(ulcerous conditions; and in old people)*; Phos. *(consumptive patients)*; Tellurium *or* Sepia *(Herpes circinnatus)*.

3. *Pleurodynia.*—Ranun. Bulb.; see Section 53.

4. *Additional remedies.*—Mang., Staph., Cistus Can., Comacladia.

ACCESSORY MEASURES.—The daily bath; plenty of out-of-door exercise; and the "Accessory Measures" suggested in Section 53. For local application, see article "Glycerine," in Part. IV.

141.—Eczema *(Eczema)*—Catarrhal Inflammation of the Skin—Scalled-Head—Milk-crust.

DEFINITION, NATURE, AND SYMPTOMS.—Typical Eczema, according to Dr. Fox, is an acute inflammatory disease, "a catarrhal inflammation," characterized especially by an *eruption*, in connection with more or less superficial *redness*, of small *closely-packed vesicles*, which run together, burst, and are replaced by a slightly excoriated surface that pours out a *serous fluid*, which dries into *crusts of a bright colour*, and of moderate thickness. *The discharge has the property of stiffening linen.* The vesicles *appear in successive crops*, may prolong the disease for an indefinite time, and are attended with *itching* and local *heat*. The skin is irritable; occasionally excoriations or crackings of the part occur, and sometimes the parts around the patch inflame, probably from the irritating nature of the discharge.

The patches form on various parts of the body,—the head, behind the ears, the face, breasts, etc.,—are of variable size, and mostly symmetrical. If the disease be extensive, there may be considerable fever, a pallid appearance, headache, loss of appetite, etc. The mucous surfaces may become the seat of inflammation, either by the spread of the disease from the skin, or as a consequence of the general condition.

Eczema is the most common of all skin-diseases; it lasts a varying time, in consequence of successive local developments, and its tendency to spread. After its disappearance it leaves behind no traces of its former presence. Its retrocession may be followed by grave symptoms.

VARIETIES.—There are four varieties of Eczema—*E. simplex* is the simple form, often resulting from exposure to the sun's rays; it may also be caused by irritants of all kinds—heat, cold, soap, etc. If it occur in hot weather, the patient complains of fever, a "heated state of the blood," etc., and the eruption follows, appearing on the exposed parts of the body—the face, neck, arms, back of the hands, etc.: this condition is what is commonly called "*heat-spots*." In *E. rubrum* the eruption is *very red* and shining, and there is much general disturbance; the *burning* is severe; brownish scabs are formed; and the parts usually affected are the *flexures* of the body—the inner side of the thigh, groin, elbow, wrists, etc.: it is apt to become chronic in old people, and, when it occurs about the legs, often leads to ulcers. *E. impetiginodes* is the variety which occurs in lymphatic and debilitated children, especially those who have a tendency to the formation of *pus;* it is similar to *E. rubrum*, but is more severe; the discharge is soon mixed with pus, which forms greenish-yellow thick scabs: it is commonly seen in the heads of infants *(porrigo capitis, scalled- or scaled-head)*. *E. chronicum* is the chronic form of any of the foregoing kinds of the disease; it often oscillates between cure and recurrence; and the skin becomes harsh, dry, red, and thickened.

CAUSES.—Eczema usually depends upon, or is associated with, debility; hence trivial exciting causes are sufficient to develop the disease—heat, cold, etc. In adults, it is a common sequel to over-work, anxiety, irregular habits, etc.; and in infants, to improper food, impoverishment of the mother's milk, or want of attention to her general health.

EPITOME OF TREATMENT.—

1. *Earliest symptoms, and in Eczema simplex.*—Acon. in alternation with Rhus Tox.; Canth.; Sulph.

2. *E. rubrum.*—Ant. Tart.; Ars. in alternation with Bell.; Ol. Crot. *(if there be sickness or painful diarrhœa)*; Merc., Kali Bich.

3. *E. impetiginodes.*—Kali Bich., Ol. Crot., Ars., Merc., Hep. S., Calc. Carb., Silic., Nux Jug., Viola Tricolor *(milk-crust* and *porrigo capitis)*.

4. *E. chronicum.*—Similar treatment to the former variety.

ACCESSORY MEASURES.—The parts should be kept clean by frequent gentle washing with tepid water—the washing should be so done as not to spread the irritating discharge over unaffected surfaces—and afterwards well dried by "*dabbing*," not rubbing; glycerine (see article "Glycerine," Part IV) may then be used to soothe and allay irritation. Water-compresses, especially in the earlier stages of the disease, are very useful. The clothes should not be allowed to produce friction on the parts. Above all, the health must be seen to, and the "Accessory Measures" described in Sections 29 and 53 strictly carried out. *Cod-liver-oil (Möller's)* is especially recommended: see Part IV.

IMPETIGO.—We have not devoted a separate section to this disease, since its *general* treatment is similar to that of Eczema; to one form of it, however, being a common disease of infants, we briefly refer.

Impetigo is a severe, sometimes contagious, purulent inflammation of the skin, and has been described as pustular *eczema* by some writers. It is characterised by an eruption of small semi-circular, flattened pustules, grouped in clusters, having a tendency to run together, forming thick and moist yellowish scabs or incrustations; and attacks the ear, nose, scalp, and face. In children, the eruption and its yellow tenacious secretion sometimes cover the face or head like a mask, the discharge matting the hair together into a sour-smelling mass, beneath which the surface is red and tender. It is this form of the disease to which the term *crusta lactea* (milk-crust—*porrigo larvalis*) is most correctly applied.

The ill-fed and the scrofulous are those who chiefly suffer from Impetigo.

TREATMENT.—*Viola Tricolor* for simple crusta lactea; *Ant. Tart.*, *Kali Bich.*, *Ant. Crud.*, or *Ars.* See also the treatment for Eczema.

142.—Acne (*Acne*)—Pimples.

DEFINITION.—"A chronic inflammation of the sebiparous glands, and of their excretory hair-follicles, characterized by an eruption of hard, conical, and isolated elevations of moderate size, and various degrees of redness."

NAMES AND VARIETIES.—The word "acne" (which in all probability was given in error for *acme*), was intended to signify the occurrence of the disease at the *acme* of man's development (puberty), when, indeed, the simple form is most common. In *A. punctata*, there is simply a collection of sebaceous *(suety)* matter in the form of a pointed eruption: this collection, when squeezed out of the skin, is emitted in a cylindrical form, having the appearance of a small grub or maggot *(comedones)*, hence it is sometimes called "maggot-pimple," or "whelk;" it is most frequent in young females. *A. indurata*—sometimes called "stone-pock"—describes the disease when it is chronic and indolent, and when the pimples are become *hard*, with a dusky-red base; they are often painful, and produce a sensation of tightness about the face, the skin being congested and thickened. *A. rosacea* is seldom seen in young persons, but sometimes occurs in women in whom the catamenial function is imperfect; the redness is bright, there being much congestion; the veins are varicose, the face is much disfigured, the surface is red and dotted over with pustules, the skin is thickened, and food and stimulants produce great burning and flushing of the face. This is the variety which is favoured with the names of "rosy-drop," "copper-nose," "carbuncled face," "bubunkle," and "grog-blossom;" though it must be remembered that the disease is not necessarily connected with the use of alcoholic liquors, since it is not infrequent in total abstainers. *A. strophulosa* (*strophulus albidus*)—"white gum-rash"—consists of small *white* pimples, chiefly about the face and neck.

Occasionally, in uncleanly persons, an *acarus* is discovered in the sebaceous follicles, called the *Demodex folliculorum*.

CAUSE.—Congestion of the sebaceous follicles. This condition may be induced by various internal and external agencies; by the stomach, which has a great reflex action on the face, as seen in flushings after food, etc.; by menstrual irregularities, constipation, physiological changes (as puberty), enervation, intemperance; cold, the use of cosmetics, want of cleanliness, etc.

Dr. Tilbury Fox thinks the lymphatic, and persons of a phthisical *tendency*, are most prone to acne.

EPITOME OF TREATMENT.—

1. *Acne punctata in young people.*—Bell. (*bright-redness of the pimples; and in persons of plethoric habit, or subject to scarlet flushings of the face*); Puls. (*females with usually cold and pale face, and menstrual irregularities*); Phos. Ac. (*weakly persons*); Baryta Carb. (*maggot-pimple*); Borax.

2. *A. indurata.*—Sulph.; Calc. Carb. (*with chronic acid dyspepsia*).

3. *A. rosacea.*—Ant. Crud., Rhus Tox., Carbo An.; Opi. (*dusky-red, bloated appearance*); Nux Vom. (*dyspepsia, constipation, etc.*); Ars. (*chronic cases, with debility; and when the eruption takes on a severe character*); Agar. Musc. The last four remedies are also well adapted to the condition when produced by alcoholic toxication.

4. *A. strophulosa.*—Ant. Crud., Calc. Carb., Hep. Sulph.

ACCESSORY MEASURES.—Hygienic measures are of the first importance in chronic acne. Indigestion, menstrual derangement, debility, or any other constitutional or local affection associated with acne, must be treated according to the instructions in the Section appropriated to it. Sudden and severe changes of temperature should be avoided, if cold be an exciting cause. *Strict cleanliness* is also necessary; besides the general morning cold-bath, the parts should be frequently washed or douched with hot water. All cosmetics and other external applications must be avoided.

A lotion of one of the following drugs, as may be indicated,

143.—Sycosis (*Sycosis*)—Mentagra—Barber's Itch—Chin-whelk.

Definition.—Inflammation of the hair-follicles of the beard and whiskers, not associated with syphilis.

It is a kind of "acne of the beard" (see previous Section). The name *sycosis* was given to the disease from its supposed resemblance, when fully developed, to the inside of a fig.

Symptoms.—It is a disease of adult life; it commences insidiously, a red itchy patch being first noticed, which, after rubbing or scratching, and the lapse of a little time, becomes much more troublesome, as the follicles enlarge and pustulate; there is considerable sensation of burning, and shaving is very painful. Successive crops of pustules appear, often grouped together, the fluid exuded becoming dry, and forming into crusts. The hairs become dull, brittle, and easily removed; and much discomfort, and sometimes disfigurement, is the result. The disease is very apt to become chronic, recurring at certain seasons.

In some cases a parasite is discovered, which may be either the *Microsporon mentagrophytes*, or the *Demodex folliculorum*. Dr. Fox and others hold that sycosis is altogether a parasitic disease, and hence call it *Tinea sycosis*.

Treatment.—The disease is often very obstinate. The remedy which has been found most curative is *Antimonium Tartaricum*, used internally and externally. *Lyco.*, and *Ant. Crud.* have been suggested. For an external application the following formula is suggested: *Ant. Tart.* ½ gr., *warm* water ℥ss; when the antimony is fully dissolved add Glycerine ℥ss, and apply to the affected parts, *after first washing and well drying*, twice or thrice daily. (See also the article "Glycerine," Part IV.)

Should the disease persist notwithstanding this treatment, leading to the supposition of the existence of a parasite, *Sulphurous Acid* should be used, externally, several times a day.

NATURE.—A low kind of inflammation of the skin, generally affecting the hands or feet, attended with itching, tingling, burning, swelling, and, sometimes, ulceration.

CHAPPED HANDS.—This affection consists of slight inflammation of the skin of the back of the hands, which becomes cracked or "chapped." It occurs in frosty weather, when it sometimes gives rise to much inconvenience and pain. It requires similar external treatment to *Chilblains*.

CAUSES.—Exposure to cold, damp, or to sudden changes of temperature; warming the hands and feet by the fire when cold or damp. Delicate persons, with a constitutional predisposition to skin-disease, are affected chiefly.

EPITOME OF TREATMENT.—

1. *Simple Chilblains.*—Arn.; Tamus Communis φ as a paint; Bell. *(bright-red shining swelling, and pulsative pains)*; Puls. *(blue-red appearance, pricking-burning pains, worse towards evening)*; Rhus Tox. *(inflamed chilblains, with excessive itching)*; Canth.; Sulph. *(great itching, increased by warmth; obstinate cases; and to remove the predisposition)*.

2. *Broken or cracked chilblains.*—Petroleum *(general unhealthy state of the skin with a tendency to fester)*; Bell.; Agaricus; Rhus Tox.

3. *Ulcerated.*—Ars. *(burning pains)*; Petroleum; Phos. *(fœtid discharge, and when occurring in unhealthy subjects)*; Krea.; Nit. Ac.

4. *Frost-bite.*—Rub the part well with snow, afterwards with cold water, in a room without a fire, to prevent too sudden reaction.

LOCAL AND GENERAL TREATMENT.—All the remedies prescribed may be used both internally—in the dilutions marked, pages 72-3,—and externally—in strong tincture or a low dilution, according to the power of the drug, either in the form of lotion or cerate. *Arnica*-lotion or cerate should never be used for broken chilblains. *Glycerine* (see Part IV, article "Glycerine"), *Glycerine of starch*, or one part of *Glycerine* mixed with two parts of *Eau-de-Cologne*, is an excellent remedy for chilblains, chapped-hands, *fissures* or *cracks*. It removes the stinging, burning sensations, and makes the parts soft and supple. Ulcerated chilblains require a poultice, or other mild application, until relieved. The soreness of chilblains and chapped-hands may be removed or mitigated by applying soft linen rags squeezed out of cold water, and then covered with oiled-silk. This compress should be applied on going to bed; it equalizes the temperature of the part, improves the nutrition of the skin, and diminishes the tendency to the re-formation of chilblains.

Extremes of temperature are to be avoided; also cold stone floors, suddenly approaching the fire after coming in from the cold, warming the feet on the fender, or the hands close to the fire, etc.

As chilblains generally occur in persons whose circulation is defective, plenty of exercise in the open air, the free use of the skipping-rope, and wholesome nutritious diet, are necessary to prevent their recurrence. Pork, salted meats, and all irritating or indigestible articles of food, should be excluded from the dietary.

145.—Ulcer *(Ulcus)*.

Definition.—A chasm on any part caused by the stripping off of its proper cuticle or epithelium, or by the destruction of a portion of its substance by disease or injury. *Ulceration* is the progressive softening and disintegration of successive layers of the *ulcerating* tissue, and is attended with a secretion of pus, or other kind of discharge.

VARIETIES.—The *healing ulcer*, is that in which the granulating process goes on uninterruptedly to reparation; the *inflamed ulcer*, is hot and painful, with a red, bleeding surface, and a thin ichorous discharge; the *indolent ulcer* is marked by an imperfect form of organization, so as to be incapable of healing; the *fistulous ulcer* consists of a narrow channel, with a false mucous membrane, produced by abscesses which have not healed from the bottom; the *spreading ulcer* is that in which the destructive process which formed it, still existing, causes it to extend; the *varicose ulcer*, which generally forms on the lower extremities, is the consequence of a varicose condition of those parts. There are also other varieties.

CAUSES.—A bruise, burn; constitutional derangement from inflammation, improper food, etc.; or, ulcers may be openings by which nature rids the system of products, which, retained, would produce serious disturbances. "The constitutions most liable to ulceration are those which are debilitated by intemperance or privations, tainted with syphilis or scrofula, or broken down by the excessive use of mercury, or in which the blood is impure from inaction of the liver, skin, and kidneys. The parts most disposed to it are those whose circulation is most languid, such as the lower extremities. On this account, tall persons are more frequently affected with ulcers than short" *(Druitt)*. Ulcers over the sub-cutaneous surface of the tibia are more difficult to heal than similar ones situated over the fleshy parts of the leg.

TREATMENT.—Strictly *constitutional* treatment is generally necessary. This may be illustrated by the fact that the appearance presented by a sore often furnishes an excellent barometric test of a patient's health; a weak or indolent ulcer rapidly assumes a healthy aspect on any improvement of the constitutional powers of the patient; on the other hand, a healthy sore immediately becomes indolent, or sloughs, when any extreme depressing cause comes into operation.

LEADING INDICATIONS.—*Belladonna.*—Painful ulcer with surrounding redness.

Silicea.—Simple ulcer; and in chronic cases.

Kali Bich.—Ulcer on the leg, deep, with hard base and overhanging edges. This remedy may also be used externally (gr. j. ad aquæ ℥viii.).

Hydrastis Canadensis.—Unhealthy ulcers; ulcerations of mucous surfaces—the mouth, throat, nose, eyes, etc. It should be administered internally and applied locally as a gargle or wash, as the case may require.

Arsenicum.—Inflamed ulcers with *burning pain*, raw surface, or presenting a livid appearance, and easily discharging blood or thin matter.

Hepar Sulph., *Calcarea*, or *Sulphur.*—For constitutional ulcers, and to improve the general health (see also Section 29).

LOCAL TREATMENT.—The ulcer may be covered with a little soft linen or lint, wetted with cold or tepid water, as is most agreeable to the patient, covered with oiled-silk, and lightly bound over with a bandage. Sometimes it will be desirable to use *Calendula-lotion* (thirty drops of the tincture to a teacupful of water), or some other soothing application; but in the majority of cases the simple water-dressing is sufficient. In addition to the above treatment, bandages are more or less necessary in all ulcers on the legs, unless absolute rest, with the elevation of the foot above the level of the hips, can be enforced. Laced-stockings or elastic-stockings are very convenient substitutes for the bandage, and are more easily applied. The frequency with which the dressings should be changed depends on the amount of the discharge. If that is considerable, they should be changed every day; otherwise three or four times a week will suffice. In the treatment of ulcers on the leg, as, indeed, on every other part, perfect *cleanliness* is most essential. The filthy habit of many persons, who allow their feet and legs to remain unwashed for weeks together, induces an imperfect vitality of the skin, which favours the formation of ulcers and renders them disagreeable and obstinate in their results. Washing the lower extremities daily is one of the most potent means of preventing and curing the disease, and restoring the lost vitality of the parts.

As much out-door exercise should be daily taken as is consistent with the patient's strength; but he should not stand much, nor sit with the legs hanging down.

146.—Boil (*Furunculus*).

DEFINITION.—A hard, conical, painful tumour, involving the under surface of the true skin and the subcutaneous areolar tissue, which suppurates imperfectly, and contains a central slough or core, arising from deposit of unhealthy lymph in the part.

SYMPTOMS.—A small, tense, inflamed and painful swelling, the size of a split-pea; this hardens, and the red blush around its base changes to purple. In a few days the swelling enlarges, owing to the formation of pus, and the pain becomes throbbing; the tumour bursts, and the core is discharged.

A *blind-boil* does not suppurate, but slowly subsides. Boils often appear in crops, or one appears as soon as the preceding one has healed. They generally occur in the thick skin of the neck, back, nates, or arms, especially in the young.

CAUSES.—A disordered condition of the blood, from unwholesome food, from some unknown atmospheric causes, or from depressing influences generally.

TREATMENT.—*Belladonna.*—Painful, hot, shining, erysipelatoid swelling, with inflammation round the base. Dr.

Hughes states that a boil in the stage of inflammatory engorgement, before matter has formed, may almost always be blighted by repeated doses of *Belladonna* (1st. dec.). Later still, states Dr. Madden, its progress may be arrested by *Silicea* (3rd dec. trit.).

Hepar Sulphuris.—Should a boil not have been blighted as above, this medicine will facilitate the suppurative process, and, to a great extent, prevent its subsequent extension.

Silicea.—Indolent boils; and where the disease is chronic.

Nit. Ac.—In some debilitated persons this remedy is required; it is very valuable in wounds which fester, and when fungoid excrescences *(proud-flesh)* form. An aqueous dilution may also be applied topically.

Sulphur, night and morning for eight or ten days, to prevent a return of boils. Dr. Hughes states that if boils recur again and again, the constitutional tendency may be checked by a course of *Sulphur*, and that he finds no need for any other medicine for boils than *Bell.* and *Sulph.*

General Treatment.—As soon as the swelling points, indicating suppuration, a poultice, covered with oiled-silk, should be applied and renewed twice or thrice daily, until suppuration is completed. In the early stage, a cold compress should be used. When boils are of an acute variety, and the skin covering them is very thick, a free incision over them with a sharp lancet will do good service. For treatment of *proud-flesh* see *Nit. Ac.* above.

In order to prevent a recurrence of boils, attention must be directed to the constitutional causes which originated them. If, as is often the case, they arise from derangement of the digestive organs, abstinence from meats, gravies, pastry, sweetmeats, etc., is imperatively necessary. Correct diet, cleanliness, and healthful exercise, will do much towards eradicating a predisposition to boils and other skin affections.

Symptoms.—As the red swelling gradually increases, the skin covering it assumes a purple or brownish-red tint, and, in a few days, softens, suppuration taking place at *several points*. The matter is thin, watery, and scantily discharged; but if pressure be made, a thick glutinous fluid may be squeezed out. It is generally attended by considerable constitutional disturbance and depression; if large, and especially if seated on the head, there is violent fever, and great and even fatal prostration may result.

Diagnosis.—Carbuncle differs from a boil in its greater size; its broad, flat shape; in usually appearing singly; in giving way and discharging from *several openings*; in the dusky redness of the inflamed integument; and in the great constitutional disturbance and irritation which accompany it.

Causes.—A disordered condition of the blood, usually met with in individuals in a debilitated state of the constitution, as the result of chronic, exhausting diseases, or severe acute maladies; great alteration in habits or diet; long-continued fatigue; etc. In the cholera year of 1854, there were in England nearly 400 deaths from carbuncle. Unlike boils, carbuncle is rare in young people, being usually met with in debilitated persons who have passed the middle period of life; and more frequently in males than in females.

Treatment.—The chief remedies are—*Ars.*, *Lach.*, *Bell.*,

LEADING INDICATIONS.—

Aconitum.—Severe inflammation and fever. *Acon.* may precede, follow, or be alternated with any other remedy.

Arsenicum.—Large, painful, malignant carbuncle, with great constitutional prostration.

Lachesis.—Low, inflammatory type of the disease, with evidences of the poison of the tumour extending to the blood; cerebral symptoms.

Apis.—Continuous extension of the erysipelatoid inflammation.

Silicea.—Promotes healthy granulations, etc.

LOCAL TREATMENT.—Early fomentations, followed by a linseed or bread-and-milk poultice, will mitigate pain by relieving tension, and hasten the cure. In many cases, the simple cold-water compress will be the best local application. In some cases, incisions are necessary; but in the absence of great tension, severe pain, or extension of the inflammation, the care of these tumours may be safely confided to nature, attention being directed to such constitutional treatment and soothing applications as each particular case may require.

If there be any signs of putrescence, a yeast poultice should be applied, and sprinkled over with a powder of the first trituration of *Carbo Vegetabilis.* This should be renewed every six hours, till the parts have a more healthy appearance.

DIET.—The diet should be nourishing, and include Tooth's Essence-of-Beef, Cod-liver-oil (Möller's: see Part IV, art. "Cod-liver-oil.") In very debilitated cases, the brandy-and-egg mixture may do good.

148.—Whitlow *(Paronychia)*—Gathered Finger.

DEFINITION.—A painful inflammatory swelling at the end of one of the fingers or thumbs, having a tendency to suppurate, and, in debilitated constitutions, to recur.

VARIETIES.—The *cutaneous* whitlow is inflammation of the surface of the skin with burning pain, and formation of a serous or bloody fluid, which raises the cuticle like a bladder. The *subcutaneous* is attended with great pain and throbbing, and suppuration under the skin at the root of the nail, which often comes off. *Tendinous whitlow* or *thecal abscess* is inflammation of the *tendinous sheath* of the finger. When whitlow is malignant, pressing on to the periosteum, it is sometimes called *felon*.

CAUSES.—Cutting the nail to the quick; a bruise, burn, or other mechanical injury; the introduction of poisonous or acrid matter into scratches on the finger; unhealthy constitution.

SYMPTOMS.—Heat, pain, throbbing, and redness at the end of the finger; as the symptoms increase, there is swelling and tension, and the pain may extend up the arm; the surface becomes livid, and shortly assumes a palish cloudy appearance. If suppuration occur, a dirty-looking fluid is discharged; by and bye the nail falls off; and, if the finger be kept at rest, and the health be not very defective, a new nail is produced, and the finger is well. Under unfavourable conditions, however, the part may ulcerate, the finger inflame, the bone become diseased, and phlegmonous inflammation attack the arm.

TREATMENT.—As soon as the first indications of whitlow are noticed, the finger should be held in a raised position in water as hot as can be borne, for two or three hours or longer, and a dose of *Silicea* taken every three hours. Thus its formation may often be prevented. Should these means not succeed, a warm bread-and-milk poultice should be applied, and *Silicea* continued every four hours, in alternation with *Acon.* if there be much feverishness, or *Bell.* if the inflammation have a marked erysipelatous character. Hot fomentations will relieve pain. *Merc.* or *Hep. Sulph.* are also good remedies.

ACCESSORY MEANS.—Hot fomentations to relieve pain. If inflammatory action persist, the finger becoming hard, and there be no signs of early suppuration, a free incision should be made by a surgeon, to relieve tension and prevent sloughing, and, possibly, disease of the bone.

ONYCHIA is inflammation of the nail-matrix *(the substance from which the nails grow)*; it may be induced by similar causes to those of whitlow, and especially by an ingrowing nail, or cutting the nail down to the quick. *In-growing of a nail (Unquis involutus)* may be remedied by softening it in warm water, then paring it thin on the upper surface, and cutting it down as far as may be at the middle part of the extremity, *avoiding cutting the parts which tend to grow in.* By these means the growth is diverted from the sides; since *the nail will grow most which is cut most.*

149.—Corn *(Clavus)*.

NATURE.—A small thickened mass of epidermis accumulated on the dermis in situations where the papillæ, subjected to undue pressure, or friction, or both, have acquired unnatural proportions. It not only lies upon the dermis, but penetrates into it. A corn may be *hard*, dry, and scaly; or, if situated in places where the secretions of the skin are confined, *soft* and spongy. When inflammation or suppuration takes place underneath a corn, it becomes excessively painful.

CAUSES.—Pressure from tight-fitting boots or shoes;* hereditary predisposition sometimes seems to favour their development.

* There is no member of the extremities which has been more disgracefully used than the foot. This wonderful organ, by the perfection of which God has "made man upright," and whose structure so pre-eminently distinguishes him from his recently so-called "great-grandfather," the gorilla, has been made to suffer from compression more generally than any other organ. The

TREATMENT.—*Arnica.*—As soon as corns appear, the surrounding skin should be softened by a warm foot-bath, the hard head of the corn gently extracted with the finger nail or some other convenient instrument, and the thickened skin pared off, wounding the adjacent parts as little as possible. The corn should then be dressed with a lotion prepared by adding thirty drops of the strong *Tincture of Arnica* to a wine-glassful of water, and next morning a piece of *Arnica-plaster*, or an *Arnicated corn-plaster*, applied. The dressing may be repeated several times, till the inconvenience is removed. The *Arnicated amadou-* or *felt-plaster*, having a hole punched in it to receive the corn so as to relieve it from pressure, is a very useful contrivance.

If internal treatment be necessary, *Calcarea* and *Sulphur* will be the most suitable medicines. *Calcarea* may first be administered every night and morning for a week or ten days; and then, after waiting a few days, *Sulphur* in the same manner. After pausing several days, if necessary, the course may be repeated. See *Verat. Vir.* in next Section.

SOFT CORNS.—These are best treated by cutting off the thickened skin with sharp scissors, taking care to wound the surrounding parts as little as possible, then applying a drop or two of diluted tincture of *Arnica*, and always wearing a layer of cotton-wool between the toes, changing the wool daily.

ACCESSORY MEANS.—Corns can only be *permanently* cured by wearing *easily-fitting boots*, often washing the feet with tepid water, and frequent change of stockings.

thought at once suggests the cruel practice of the Chinese, who prevent the growth of the female foot, by placing it in infancy in an unyielding shoe. This fact has had the universal testimony of travellers in China, and if anything more were wanted to prove it, a collection of the feet of Chinese women is at present to be seen in the Museum of the College of Surgeons of England, in which, by careful dissections, the sad havoc to natural growth produced by this heartless custom is scientifically demonstrated (*Lankester*).

150.—Bunion* *(Bunion)*.

Definition.—An enlargement of the bursa at the inside of the ball of the great toe; or the formation of a new serous sac on the inner and posterior part of the metatarsal bone.

Cause.—The *pressure of narrow-pointed boots or shoes*, throwing the great-toe over or under the contiguous toes; in this way a sharp angle is made on the inner side of the joint of the great toe on which the bunion is formed.

Symptoms.—Pain, redness, and swelling of the part, which soon subside on removal of the cause. Should, however, undue pressure be continued, the symptoms increase until pressure becomes unendurable. After this, on discontinuing the offending boot or shoe, the pain subsides; nevertheless, a permanent bunion has been formed, and inflammatory symptoms are at any time liable to recur from irritation.

Treatment.—The direction of the toe must be changed by wearing properly-shaped boots, made with the inner side of the sole straight from the toe to the heel. If irritation be accidentally excited in the part, the warm foot-bath should be used, and afterwards a lotion (twenty drops of *Arnica* ϕ to two tablespoonfuls of water), continuously applied, for two or three days. If *Arnica* be unsuitable to the patient, *Ruta Grav.* may be substituted. Should the inflammation be followed by the formation of matter, a linseed-meal poultice will be more suitable; at the same time a dose of *Hepar Sulphur* may be given every four hours.

Veratrum Viride, painted on bunions, generally gives rapid and perfect relief. There is no agent comparable to *Verat. Vir.* for bunions or inflamed corns *(Dr. J. G. Wilkinson)*.

Ganglion,* Housemaid's-Knee, and Miner's Elbow, require similar treatment.

* In the "New Nomenclature" *Bunion* and *Ganglion* are amongst "Diseases of the Appendages of the Muscular System."

PREVENTION.—If the *Arnica* or *Verat. Virid.* lotion be used immediately the first inflammatory symptoms arise, and all undue pressure at once and permanently discontinued, the formation of a bunion may be altogether prevented.

151.—Nævus *(Nævus)* Port-wine-Stain—Mother's Mark; and Nævus Pilaris *(Nævus Pilaris)*—Mole.

DEFINITIONS.—*Nævus* is a hypertrophied state of the blood-vessels of the skin, forming slight flattened elevations of a bright-red (if arterial) or purplish (if venous) colour, occupying a greater or less extent of surface, from the size of a pin's-head to many inches.

Nævus pilaris is a nævus covered by hair of variable length, and, like ordinary nævus, is liable to occur on all parts of the body.

Nævi are usually congenital; they are popularly called "Mother's marks" from a supposition that they are produced on the child before birth through some fear or fancy of the mother; and are variously named, according to their apparent resemblances,—"cherry-," "strawberry-," or "mulberry-stain," etc.; and if the nævus be hairy, it is called a "mouse-mark," etc.

In many cases no inconvenience results except the deformity; but occasionally, more especially when the growth is at all prominent, there is a great disposition to ulceration of an unhealthy character. When bleeding occurs, it is usually in a trickling stream, and without any degree of force *(Erichsen)*. Nævi sometimes die away without interference.

TREATMENT.—When treatment is desirable, the internal and external use of *Thuja*, as recommended for warts (see Section 153), is sometimes successful. Dr. Hempel says that nævi may be removed by the external use of *Kreasotum*, one drop of the tincture to eighty of water, applied two or three times a day, the effects being excoriation, ulceration, and cicatrization, with scarcely any disfigurement remaining.

152.—Sebaceous Tumour *(Tumor Sebaceus)*—Wen.

Definition.—A tumour composed of suety or fatty (*Steatoma*) matter, and enclosed in a sac beneath the skin, occurring from obstruction of the secretory ducts.

These tumors arise on various parts of the surface of the body, are smooth, non-elastic, pendulous, and moveable; they slowly increase without pain, often to a very great size; attain their greatest development in warm climates, in the Hindu and Negro races, where they have been met with of an enormous weight and size.

Treatment.—If wens are likely to be amenable to medicinal measures, *Baryta Carb.*, *Silic.*, *Calc.*, and *Sulph.*, are probably the most appropriate remedies. See Section 142. But *excision* is generally needful.

153.—Warts *(Verrucæ)*.

Nature.—A vegetation consisting of elongated and enlarged papillæ of the cutis vera, clothed with a strata of hypertrophied and hardened cuticle, chiefly affecting the hands and face of young people, appearing and disappearing without any particular known cause.

Treatment.—*Thuja.*—The warts should be painted twice daily with the matrix tincture; at the same time a dilution (6. dec.) of the same medicine may be taken internally, morning and night. The latter use of *Thuja* is especially necessary when the warts appear in crops. This course may be followed for a week or two, and if improvement ensue, a-it generally does, the treatment should be continued longer. If *Thuja* do not succeed, *Rhus Tox*. may be substituted, and used internally and externally in the same way.

Sulphur, once a day for a week or two, is an excellent remedy for numerous and obstinate warts upon the hands. It is also useful after other medicines, to eradicate the tendency to recurrence.

154.—Parasitic Diseases of the Skin
(*Morbi cutis parasitici*).

Of the *Ectozoa* there are, as we have before remarked (see Section 112), several members, the most common of which (except *Scabies*, see the next Section) are the following:

TINEA TONSURANS (*Tinea capitis*), the common scurfy *ring-worm of the scalp*, is generally seen only in children, is contagious, but not necessarily associated with impaired health, though it is common in lymphatic persons. It consists of circular patches varying from half-an-inch to several inches in diameter, the hairs of which look dry, withered, and as if nibbled off at a short distance from the scalp. The parasite is the *Achorion Lebertii*.

TINEA DECALVANS (*Alopecia areata* or *Porrigo decalvans*), consists of smooth, circular *patches of perfect baldness*, quite pale, of variable size—one to two inches or more in diameter, and of which there may be several; the disease is sometimes seen in young persons, chiefly in girls, but is most common in adults. The parasite is the *Microsporon Audouini*.

TINEA FAVOSA (*Favus* or *Porrigo favosa*) is the *crusted* or *honey-comb ringworm*; it is uncommon in England, but is seen in some parts of Scotland—Edinburgh, etc. It commences when the patient is about seven years of age, and is characterized by the presence of small straw- or sulphur-coloured cupped crusts, which coalesce and give rise to a honey-comb appearance; or remain separate. It is contagious. Its parasites are the *Achorion Schœnleinii* and the *Puccinia Favi*.

TINEA VERSICOLOR *(Pityriasis versicolor* or *Chloasma)* commences as small erythematous points, with itching, which is increased by warmth; slightly-elevated, dry, rough patches of a fawn-colour arise, somewhat scaly at the edge, and from which branny scales can be rubbed off; they occur on the chest, abdomen, and arms, vary in size from that of a three-penny piece to that of the palm of the hand, and are much irritated by flannel. It is sometimes called *variegated dandriff*, or *liver-spots*. The parasite is the *Microsporon furfur*.

PHTHIRIASIS is the condition of the body favourable to the existence of *pediculi* (lice).

IRRITATION OF THE SKIN caused by various parasites, etc., is also classed as a parasitic disease. Thus there is the irritation caused by the *Pediculus capitis* (head-louse), often associated with Eczema and other skin-diseases; the *P. palpebrarum* (louse of the eye-lids); *P. vestimenti* (body-louse); *Phthirius inguinalis* (crab-louse); *Pulex penetrans* (Chigoe), an insect of the West Indies which chiefly attacks the toes or intervals between them, is black, causes extreme itching, and even ulcers; *Pulex irritans* (the common flea); *Cimex* (the bug); *Leptothrix autumnalis* (harvest-bug), which is common in grass in autumn, and, getting on to the body of man, though exceedingly small, produces extreme irritation of the skin; etc.

Under this head also comes irritation from the stings of *Wasps*, *Bees*, etc., the treatment of which may be found in Section 156.

TREATMENT.—There is no great difficulty in the treatment of the Ectozoic or Epizoic class of parasitic diseases, except when associated with true skin-disease. Even then, correct treatment is successful.

Strict cleanliness, the free use of soap and water, i *qua non*, and in some cases may be alone sufficient; seconded by the local application of *Sulphurous Acia* as a lotion or by spray, a cure will certainly be effecte

Sepia is the best internal remedy for ringworm scalp, and if given early will often prevent the increas disease. *Calc. Carb.* and *Sulph.* should also be reme as useful remedies, combined with hygienic meası procuring and retaining a healthy condition of the ski

The irritation from flea-bites, etc., is amenable necessary, to the treatment directed in Section 156.

PREVENTIVE MEANS.—*Perfect habitual cleanlines* proper attention to health.

155.—Scabies (*Scabies*)—Itch.

NATURE.—A contagious disease, characterized by a lar eruption, presenting numerous watery conical p with violent itching, aggravated by scratching and at depending essentially on the burrowing in the ski minute parasite—*Sarcoptes Scabei*, or itch-insect.

The violence of the symptoms depends on the nur the parasites present, the length of time the patient h affected, and the degree of sensibility of the skin. disease may occur on any part of the body, but the a cules generally prefer delicate parts, such as the thin the flexures of the joints, especially the wrists and b the fingers.

TREATMENT.—In our own practice we have found t application of *Sulphur-ointment* rapidly effective in dest the insect and its ova. After thoroughly rubbing the body with soft-soap and water, then washing in bath, or with hot water, and wiping thoroughly dı superficial and effete cuticle is removed, and the burro parasites freely exposed; the ointment should then be well rubbed in and allowed to remain on the body all night. On the following morning a tepid bath, using yellow soap, to wash off the ointment left on overnight, completes the cure. If the application of the ointment and the ablutions be not thorough, the processes should be repeated once or twice. *Sulphur-ointment* must not be continued too long, or it will produce an irritable state of the skin, which is often mistaken for a persistence of the disease. The administration of *Sulphur*, during the use of the ointment and for two or three days subsequently, is recommended. All contaminated linen should be put into boiling water; other garments should be well ironed with a hot iron, or exposed to hot air at a temperature not less than 150° or 180° Fahr., or well fumigated with the vapour of sulphur, to destroy any insects or ova concealed in the texture of the linen. The cure is often retarded, and the disease conveyed to others, by neglecting to carry out these suggestions as to clothing.

156.—Irritation caused by Stinging-Insects and Plants (*Irritatio orta ex insectus et plantis aculeatis*).

The most common insect-stings and bites are those of the Wasp, Bee, Hornet, Gnat, and Musquito. These, though painful, are not serious, except when a tender part or sensitive or important organ of the body is attacked; or when the multiplicity of the wounds is so great as to produce general or venomous symptoms. Thus a man has been stung to death in a short time by a swarm of bees; when the eye is stung the consequences are liable to be serious; and a sting in the pharynx, as from swallowing a piece of honey-comb with a bee concealed therein, may be very dangerous. Musquito-stings are peculiarly irritating, and, when numerous, poison the blood, producing nervous depression and great febrile irritation. Some insects, as scorpions, or the tarantula in Italy and Russia, give rise to more serious and even fatal disturbance or stupor by their bite.

In India and other hot countries, various other insects, besides the musquito, attack man, and are a source of irritation and annoyance; "for every animal, insect, or reptile, in the warmer lands, is distinguished by its ferocity and pugnaciousness." The *ant*, especially the *black-ant*, and the *cockroach*, are common and troublesome—the latter especially on board-ship. It attacks the toes of persons asleep, and this so insidiously that the sleeper is not awoke until the quick is reached and the blood flows. The eye-brows, as well as the toe-nails, are also liable to suffer, unless protected. "There is a small *black-beetle* in India, found in the short grass and herbage, which is dangerous to persons lying on the ground, as it attempts, if possible, to enter the ear. Children are frequently attacked by it, and the agony caused by it is extreme. The only effectual remedy, and it is effectual, is to pour a little oil into the ear, which so disgusts the beetle that it backs out, leaving the person uninjured. Such, however, would not be the case if force should be attempted in the extraction."*

Nettle- and other stings of plants do not cause much disturbance besides the local irritation.

TREATMENT.—*Ledum Palustre* is the most useful remedy for common stings and bites. It should be applied locally, in a diluted form—twenty drops of the tincture to half a wine-glass of water. Should *Ledum* not be at hand, *Rhus Tox.* may be used. If neither of these remedies be available, *Allium Cepa* (the common onion) should be promptly applied: a piece cut off and at once placed on the wound. Indeed, Dr. Hill uses no other remedy than this for stings, etc.; if the pieces of onion are changed every few minutes, the pain,

* From the *Leisure Hour*, June, 1869.

he says, diminishes immediately. If there be much swelling, *Apis* should be given. *Acon.* will speedily cause febrile symptoms to disappear. For Venomous and Poisoned Wounds, see next Section.

ACCESSORY MEASURES.—If a wasp or other stinging-insect be the cause of the trouble, examination must be made for the sting, as this is often left in the wound; if present, it must be carefully extracted by the fingers or by a pair of fine-pointed forceps. If this cannot be done, and the sting has entered the skin perpendicularly, the pressure of a small key may be tried: the centre of the hole should be placed over the wound, enclosing it, and gentle pressure should be used; when, probably, the sting will be squeezed out. The wound should then be sucked well, to extract the venom as directed in the next Section. After this, the lotion should be applied; or, if pain be very great, hot fomentations.

Musquitoes may be prevented from troubling in the night, by taking the precaution of rubbing a little soap on the hands before going to rest. This is said to be a certain remedy. Honey is also good, but from its sticky nature is more disagreeable than the soap. *The cockroaches* of hot climates may be got rid of by burning the bodies of two or three, and letting them lie about; the smell drives the rest away.

157.—Poisoned Wounds—(*Vulnera Veneno Infecta*).

DEFINITION.—"Wounds inoculated with foreign matter, producing general symptoms, or propagating inflammation to other parts of the body."

VARIETIES.—Poisoned wounds may be made by venomous animals—snakes, scorpions, etc.; by animals having infectious disease; by dead animal matter; by morbid secretions; by

vegetable substances; poisoned arrows; [illegible]
tion, etc.; or by mineral substances.

SERPENTS are venomous in a variable degree, ac
their nature, size, or vigour; some cause immediate
convulsions; others produce inflammation of th
others again induce death by slow poisoning, or b
healthy or diffuse inflammation which they excite.

The *Viper* is the only poisonous snake in the Brit
and its venom does not often produce death in [illegible]
when the victim is a child or very weak person.

The *Rattlesnake* and *Cobra di Capello* are two of
deadly reptiles, their bites being frequently fatal.

TREATMENT.—The *immediate* treatment of poisone
is highly important; especially if they result from
of venomous reptiles.

(1.) The first object to be attempted is arrest of
culation of the poison. A handkerchief, rope, or
else to serve the purpose, should be tied tightly r
limb, between the wound and the heart. While this
done, if possible a second person should extract the
suggested in the next paragraph.

(2.) The wound should be sucked with all the
patient can command; or, if unable to do it hi
attendant should do it for him. No danger attach
person thus sucking the wound so long as the poison
come in contact with any abraded or otherwise i
surface of the mouth or other part of the body.

(3.) *Alcohol*, in any of its forms—brandy, whis
etc., according to Dr. Hill's testimony, should b
largely by the patient. He says: "Let him drink
a gill or more at a time, once in fifteen to twenty
(or small doses oftener), until some symptoms of int
are experienced. . . . . It is remarkable ho
alcohol a patient suffering from the poison of the Ra

will bear. A little girl of ten years, who had been bitten by a Rattlesnake, took over three quarts of good strong whisky, in less than a day, when but slight symptoms of intoxication were produced. She recovered from the intoxication in a few hours, and suffered no more from the poison of the serpent. Instances of cures with whisky are numerous, and I have never heard of a failure, when it was used as here directed. I presume it will do the same for the poison of other serpents." Alcohol so prescribed is not given with a view of "combating the depression," but as a material antidote to the material poison.

Ammonia seems also to be potent, and may serve as an alternative.

Arsenicum, in a low potency (1st or 2nd dec.) may be given if symptoms of rapid prostration occur. Thus administered it tends to correct the poisoned condition of the blood and acts strictly homœopathically.

Excision of the wounded part may be required in some cases; but unless this be done at once it is of no use. It may be performed as directed for Hydrophobia, page 252.

OTHER POISONED WOUNDS should be treated, according to their nature, by appropriate antidotes. In the case of wounds from the introduction of mineral substances under the skin, those to which workmen—mechanics, founders, and others,—are liable, the offending material has generally lodged in the body and produced disturbance in the part before its presence is suspected. Inflammation is the result, and suppuration should be encouraged, as this is generally the only method of eliminating the poison. The treatment recommended for abscess is appropriate to this condition, with, in some cases, the aid of *Arsenicum*.

CHAPTER XII.

MISCELLANEOUS DISEASES.

158.—Morbus Coxæ (*Morbus Coxæ*)—Scrofulous Disease of the Hip-Joint.

This is a slow and serious disease, of a very insidious character. So soon as the earliest symptoms are noticed, it should at once be placed under the care of a homœopathic practitioner, who may be able to arrest the progress of the malady. The child is supposed to be suffering from "growing-pains" for months before the disease assumes an active form.

SYMPTOMS.—The first distinctive symptoms are—slight pain, *chiefly referred to the knee*, lameness, and weariness. There may be even slight swelling in the knee-joint, so that remedies are often applied here, but the disease is in the hip. This may be proved by pressing either in front or back of the hip-joint, or by jerking the thigh-bone against the joint, as by a sharp tap on the heel, when pain will be felt in the hip. As the disease progresses, the *nates* (buttocks) waste and become flabby; the limb is shortened, either by caries of the neck of the *femur* (thigh-bone), or by destruction of the ligaments of the joint and consequent dislocation of the joint upwards on the *dorsum ilii*. There is increased fulness about the limb, the pains increase in severity, especially at night, and there are often startings of the limb during sleep;

abscesses form, and afterwards burst on the nates or groin, or burrow deeply and discharge their contents into the rectum.

The *duration* of the disease varies from two or three months to several years. But it is much modified, both as to its duration and results, by recent skilful contrivances.

Adults rarely recover; but, in children, when the strength is not too much exhausted, and the lungs are unaffected, the disease frequently terminates in *ankylosis* (stiff joint).

White swelling of the joints is a disease of similar character.

TREATMENT.—The medicines most likely to prove beneficial are—*Acon.*, *Bell.*, *Coloc.*, *Hep.* S., and *Ars.*, in the early stage of the disease, and for special symptoms, *Calc.*, *Silic.*, and *Phos.* When abscesses have formed and suppuration is established, see the next Section.

ACCESSORY TREATMENT.—REST, with the limb in a straight position, and absence of articular pressure, the latter being, probably, the more important element: surgical appliances are necessary to ensure it.

The *diet* should be nourishing, and include *Cod-liver-oil* (see Part IV, art. "Cod-liver-oil"), etc. The Sections on "Scrofula" and "Abscess" should also be referred to. Pure air, and especially residence by the sea-side, will expedite the cure.

159.—Abscess (*Abscessus*).

DEFINITION.—A collection of matter in any tissue or organ, deposited within a sac or cyst of organized lymph, and supplied with absorbent and secreting vessels.

a. *Acute Abscess* commences with throbbing pain, bright redness, and swelling of the part; these symptoms are soon followed by suppuration, which is marked by an alteration in the colour of the skin, and a change in the character of the pain, the former becoming livid, and the latter less acute, being rather felt as a sensation of weight and tension. "After this, the parts between the abscess and the surface become successively softened and disintegrated. The tumour becomes more and more prominent; the centre exhibits a dusky-red or bluish tint, the cutis ulcerates, the cuticle bursts, and the pus escapes. But where pus is formed under dense fasciæ, or deep in the breast or pelvis, and cannot quickly make its way to the surface, the pain is not relieved, but much aggravated by the increase of distension; and the constitutional fever and chills are much more intense." (*Druitt*).

b. Chronic Abscess first appears as an indistinct tumour, the fluctuation being more or less marked according to the distance from the surface. The inflammatory symptoms of the acute variety are altogether absent, unless far advanced, or accidentally irritated.

Abscess and Diseased Bone.—Chronic abscess is sometimes a consequence of *inflammation of bone*. This may be suspected whenever permanent inflammatory enlargement and tenderness exist, especially if it can be traced to an injury, and there is a fixed pain at one particular spot, which is increased at night. The long persistence of such symptoms, in spite of remedies, although there may be occasional remissions, almost certainly indicates the existence of a circumscribed abscess in the bone, which requires surgical measures for its relief and cure.

Mammary Abscess—gathered breast—is fully treated of in "The Lady's Manual," pp. 158–161.

Causes.—Abscesses, with few exceptions, are indicative of constitutional debility, and are a frequent sequel of low exhausting fevers. They may, however, result from blows, or from foreign bodies introduced into the skin or flesh, such as splinters, thorns, etc.

Diseased bone, as stated above, may cause abscess, or inflammatory enlargement of a part.

EPITOME OF TREATMENT.—

1. *Before suppuration.*—Acon., Bell., or Mercurius. At the same time lint saturated with water, to which a few drops has been added, of the same remedy as taken internally, should be used locally.

2. *During suppuration.*—Hep. Sulph., Silic., Ars.

3. *After suppuration.*—Calc. C., China, Sulph., etc.

TREATMENT.—*Hepar Sulphur.*—This remedy is often serviceable in promoting the suppurative process in acute abscesses, and is generally sufficient when the discharge is healthy. At the same time, local measures should be adopted, as pointed out further on.

Silicea.—Tardy, long-continued, or unhealthy discharge; especially useful in chronic abscesses and abscess of bone; it facilitates suppuration, or moderates it when excessive.

Mercurius.—Painful abscess, attended with chilliness and thirst, and a copious discharge of thick matter; with aggravation of the pains at night.

Belladonna.—Severe pains, headache, and much constitutional disturbance.

Arsenicum.—Severe *burning* pain, with symptoms of general vital depression; abscess having a gangrenous appearance, or pus tinged with blood.

China.—Abscesses following prolonged disease, with prostration from excessive discharge of matter or blood, diarrhœa, etc.

Calcarea.—After suppuration is completed, this remedy will assist the healing of the abscess, and the elimination of the disease from the constitution.

Aconitum.—Well marked, feverish symptoms, during any stage of the disease.

LOCAL TREATMENT.—Abscesses arising from local injury should be freed from all sources of irritation, such as thorns, splinters, etc. Poultices (See Part IV) are valuable from several points of view; they relax tension, and, consequently, relieve pain; if applied directly an abscess begins to develop, a poultice will either disperse or restrict the formation of pus. If suppuration have proceeded too far to be arrested, poultices facilitate the progress of the pus to the surface and its ultimate expulsion. *Fomentations* with hot water, frequently repeated, are valuable adjuncts to poultices. Generally, when pain has subsided, a *water-dressing* should be substituted. *Spongio-piline* in some cases may be employed instead of a poultice.

Opening of Abscesses.—Acute abscesses seldom require the lancet, especially when they point and become pyramidal, without enlarging in circumference. The formation of an abscess under strong fasciæ or ligamentous textures, which ulcerate with difficulty, require an artificial opening to prevent burrowing of the pus, and the setting up of great constitutional disturbance. When an abscess occurs on an exposed part, and it is desirable to avoid the scar which generally ensues when it bursts spontaneously; or when it is so situated that it may discharge into some internal cavity, —the chest or windpipe, an opening should be made by a surgeon. When an artificial opening is required, the operator should be certain that the knife enters the cavity of the abscess to let out the pus freely, and that the opening be made at the most dependent part. For those who dread pain even in the trifling operation here referred to, the use of local anæsthetic agents renders all such operations almost painless.

After an abscess has been opened, and its contents discharged, the *Calendula lotion* (one teaspoonful of the tincture to three tablespoonfuls of water), will greatly expedite recovery. It may be applied by saturating a piece of lint, or two or three thicknesses of linen, with the lotion, and covering it with oiled-silk. The dressing should be repeated two or three times a day.

Diet and Hygiene.—As abscesses are generally indications of debility, a liberal allowance of nourishing food is of great importance; it should include good animal broths, broiled mutton chops, chocolate or cocoa, and, in some cases, good beer or wine. Change of air, with residence at the sea-side or in the country, forms an important part of the hygienic treatment.

160.—Obesity (*Obesitas*)—Corpulence.

Definition.—The excessive accumulation of fat under the skin and around the organs of the body, so as to exercise a prejudicial influence on the health, usefulness, or comfort of the patient.

Obesity may be said to exist only when fat is present in such large quantities as to disqualify the person for performing the various duties of life, by occasioning difficulty of breathing, panting on slight exertion, deranging the circulation, and causing various functional disturbances, with diminution of mental and bodily activity. The term *Corpulence* is restricted to cases in which the quantity of fat is not so great as to amount to positive inconvenience or discomfort.

Causes.—*Hereditary* tendency or constitutional predisposition can alone account for the excessive accumulation of fat in many instances. Some persons are naturally fat, others lean; some become corpulent on a moderate diet, others spare in the lap of luxury. These are matters of common observation, but of which we can offer no explanation. *Age* exercises considerable influence; children are usually fatter than adults; after the middle period of life, fat often accumulates in considerable quantities. In old age, however, the adipose tissue, and the fat it contains, generally diminish. *Race*, again, is an important element in the question. The Americans are remarkable for their leanness, and the Arab is almost destitute of fat; Europeans, and especially the English and the Dutch, on the other hand, are proverbially fat; hence John Bull is always pictured excessively corpulent.

Besides individual or accidental causes of corpulency, the following circumstances directly influence the production of fat. *Food*, rich in hydro-carbonaceous matter; for although a certain amount of such food is necessary to maintain the temperature of the body, if it be taken in excess, such excess is often stored up as fat. *Ease of mind*, and *repose of body*, are conditions highly favourable to the formation and accumulation of fat; whereas, anxiety, fretfulness, night-watching, etc., have a directly opposite effect. Thus science proves the truth of the adage—"A contented mind is a continual feast." A *comfortable temperature* is an important element in the production of corpulence; for although a high temperature does not directly engender fat, it is a condition in which less is consumed.

TREATMENT.—The treatment of corpulency brought prominently before the public by Mr. Banting,* in the simple story of his remarkable experience, proves that a proper diet alone is sufficient to remove the condition, with its long train of evils, without the addition of nauseous drugs, or of those active exercises which it is in vain to instruct unwieldy patients to take.

The chief feature in the *Banting dietary* is the exclusion of two elements—starch and sugar—from the ordinary food of a well-to-do gentleman:—*Bread* (except toasted, or the crust off a common loaf), *potatoes*, *sweet roots*, *butter*, *sugar*, *cream*, *beer*, *port*, and *champagne*.

These articles of food and drink contain starch or saccharine matter, and are the chief fat-producing elements in our dietary, and to relinquish them is to escape the thraldom of

* See Review of the Fourth Edition of Mr. Banting's pamphlet in *The Homœopathic World*, August, 1869.

corpulence. In one year, on this diet, Mr. Banting reduced his weight 46lbs., and his bulk about 12 inches; at the same time his numerous corporeal infirmities were greatly mitigated or altogether removed. This is some six years ago, and in the fourth and enlarged edition of his pamphlet, he brings the history of his experience down to May in the present year (1869).

"I can conscientiously assert," he writes, "that I never lived so well as under the new plan of dietary, which I should formerly have thought a dangerous, extravagant, trespass upon health; I am very much better, bodily and mentally, pleased to believe that I hold the reins of health and comfort in my own hands."

The "plan of dietary" suggested in a previous portion of this work, page 25–8, with the sugar, butter, superfluous bread, potatoes, etc., eliminated from it, would meet the requirements of most corpulent persons admirably. A *Banting* diet cannot, however, be recommended indiscriminately. Persons who may deem it necessary to make great changes in their diet should consult a physician.

161.—Old Age *(Senectus)*; and Senile Decay.

Human life may be divided into three great epochs,—the period of development, that of middle life, and that of physical decay.*

Under the first division is included the whole time from birth up to about the twenty-fifth year, during which the vegetative organs and those of the lower animal life are consolidating. The central nervous system is more slow in reaching its highest development, and the brain especially is many years later in acquiring its maximum of organic consistency and functional power.

* See Dr. F. E. Anstie on Neuralgia, in *Reynolds' System of Medicine*, Vol. II.

The middle period of life—between about the twenty-fifth and the forty-fifth year—is the time that the individual is subjected to the greatest pressure from external causes. The industrial classes are absorbed in the struggle for maintaining themselves and their families; the rich and idle are immersed in dissipation, or haunted by the mental disgust it entails. At the same time, the women are going through the exhausting process of child-bearing, and are either surrounded with the cares and duties of a poor household, or equally pressed with anxiety to attain position for themselves and their children in fashionable life; or they are idle and heart-weary; or forced to an unnatural celibacy. Frequently they are both idle and anxious.

The period of decline may be said to commence when the first indications of distinct physical decay manifest themselves, and when a new set of vital conditions come into force.

There is not, however, any sharp lines of demarcation between the epochs thus sketched, the one insensibly grows into its successor.

Youth and Age.—Although the activity of the growth of the organs in childhood and youth offers a striking contrast with their decline in old age, there is, notwithstanding, a resemblance in the diseases of the two extremes of life, like the tints of the rising and setting sun. Infantile convulsions, and senile convulsions; infantile diarrhœa, and senile diarrhœa; infantile eczema, and senile eczema; uric acid deposits in childhood, and uric acid deposits in age, may be adduced as illustrations of the resemblance of the diseases affecting the two extremes of life. In the early period, the constitution has not acquired its vigour; in the closing, it is losing it.

To the mere worldling, old age is repulsive. But if life have been spent wisely,—errors corrected, the heart disciplined, and the intellectual and moral powers are in the ascendant—old age—moderated, chastened, elevated—presents a spectacle happily described as a "Crown of glory." A human being who, after fulfilling all the duties of life, is still living in a "green old age;" "whose eye is not dim, nor his natural force abated," though ripened for the future, may well command our admiration and veneration.

A brief reference to the changes and dissolution of man's material frame will form an appropriate conclusion to this portion of our work.

The decay of nature is gradual, and does not affect all the structures of the body equally at the same period; it also begins in some at a comparatively early, and in others not until a considerably advanced period of life. As illustrations of the changes attendant upon old age, and which exercise an important influence in accelerating that final one which is the common lot of humanity, we may note the following:—

I. The Bones.—As old age advances, the bones undergo very characteristic changes. In infancy and childhood the *animal* element predominates; hence we can explain why the bones are then so pliant and fracture so rare. In adult life, the relative proportions of bone may be approximately stated as consisting of one-third of animal and two-thirds of earthy matter. In advanced age, the earthy matter is in excess. This alteration in their composition renders the bones extremely brittle and liable to fracture. Fractures are then more oblique and comminuted, and also more inapt to unite firmly again, than those occurring at an earlier age.

II. The Muscles.—The minute cells, aggregated in the form of fibres, of which the muscles of the body are composed, are rapidly destroyed by the contraction of the muscles; but in vigorous life, by the digestion and assimilation of food, they are as rapidly reproduced. In old age, on the contrary, the disintegrated cell-tissue is but tardily repaired, and the muscles become soft, flabby, and pale, from an insuffic-

supply of blood; they are consequently unequal to severe or protracted exertion; muscular debility is easily excited, and the strength but slowly and imperfectly restored. The tendinous portions of the muscles are also liable to earthy deposits in them; thus their resisting forces become weakened, and they are in constant danger of rupture if subjected to any undue tax.

III. The Heart.—Another most important and frequent change is one that takes place in the textures of the central organ of circulation. The heart becomes weakened from senile softening, and degeneration of its muscular structures into a fatty tissue; its pulsations are thus rendered less and less efficient to propel the blood to the extremities. The blood failing to complete its circuit, the hands and feet become cold, the decline of temperature gradually extending to the central organs of the body. This reduced power of the heart, with the disposition to *atheromatous* deposits in the coats of the blood-vessels, referred to in the next paragraph, with subsequent ossification of the valves of the heart, is one of the most common and fatal changes attendant upon old age.. These changes as they proceed are generally hidden and painless.

IV. The Blood-Vessels.—In the silent progress of years the arterial system is liable to undergo changes which are incompatible with the performance of its important functions. The arteries gradually become converted into ossific or bony patches of greater or less extent, often so considerable as to lead to changes of a vital character by destroying the elasticity of the arterial tubes, and deranging the circulation of the blood in the parts to which they conduct. Thus the nutrition of the body is impaired, and the functions of the nervous and muscular systems are only imperfectly performed. Further, the ossific patches in the coats of the arteries may lead to their rupture, or become causes of aneurism, gangrene, apoplexy, etc., forms of disease to which the aged are especially liable. Apoplexy, from this cause, is one of the most frequent causes of death in old age. The cerebral arteries become diseased, and as the blood is driven into them they give way. Even thin persons, whose blood-vessels and heart are diseased, die from apoplexy.

An observation on the two last paragraphs may not be here inappropriate. Petrifaction of the coats of the arteries, and fatty degeneration of the heart, usually occur at the same time of life, and the one condition, happily, counteracts the consequences of the other. The life of an aged person would be in far greater jeopardy, if, while the walls of his arteries were decaying and rotting, his heart retained all its original force. As it is, however, the loss of resisting power of the coats of the arteries finds its counterpart in the fatty metamorphosis of the muscular tissues of the heart.

V. The Vertebræ.—The changes in the spinal column are very considerable; they alter the external form of the body, and more or less derange the functions of the chief organs. The three graceful curves in the spine, so exquisitely arranged, both to give space and protection to the internal viscera, and for the transmission of the weight of the head and trunk in the line of gravity, become more or less obliterated in advanced life, and the centre of gravity disturbed. The vertebral column also loses its *elasticity;* the disc of cartilage placed between each vertebra, to break the force of shocks and prevent jarring of the brain, partly disappears or ossifies; the mobility of the spine is likewise diminished, and thus a false step or a trifling accident may be converted into an occurrence of grave importance. The alteration in the curves of the spine produced by the above causes, gives that change to the *external form* which is so characteristic of old age. Corresponding with these changes in the spine, as affecting the external form, are others which affect the bones generally. Owing to the diminishe the muscles, and the absorption of fat from beneath points of bone in various parts become more ang prominent, and the limbs lose that graceful and roti which was the pride of earlier years.

VI. The Eyes, etc.—The special senses, as sight and hearing, frequently, and sometimes at paratively early period, give evidence of approachin The *arcus senilus*, a circumferential opacity of the resulting from fatty degeneration, and generally a with a like degeneration of the heart, is, as its name an affection incident to the aged. *Cataract*—opacit crystalline lens, or its capsule, or both—seems to consequence of impaired nutrition, and is met with ir persons only, except as the result of inflammation o But the most frequent cause of impaired or perverte is alteration in the form of the lenticular bodies of tl the cornea and the lens—which, losing their natu vexity, interfere with the correct impression on the the proper fixed point of the object of vision.

Defective hearing is another not infrequent attenda old age, and may result from various causes, the n quent being impairment of the acoustic nerve.

Gradual Decay.—The varied forms of man's de gradual and progressive. Death may take place s from *heart-disease*, apoplexy, rupture of an aneurism but it is only the termination, not the disease, that is For years before the fatal issue the organ undergoes ration of structure. Death under such circumstances compared to the fall of some towering cliffs, whic everything beneath. The catastrophe is terrible, an unexpectedly; but it was the slow disintegration many preceding winter's frosts that hurled it down th

Sudden death is a misnomer in language, except as it takes place from accident or poison.

PREMATURE OLD AGE.—In alluding to the decay of nature, we may add that we refer rather to the vital decay of individuals than to the mere lapse of years; vital conditions cannot always "be measured by number of years." It is well known that some persons at fifty, or even earlier, are in this respect older and more shattered in constitution than others who have attained to the age of seventy or upwards.

Our present manner of life, business haste or anxieties, tend to induce premature decay (see Section 75). Probably as the result of improved sanitary measures, a more correct and general recognition of the laws of health, and of the rapid spread of homœopathy, the attainment of a vigorous old age without the premature feebleness and decay hitherto so generally observed, will be more common.

TREATMENT OF THE AGED.—There are many ailments peculiar to the approach of old age which require special medical treatment, or the application of particular measures, which we cannot enlarge upon here, but in which the timely use of appropriate remedies, and the prompt employment of judicious means, are often rewarded in seeing the flickering flame rekindled, and valuable life considerably prolonged. On two or three points only can we make general observations.

1. FOOD.—Food should be of a much less solid form than during the vigour of adult life. Just as nature provides fluid food during infancy before the teeth appears, so the loss of teeth, a common attendant upon old age, necessitates a return to a form of food which does not require mastication. Inattention to this point is, we believe, one of the most fruitful causes of the impaired digestion, weakness, and sufferings of the aged. Frequently, artificial teeth cannot

be tolerated, and the only path of safety lies in the adoption of an almost exclusive fluid diet. We have had many cases under care in which our advice on this point has been carried out with the most beneficial results.

2. Rest.—This is essential to the health and safety of the fragile frame of the aged. The sports and exercises of youth, or the exertions of maturer age, would fracture the bones, rupture the tendinous portions of the muscles, or occasion a blood-vessel to give way. To the aged, long-continued exercise and too little or broken rest, are highly unfavourable, the reparative processes being only slowly performed. Happily the activities and athletic exercises of youth become distasteful, and the burdens of mid-day life are transferred to the succeeding generation, and he now seeks and enjoys a condition of quiet and repose necessary to his present well-being.

3. Warmth.—In the winter season, when sudden changes of temperature are frequent, provision should be made for preventing the ingress of the cold night-air, and for maintaining a suitable temperature in the bed-room through the whole night. The temperature of the sleeping-apartment should be kept at 60° to 62°, and measured by a thermometer, as the sensations of persons are not a sufficient guide. A thermometer should therefore be kept in every house, and suspended out of a current of air, and beyond the direct influence of the fire, so that the facts which it registers may be accurately observed. It no doubt often happens that the lonely encounter with death takes place in the stillness of the night-season, from a sudden access of cold air, which the extreme feebleness of old age could not resist or endure. Very cold weather seriously affects the aged, and it is a fact that excites frequent observation, that soon after the setting-in of intense cold, the obituaries of persons in advanced life become unusually numerous in the public papers. "An aged

man, with a sluggish heart, goes to bed in a temperature, say of 50° to 55°; in his sleep, were it quite uninfluenced from without, his heart and his breathing would naturally decline. Gradually, as the night advances, the low wave of heat steals over the sleeper, and the air he was breathing at 55° falls and falls to 40°, or it may be 35° or 30°. What may naturally follow less than a deeper sleep? Is it not natural that the sleep so profound shall stop the labouring heart? Certainly. The great narcotic never travels without fastening on some victims in this wise, removing them, imperceptibly to themselves, into absolute rest, inertia, until life recommences out of death" *(Richardson)*.

A regulated temperature in his apartment, heat-producing kinds of food, warm clothing, and other kindred measures, such as an enlightened physician would suggest, should therefore be adopted in the treatment of the aged.

4. Medicines.—On this point we can offer no definite suggestions. The selection of remedies must be determined strictly according to the symptoms the patient may present, modified by any idiosyncrasy of constitution that may have been noticed.

Thus the physical frame decays and man passes away, death terminating the journey of life, and the traveller welcoming the long repose as he had often welcomed sleep after the fatigues of the day. We have reason to believe that dying is as painless as falling asleep. Persons who have been resuscitated after drowning, and after all sensation had been lost, have asserted that they experienced no pain. What is often spoken of as the *agony of death* is probably purely automatic, and therefore unfelt. The idea embodied by the poet in the following lines is literally true—

> "Passing through nature to eternity,
> The sense of death is most in apprehension."

There is, thus, beneficence in man's decline just as in his growth and maturity, and there is also design. The Christian philosopher not only submits with resignation to the decay of his material form, but rejoices in the assured hope that so perfect and highly endowed a structure, teeming with evidences of beneficent design, has not been constructed merely to rise, flourish, and then to disappear without a future grand result, commensurate with so costly an expenditure of wisdom and goodness. INFINITE WISDOM, which designed and called forth man into being, would, it seems, forbid that such a creation should be comparatively vain, leaving only a dark blank as the memorial of its existence. We infer, therefore, that the dissolution of our earthly form is really but a mysterious transitional process, through which the good pass from an introductory and transient state of existence to one that is immortal.

CHAPTER XIII.

INJURIES.

162.—Asphyxia (*Asphyxia*)—Apnœa (from Drowning).

DEFINITION.—The term *asphyxia* is generally used to express the effects of interrupted respiration, as in the case of drowning, hanging, or from breathing noxious vapours. In this section we restrict it to drowning.

TREATMENT.—Not a moment's time should be lost. The two points to be aimed at are—immediately to *restore breathing*, and, next, *warmth and circulation*. The wet clothes should be removed, the skin dried, the mouth cleansed, the tongue drawn forwards, and the patient placed on the back, with the head and shoulders a little raised. Both arms should be held above the elbows, and drawn gently and steadily upwards above the head, and kept stretched whilst counting, one, two. *See figure* 1. This is inspiration, or filling the chest with air.

Then the patient's arms should be pressed gently and firmly against the sides of the chest while counting, one, two. *See figure* 2. This empties the chest of air.

Repeat these movements, about fifteen times in a minute, until natural breathing takes place.

Next, not before, try to promote circulation. Rub the limbs upwards with firm pressure, to favour the return of blood to the heart.

FIG. 1.—INSPIRATION.

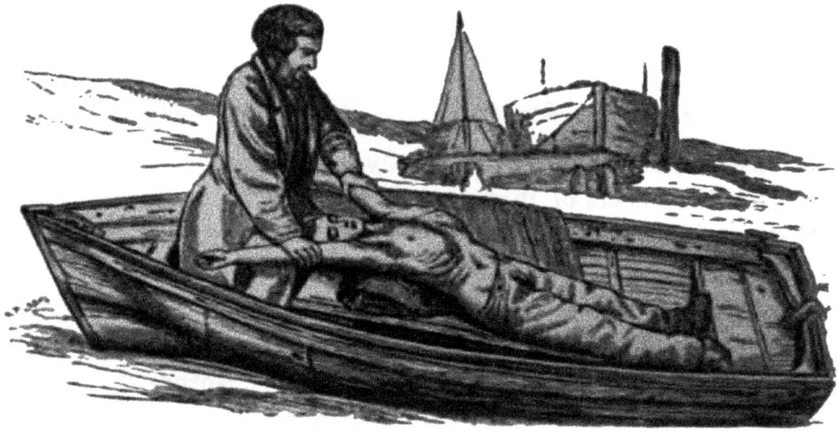

FIG. 2.—EXPIRATION.

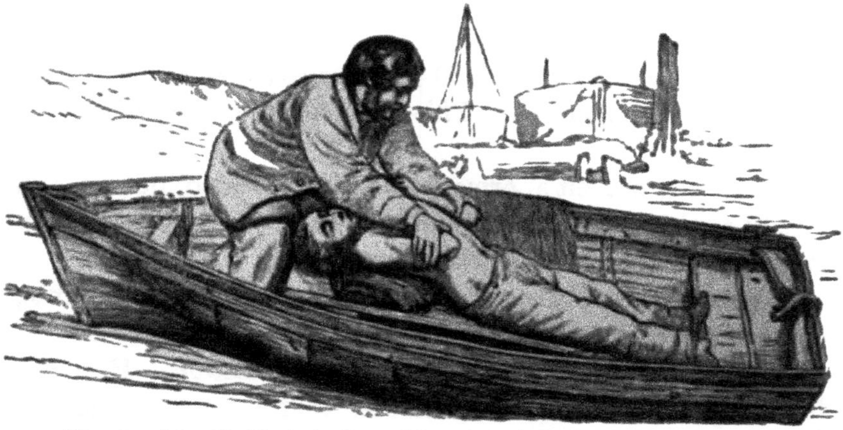

Figs. 1 and 2.—To illustrate the position of the body during the employment of Dr. Sylvester's Method of restoring Breathing.

Promote *warmth* by the application of hot flannels, hot bottles wrapped round with flannel, heated bricks, or by any means at hand, to the pit of the stomach, the arm-pits, between the thighs, and to the soles of the feet. The efforts should be persevered in for some time—if necessary, several hours.

163.—Concussion of the Brain *(Concussio cerebri)*.

DEFINITION.—An interruption to the functions of the brain, from a blow or other mechanical injury of the head; it may vary in degree from a slight stun to extinction of life.

SYMPTOMS.—Insensibility; pale face; small, sometimes imperceptible pulse; stertorous breathing; cold extremities; etc. By shaking the patient, or calling his name loudly in his ears (which, however, should never be done), he may give a surly answer, and soon become insensible again. After a time, longer or shorter according to the severity of the injury, reaction comes on, and consciousness returns, often with vomiting. At first the reaction may be imperfect; it is often several days or even weeks before the power of the mind is restored.

TREATMENT.—*Arnica.*—Place two pilules upon the tongue, or moisten it with a few drops of the tincture by means of a feather or quill, and repeat the dose every hour for several times.

Aconitum should be administered alternately with *Arnica*, if fever attend the return of consciousness. But if there be danger of cerebral disturbance—head-ache, flushed face, or other head-symptoms—*Aconitum* and *Belladonna* should be alternated. A dose every one, two, or three hours, repeated several times.

GENERAL TREATMENT.—The patient should be placed in a warm bed, with his head at first moderately low, and warmth applied to his extremities and *axillæ* (arm-pits). On no account should he be induced to eat or drink; he must be kept very quiet, and no attempt should be made to arouse him. When reaction comes on, the head and shoulders should be raised a little, and cold evaporating lotions applied to it, keeping the patient at the same time in a cool, quiet

the formation of vesicles, which, in slight cases, soon dry up and heal; or, if the skin has been much injured, may be succeeded by obstinate ulcers. (3) The *Gangrenous*, from destruction of the tissues. This variety, although probably exempt from pain, is by far the most serious.

The constitutional disturbances, and the periods of danger consequent on deep burns, have been divided into three stages: 1. Depression and congestion, during the first four or five days; 2. Reaction and inflammation, in which the patient may sink with an affection of the head, chest, or abdomen; and, 3. Suppuration and exhaustion, which may continue from the second week to the close, and is often associated with hectic, inflammation of the lungs, or pleurisy. The danger of burns often depends more upon their *superficial extent* than upon the depth of the injury. *Burns on the trunk*, *head*, or *neck*, are far more perilous than those of an equal extent on the extremities. Children appear to suffer much more severely from burns than adults.

Treatment.—A most important object to be attained is to cover the injured part with some suitable material that shall *exclude atmospheric air*, which should not be removed till the cure is complete. The following are the local applications most frequently used:

1. *Cotton Wool.*—This should be immediately used to thoroughly cover the burnt part, after it has been first well saturated with oil. It must be so closely applied, and in such layers, as to preclude the access of air. If the wound be large, and the cotton becomes hard and uncomfortable, it should be softened by pouring a little oil upon it, without removing it.

The application of a lotion of *Urtica Urens* (twenty drops of the tincture to an ounce of water) in the simplest cases, or of *Cantharides* (ten drops of the tincture to an ounce of water) when blisters are forming, under the cotton-wool, is of great service. *Kreas.* is also sometimes useful.

2. *Soap.*—Moisten white or brown soap in water, and rub it on a piece of linen so that the soap forms a coating on the linen as thick as a shilling, and larger than the wound it is intended to cover, so that it may the more perfectly exclude the air.

3. *Flour or Starch.*—One of these may be used as a substitute in the event of either of the above not being at hand. Wheaten flour or finely-powdered starch, should be uniformly and thickly applied by an ordinary dredger, so as to form a thick crust by admixture with the fluids discharged from the broken surface, thus excluding the air; and repeated when any portions fall off. Flour is, however, inferior to wool or soap, and its after management is more difficult. The points of greatest importance are, *immediate application* of the local remedy, complete *exclusion of atmospheric air*, and *infrequent* changing of the dressings, not, indeed, until they have become loosened or fetid from the discharges. A *complete* change of dressing often causes pain, depression, and the detachment of portions of the new skin, and so retards the cure.

165.—Contusion (*Contusum.*)—Bruise.

DEFINITION.—An injury inflicted on the surface of the body by mechanical violence, without laceration of the skin. It may be either slight, involving only the rupture of minute *subcutaneous* blood-vessels, and perhaps the tearing of some muscular fibres; or a large blood-vessel may be torn; or even disorganization of the tissues beneath the skin may be caused, as from the dull force of a spent cannon-ball. The remarkable properties of elasticity and toughness possessed by the skin often permit serious damage to its underlying structures while it remains entire.

CAUSES.—A blow from a hard, blunt body; forcible pressure between two forces, as a wheel passing over a limb and crushing it; or indirectly, as when the hip-joint is contused by a person falling on his feet from a height.

TREATMENT.—In the less severe form of bruises, which alone come under domestic treatment, the object should be to excite, as speedily as possible, the absorption of extravasated blood. To this end the bruised part should be raised, and a *warm Arnica* lotion *immediately* applied (one part of the strong tincture of *Arnica* to ten of water) by saturating lint with the lotion, and covering it with oiled-silk, to exclude the air. The value of this application is undoubted, and happily is now becoming generally recognised. In contusions involving glandular structures, as the female breast, *Conium* is recommended in preference to *Arnica*; or when the covering of bone, as of the shin, is involved, *Ruta*. When pain or tenderness has subsided, a bandage should be applied. Leeches or punctures, where there is any chance of procuring absorption by other means, should never be resorted to, as air would thus be admitted to the part, and suppuration be set up.

ECCHYMOSIS.—This is discoloration of the skin following a bruise, and is produced by extravasated blood under the skin. It is first of a reddish colour, but speedily becomes black. During recovery, the parts change, first to a violet colour—the line which defined the bruise becoming indistinct—afterwards to a green, then yellow; and thus, sooner or later, according to the health of the individual, or the quantity of blood poured out, the discoloration disappears.

Black-eye is a common instance of *ecchymosis*. *Arnica-Lotion* has great power in *preventing* this condition if used *immediately* after an accident. If extravasation have already occurred, *Hamamelis* lotion (one part to six of water) will be more appropriate.

166.—Wound *(Vulnus)*.

DEFINITION.—A solution of continuity, or separation by external violence, of parts naturally united.

Wounds are termed *incised*, when made by clean-cutting instruments; *punctured*, when the depth exceeds the breadth, as stabs; *lacerated*, when the parts are torn and the lips of the wounds irregular; *contused*, when effected by bruising (see previous section). We may also add, *gun-shot* wound,.

which is termed *penetrating*, when the shot is lodged in the part; *perforated*, when it passes through it; and, according to law, *burns*. For *poisoned* wounds, see Section 157.

TREATMENT.—The following are the chief points:—1st. *To arrest the bleeding*. In most cases, the elevation of the part, keeping the bleeding surface uppermost, the application of cold, moderate pressure, and the coaptation of the edges of the wound, will suffice. A *Calendula* lotion will serve to arrest hæmorrhage, and check suppuration. In severe wounds involving *arteries*, the parts should be laid open by a surgeon, and the wounded vessels ligatured. See also further on.

2nd.—*The removal of foreign bodies.*—Dirt, hairs, glass, clots of blood, etc., should be speedily removed by the fingers, forceps, or sponge and water.

3rd.—*To bring the injured parts into nice apposition.*—Any muscular fibres likely to prevent complete union should be

instrument. If the blood flow in a *steady stream*, and is *dark-coloured*, it is from a vein, and can generally be checked by applying cold water, and exposing the cut surface to the cold air. But if large veins be wounded, they should be compressed with the fingers, or by a bandage. A few thicknesses of linen, with steady compression, are more efficient than heaping on a large quantity. If the blood be *bright-red*, and flows in *jets*, it is *arterial*, and the same means must be adopted as just pointed out, unless the bleeding be excessive, in which case a handkerchief should be tied round the limb, near the wound, and between it and the heart; a stick inserted under the handkerchief, and a firm compress over the course of the blood-vessel; the stick should then be twisted until it stops the circulation, and, consequently, the bleeding. But such means are only temporary, as wounded arteries of size require to be *ligatured* by a surgeon before bleeding can be permanently arrested. If no surgeon can be obtained, a clever manipulator should grasp the wounded artery with a pair of forceps, and draw it slightly and gently forward, so that it may be securely tied by means of a strong ligature of silk.

7th.—Should a wound or bruise be followed by constitutional disturbance, fever, chills, and throbbing in the parts, internal medicines should be administered.

Arnica (as prepared for internal use) and *Aconitum* will generally meet the requirements of such cases, and should be administered every three hours, in alternation, for several times; or if the injured part be very painful and swollen, with congestive head-ache, etc., *Bell.* may be alternated with *Acon.* *Hepar Sulph.*, when suppuration is established, or *Silicea*, if there be unhealthy suppuration.

Cuts.—The treatment of this variety of wounds, if only of moderate size, is generally simple. The edges of the cut should be brought together and maintained so by narrow strips of *strapping-plaster*; then, if necessary, a bandage applied over the plaster. If, however, inflammation and pain occur, the application of *lint*, saturated with *Calendula lotion*, covered with oiled-silk, and a bandage over all, is necessary. In two or three days the plaster should be removed without disturbing the union, and replaced by new.

167.—Foreign Bodies (*Corpora adventitia*).

TREATMENT.—Any foreign body in the flesh,—glass, a thorn, splinter, broken needle, etc.,—should be removed as quickly as possible, by the fingers or by forceps, or sponge and water if there be a lacerated wound. Foreign bodies in the eye and ear require distinctive notice.

FOREIGN BODIES IN THE EYE.—If sand, flies, or hairs, are between the lids and the globe, they should be removed immediately by bathing the eye; but if the substance cannot be removed in this manner, the eye should be gently wiped with a soft, moistened handkerchief, or with a feather, or a bent bristle may be used, the two ends being held by the finger and thumb. In one of these ways, with a little perseverance, the offending substance may generally be removed.

If small pieces of *flint or iron* become fixed in the front they may continue a long time, till difficulty of hearing or uneasiness in the ear, leads to an examination of the tube. Any such body should be removed as speedily and as gently as possible, either by syringing the ear with warm water, or by means of small dressing forceps, or other suitable instruments. If it cannot be removed by gentle means, the case should be submitted to a surgeon, so that a careful examination may be made by means of the ear speculum, and the aid of sunlight or a lamp. This examination is necessary for two reasons; for although a foreign body, if present, may generally be seen without such means, still the absence of such body cannot be affirmed without a complete exploration of the tube. Further, instances often occur in which surgeons are requested to remove a foreign body when none exists, and a proper examination with the speculum would often prevent any injudicious meddling of the ear with instruments. A late eminent hospital surgeon is said to have dragged out the little bones of the ear *(stapes)* whilst attempting to find a small nail, which was not in the ear at all! A careful exploration of the canal, as above suggested, would have prevented such a serious practical mistake. Any soreness or inflammatory symptom that may ensue from the foreign body, or the attempts at extraction, should be met by washing the ear with a weak *Arnica lotion* (six drops of *Arnica* φ to two tablespoonfuls of water), and afterwards enveloping the ear with a rag wrung out of the lotion, and covered with oiled-silk.

168.—Fracture *(Fractura)* Broken Bone.

A few words on the immediate management of cases of broken bones seem necessary in this manual, as a surgeon is not always just at hand, and it is necessary to be prepared to act till surgical attendance can be had.

SYMPTOMS.—A fractured bone may generally be detected by having felt or heard it *snap*; there is also some *deformity*, such as bending or shortening, and if the upper end of the bone is held firmly by the hand, the lower part may be moved independently; also, if the broken ends are rubbed against each other, a grating noise *(crepitus)* may be heard. There will, further, be pain, loss of power of the broken part, and other symptoms. Fracture is said to be *simple* when there is no wound of the skin communicating with it; *compound* when there is such a wound.

CAUSES.—*Mechanical violence* is the most frequent; but muscular contraction is sometimes a cause. Old age, some diseases, and prolonged disuse of a limb, render bones liable to fracture from trifling causes.

IMMEDIATE TREATMENT.—The patient must be moved *gently*, and special care taken to prevent the broken bone from being forced through the flesh and skin. He should be placed on a stretcher or litter, and taken to his home or to a hospital. A litter may be made of a couple of poles and a horsecloth or sack; even a door or hurdle may serve the purpose. Placing him on this, and carrying him by two men, is much better than removal in a cart or carriage. It is important *not to be in a hurry*, as an injury is often greatly aggravated by carelessness or too hurried measures. When a surgeon is within a moderate distance, after making the patient as comfortable as possible, it is better to wait a little, so that he may superintend the moving.

If there be a wound in the skin and much bleeding, treat as directed in Section 166.

When the patient has been placed on a firm bed or mattress, and the injured part examined, the surgeon will bring the broken ends of the bone into close apposition, and in their natural form, and having done so, maintain them in perfect contact, and at rest, till firm union has taken place. To maintain the proper shape and length of the limb, *bandages*, *splints*, and other apparatus are required. Little can be done, however, beyond the mere management of such accidents, until the surgeon arrive, as these cases can only be properly treated by a skilful practitioner.

A BROKEN LEG should be fastened to the whole one by handkerchieves at the ankle, and above and below the knee, before the patient is removed.

FRACTURE OF THE ARM requires the immediate support of a sling, which may be made by a handkerchief and fastened round the neck.

BROKEN RIBS require a *flannel* bandage, about two hands broad, round the chest, with shoulder straps to keep it up. A rather tight-fitting bandage lessens the movement of the chest in breathing, and is a great comfort.

169.—Sprain (*Stremma*)—Strain.

DEFINITION.—An overstretching of the ligaments and tendons, generally with a rupture of some of their fibres.

TREATMENT.—In bad cases the chief points are, keeping the parts at perfect rest, by means of a roller nicely applied, and controlling the motions of the joint by a splint. In simple cases the application of cloths saturated with *Rhus-lotion*, and covered with oiled-silk, hastens the cure, especially if the same remedy be also taken internally.

Aconitum, in alternation with *Rhus*, may be administered, if the joint become swollen and painful; and, especially, when constitutional disturbance attends the injury.

When the pain and swelling subside, the joint may be partially liberated, and gentle motion allowed; but great care must be observed for several weeks in using the limb, as the injury may easily be re-induced, and then the cure becomes difficult and tedious, especially if the patient be rheumatic.

170.—Exhaustion of the Muscles (*Exinanitio virium*)—Fatigue—Over-exertion.

DEFINITION.—A condition of the *muscular system* induced by an undue drain on its strength.

TREATMENT.—If the feet be swollen or blistered, or the ankles ache after walking, a warm foot-bath may be used, to which a teaspoonful of the strong tincture of *Arnica* has been added; the relief afforded is immediate and permanent. If the hands or wrists ache from excessive or unaccustomed exertion, they may be bathed in about a pint of water, to which twenty or thirty drops of *Arnica* have been added. If necessary, in one or two hours, the application may be repeated. In muscular fatigue from long-continued, or short but severe, exertion, affecting the hips, thighs, etc., a hip-bath, to which a drachm of the strong tincture of *Arnica* has been added, is an excellent remedy. The patient should remain in the bath about five minutes. Whatever kind of bath is used, and to whatever part applied, it should be *warm* if used in the evening or immediately after exertion, but *cold* or *tepid* in the morning.

ACCESSORY MEASURES.—When suffering from fatigue, a light repast only should be taken; a full heavy meal might occasion serious embarrassment to the digestive organs, as they suffer from the general weariness.

171.—Poisons* (*Venena*).

When it is known that a deleterious substance has been swallowed, as *arsenic* and other *mineral poisons*, *opium*, *poisonous fish*, *alcohol*, etc., vomiting should be immediately excited, by tickling the back of the throat with a feather or the

* For the general symptoms and treatment of poisoning from various substances, see the chapter on "Poisons," preceding the "Clinical Directory."

finger; or if this fail, by the administration of an *emetic.* The following is a convenient emetic: for a child—a tea-spoonful of mustard in a tea-cupful of warm water; for an adult—a dessert-spoonful in a breakfast-cupful of water. This may be repeated as often as necessary, and followed by copious draughts of warm water, so as to empty the stomach as completely as possible. But if *Arsenic* be the poison, no *warm* fluids should be used, as they tend to increase the activity of the drug.

The treatment of cases of poisoning must, however, be considerably modified according to the nature of the poison, and a medical man should be summoned immediately, while the temporary measures just suggested may be resorted to until he arrive.

PART III.

Materia Medica.

Introductory.—With some exceptions, th
scribed in this manual are restricted to the f
pages 72–3; most of which, in consequence o
use, have been called *polycrests*, or many-heali

Professional homœopaths, however, as a rul
of several hundred remedies, each in differen
physician has, therefore, great advantage ov
practitioner.

A difficulty will sometimes be experienc
between two or more remedies, the symptom
many points of resemblance; still, in nearly
characteristic differences exist, which the expe
detect. Remedies which, to the superficial
identical, will be found on closer inspection
tinctive features, determining, in the *ensembl*
toms, the constitution and temperament of
which it is adapted. Indeed, it rarely happen
two remedies can be selected indifferently.

A prompt and successful use of the Mate
only be attained as the result of perseveri
and though difficulties surround, and failure
first attempts, these should not deter the stud
acquaintance with the remedies, and enlarge
using them, will enable him to be the instrum
multitudes to health who need and claim his a

1.—Aconitum Napellus—*Monk's-hood—Wolf's-bane.*

This plant is a native of Asia and of central Europe, and grows spontaneously in the damp and covered parts of almost every mountainous country, especially in Switzerland, Germany, and Sweden. On account of its beautiful flowers, notwithstanding its poisonous properties, *Monk's-hood* is cultivated, and grows readily in the gardens of our own land.

The English names are—*Wolf's-bane*, because it is said that the huntsmen of the Alps dipped their arrows into its juice when hunting wolves; and *Monk's-hood*, because its beautiful blue flowers resemble the hood formerly worn by monks. It is supposed to be fatal to every species of animal, and it has been employed in the attempt to destroy whole armies.

The parts used are—the leaves, flowers, and roots, from which tinctures are made; but it is from the root that the most active preparation is obtained.

Therapeutic Value.—As a therapeutic agent, in the hands of a Homœopathic practitioner, *Aconitum* is one of the first importance. "This medicine," says Hempel, "constitutes the back-bone, as it were, of our Materia Medica;" there being scarcely an acute disease in which it is not more or less required. Had Hahnemann's labours extended no further than the discovery and demonstration of the wide and inclusive curative power of this great remedy, they would have entitled him to the gratitude of countless myriads of his fellow-creatures in every succeeding generation. He most appropriately ranks it as first and foremost in his Materia Medica, not because its name begins with the first letter of the alphabet, but because of its transcendent power and extensive sphere of action: he terms it a "precious plant," whose "efficacy almost amounts to a miracle." Let the sceptic in homœopathic therapeutics test its power in *acute fevers* in accordance with the directions of this manual, and he will witness a curative action such as is unknown in allopathic practice, and which amply justifies the statement that "*Aconite* is the *Homœopathic Lancet*." As confirmatory of this assertion, we may cite the extensive use of *Aconite* recently adopted by allopathic practitioners of eminence as a substitute for the antiphlogistic measures formerly in vogue. Some striking instances of this adoption of Hahnemann's teachings and practice by men of the old school are given in the early numbers of *The Homœopathic World* for 1869.

PROMINENT USES.—*Aconite* is useful in all affections (*not toxæmic*) accompanied by, or depending upon, *arterial excitement* or *arterial congestion*. It is also very serviceable in some reactionary conditions—exhaustion after excitement, etc. It surpasses all other known remedies in its power of controlling the circulation, and triumphantly supersedes the lancet and the leech. "To enumerate the diseases for which it is suitable would be to mention the acute inflammation of every possible order and tissue of the body; and if it be not for all of these the sole remedy, it is almost always useful either previous to, or in alternation with, another remedy which has perhaps a more specific relationship to the part affected" (*Dudgeon*).

Although it may be often greatly abused, it is probably more frequently indicated than any other single remedy, especially at the commencement, and often during the course, of nearly all affections marked by—*pain*; a *rapid* strong *pulse*; *dry heat* of the *skin*; *chills*, followed by burning heats; restlessness; *scanty* and high-coloured *urine*; constipation; aggravation of the symptoms towards night: notably, *acute rheumatism*, *catarrhal fevers*, *erysipelas*, *hæmorrhage* from internal or external surfaces, especially of an arterial character, with full, bounding pulse. It acts by moderating and equalising the circulation, and so removing local congestion, especially when affecting mucous surfaces.

Aconite has, however, no power to control fevers depending upon a poisoned state of the blood, such as exists in typhoid, typhus, intermittent, etc. Even in the eruptive fevers—scarlatina, etc.—it cannot reduce the pulse until the eruption comes out. Again, as Dr. Hughes remarks, *Aconite* does little for a fever which is symptomatic of an acute local inflammation. In pneumonia, the pulse defies *Aconite*, but goes down quickly when *Bryonia* or *Phosphorus* touches the local mischief. "Indeed," writes the same author, "it may be laid down that unless a fever (not being rheumatic) has greatly abated within twenty-four hours of commencing *Aconite*, it is one for which the remedy is unsuited. But in some inflammations, especially rheumatic, *Aconite* alone may effect a cure, as being a specific irritant of the part affected. It is only when, in a part to which *Aconite* is not specifically irritant, true inflammatory changes have actually begun, that it ceases to exert remedial influence, and a medicine Homœopathic to the local mischief must take its place." In associating *Aconite* with the conditions mentioned in the following paragraphs, the general recognition of these observations is necessary to prevent disappointment.

Nervous System.—*Neuralgia* depending upon arterial excitement of the affected part, such as occurs in persons debilitated by anxiety, over-excitement, etc., in whom the disturbed equilibrium tends to local congestions; *congestive apoplexy* with bounding pulse; *paralysis* with painful pricking sensations, and numbness and congested skin as from needles; *paralysis* of spinal meningitis, from cold; *lock-jaw* from the shock of a sudden injury; *infantile convulsions; spasmodic croup; congestive headache* when the sensorium is not involved; nervous tremors in sensitive and weakly persons: etc.

Eyes, Ears, Face, etc.—*Acute ophthalmia*, with shooting

pains, and frontal headache; acute *otitis*, *otalgia*, and deafness, from cold; *Catarrh* in the invasive stage (see "Respiratory System" below). Nasitis; over-sensitiveness of smell; *epistaxis* from cerebral congestion. *Facial neuralgia* (see "Nervous System").

Circulatory System.—Rheumatic inflammatory affections of the *heart*; *palpitation* from nervous, hysteric, or febrile excitement, or occurring in plethoric or sensitive persons; *congestion of the heart*, with anguish, heat, depression of spirits; the *paroxysms* of *angina pectoris*; fainting-fits, with collapse of pulse; and the deadly collapse of cholera.

Respiratory System.—*Catarrh* and *influenza* in their *invasive* stages—dryness and burning of the air-passages, sneezing, burning and fulness over the eyes, headache, chills, weariness and soreness; fluent coryza; chronic catarrh, with thick mucus; acute sore throat; laryngitis; bronchitis; spasmodic, dry, hard, cough; pleurisy; pneumonia; congestion of the lungs; hæmoptysis; the paroxysms of spasmodic asthma.

Digestive System.—*Teeth.*—Rheumatic and congestive tooth- and face-ache, especially from exposure to cold and draughts of air; throbbing, pressing pains in the teeth or side of the face, relieved by cold water; fever attending dentition. *Tongue, throat, etc.*—Dryness and swelling of the tongue; white or yellow-furred tongue; soreness and dry heat in the throat; swollen, elongated uvula; rising of sweetish or acid water in the mouth. *Stomach, etc.*—Continual formation and eructation of flatulence; bilious nausea; vomiting of blood, with feverish symptoms (in alternation ith *Arnica* if from a strain or blow); inflammation of the mach, bowels, or peritoneum, from cold; constipation, with er; profusely bleeding piles; diarrhœa during *teething*, little patient's cheeks being flushed, with other febrile ymptoms; acute *congestion of the liver*, and threatened *jaundice* (alternated with, or followed by, *Mercurius*).

URINARY SYSTEM.—Retention or suppression of the urine, from inflammation or congestion; high-coloured urine, with or without brickdust sediment; burning and tenesmus of the neck of the bladder; inflammation of the kidneys; urethritis; acute orchitis; etc.

SKIN.—*Dry*, *hot*, harsh, and yellow colour; ephemeral itching and burning of the skin. *Aconitum* is well indicated in the dry, burning heat of *children*, or red rash on the skin, with thirst, etc. The occurrence of perspiration after the use of this remedy marks its favourable action, and is the token for its discontinuance.

2.—Aloe Socotrina—*Aloes.*

This remedy, so much used by the allopathic doctors, is also very valuable to the homœopathic practitioner, who uses it with much greater precision of aim and specific curative result.

GENERAL USES.—*Piles*, with profuse discharge of blood, great straining, burning and cutting pains, and rush of blood to the head; *dysentery*, with similar symptoms. *Diarrhœa*, like that produced by drastic doses of the drug, having a bilious character and foul smell, and accompanied by an uneasy sensation about the liver, a continued inclination to stool, as if diarrhœa were about to come on. *Menstruation*, when profuse, and associated with piles as above described.

3.—Antimonium Crudum—*Crude Antimony.*

This mineral exists in great abundance in Hungary, Germany, France, and England; also on the island of Borneo, from which large quantities of the crude ore are imported as ballast. The native sulphuret is generally found combined with small quantities of lead, copper, iron,

medicinal purposes. We use the crystalline
and prepare it for use by *trituration*.

GENERAL USES.—The beneficial action of
chiefly limited to the mucous membrane of
tract, and the skin, more especially when those
concurrently diseased.

DIGESTIVE SYSTEM.—The *lining membrane*,
stomach and the alimentary canal, is loaded
there are—*eructations*, foul, bitter, or tasting
nausea, and sometimes vomiting; fœtid flatul
appetite; constipation, alternating with diarrh
white tongue; slow digestion, with drowsi
strength, etc. It is an excellent remedy in
condition of the intestinal canal which favours
tion of *worms*.

Chronic catarrh of the bladder, with *turbid*,
and sometimes painful micturition.

SKIN.—Pimples or blotches; tubercular eru
the roots of the beard; nettle-rash associated
tion; ill-conditioned, unhealthy appearance. A
affection of the mucous membranes and the sk
remarked, is an additional indication for *Ant. Cr*

4.—Antimonium Tartaricum—*Tartarated* *Tartar Emetic*.

This salt is a composition of oxide of antim
and tartaric acid, boiled together in water in ar
It crystallizes in rhombic octohedrons, which los
parency and diminish in weight by exposure
Though less violent as a poison than was at o
posed, it has, nevertheless, been highly destru
For homœopathic purposes it is prepared by *trit*

General Uses.—The chief sphere of action of this medicine lies in the *mucous membranes*, the *lungs*, and the *skin*.

Respiratory System.—In large doses it produces a kind of catarrhal inflammation, beginning in the lining membrane of the throat, and extending to the trachea and bronchial tubes, and even exerting its irritant influence on the lung tissues themselves. We should, therefore, expect that *Tartar Emetic* would prove a valuable remedy in certain inflammations involving these parts. Experience has amply justified this expectation, and in *catarrhal croup*, *bronchitis*, and *pneumonia*, it has proved a most useful remedy. Also in the wheezing breathing and coughs of children, when there is much mucous which is easily expelled. Allopathic authorities now recommend *Tartar Emetic* for this same condition.

Digestive System.—The *vomiting* to which this remedy is homœopathic is nervous and sympathetic rather than gastric, and is attended by *nausea*, cold and pale skin, and great prostration.

Skin, etc.—Barber's Itch, and a variety of eruptions, are amenable to this remedy. In allopathic doses it produces a pustular eruption much resembling *small-pox*; in the latter disease, consequently, *it is very valuable*.

5.—Apis Mellifica—*Honey-bee*.

To the utility of the bee in furnishing us with honey, we may add that of its poison, which is appropriated by homœopaths as a valuable therapeutic agent. The medicine is prepared either by macerating the part containing the sting, or triturating the whole bee after drying.

General Uses.—Rapid *acute œdema* of various parts; it also affects the mucous membrane of the genito-urinary organs, producing inflammation, etc. In all affections for which this remedy is thought of, the presence of urinary difficulties, retention of urine, irritability of furnish additional indications for its adminis

THROAT, ETC.—Sore throat, with œdem the tonsils, uvula and palate, and sting swallowing; hoarseness and dry cough; the tongue, etc.

URINARY ORGANS.—*Apis* has a direct acti lining of the kidneys and neck of the l *Canth.*); inflammatory affections of these quent urging, but inability, to urinate.

SKIN.—*Erysipelas* with rapid swelling, m matory redness pointing to *Bell.*, or the forr characteristic of *Rhus*; *urticaria*, for whi remedy, especially if there be itching wi burning, and acute œdema; *carbuncles*, wit sipelatous blush; and other skin affections, i stinging, and itching are prominent sympto

---

6.—Arnica Montana—*Mountain-Arnica*—

This plant is indigenous to the mountai great part of continental Europe; also Siberia; but it flourishes particularly in medicinal properties are more especially co flowers and root. The strong alcoholic tinct ish- yellowish-green colour, yielding a stro odour, which predominates over that of the a

GENERAL USES.—*Injuries*, immediate or general, *from falls or blows*; severe concussi occur in railway accidents, without leaving of violence; concussion of the brain; *physic* ache, stiffness and soreness from walking, so-called rheumatism of the intercostal muscl from over-exertion; spasmodic cough, the violence of which causes aching and soreness of the sides, and even hæmoptysis.

Aching of the eyes through over-taxing them; epistaxis or hæmatemesis, from severe exertion or a blow. *After-pains* are generally quickly relieved by *Arnica;* angina pectoris, when the pains are brought on by slight exertion; sores of bed-ridden patients; chilblains; small boils; etc.

It is chiefly adapted to plethoric persons, disposed to cerebral congestion, and acts but feebly in those of soft flesh or debilitated constitution.

The influence of *Arnica* on all ailments resulting from injuries is wonderful.

The Hunting Field.—Hunting men now and then get falls that shake every bone in their bodies; the effects of these concussions, though no bones be broken, are generally painful: one or two drops of the 1st dec. dil. in half a wine-glass of water, repeated once or twice, works wonders in these cases. Next morning, in place of being stiff and miserable, the sportsman is ready for renewed engagements.

The Labouring Classes.—Among the labouring classes in agricultural districts, a life of heavy toil often causes a comparatively early old age, with supposed rheumatic pains, which incapacitate them from further toil. These "*misérables*" are greatly benefited by *Arnica*, from 1st to 3rd dilution, in one- or two-drop doses, three times a day.

In fact, almost in every ailment traceable to falls, hard knocks or blows, or hard work, *Arnica* becomes an essential part of the treatment, whatever the immediate symptom presenting itself. In cases of very old standing, the treatment must be commenced with a high dilution, and continued by a course of gradually lower dilutions in sequence.

Fever.—In those cases of fever consequent on excessive bodily fatigue, *Arnica*, 1st, 2nd, or 3rd, may be given in-

admirably.

Enlargement of the Heart.—Hypertrophy induced by over-exertion, in young men, is *Arnica*, even after allopathic physicians have affection incurable before it was placed under

External Uses of Arnica.—*Formula.*— made by mixing twenty drops of the strong t half a tea-cupful of water; if the skin be b should be somewhat weaker. The bruised bathed with this lotion, or it may be applied saturated with it, and covered with oiled- evaporation.

In *bruises*, *concussions*, etc., the consequen stiffness, and swelling, may be almost or ent by the *prompt* use of *Arnica*. A *black-eye* m viated. This action, however, depends very *promptitude* with which it is applied after the i

In *cuts* and *lacerations*, if *Arnica* be used, th be only half as strong as for bruises. (See "(

Aching and soreness of the feet from excessi be promptly relieved by a warm foot-bath, in ful of the strong tincture is mixed. For the of *any part*, the internal action of the remed seconded by the application of a lotion—o strong tincture to about twenty of water.

After the extraction of teeth, the mouth with a little water containing a few drops of A

* See an interesting resumé of the value of *Arnica* in D sions and Facts from Ten Years' Homœopathic Practice,' *Homœopathic World*, Vol. III., from which part of the abo

Sore nipples are sometimes cured by the use of *Arnica-lotion*. The nipple should be bathed after each nursing, taking care to gently wash the part before again suckling.

To *corns, chilblains, chapped hand or lips*, and sometimes in *rheumatism*, etc., *Arnica* is also an invaluable application.

In addition to the *tincture*, there are various useful forms in which *Arnica* is prepared;—*Arnica Cerate* and *Arnicated Balls*, for chapped hands or lips, and for chilblains; *Arnica Liniment* and *Opodeldoc*, for rubbing the parts in sprains, rheumatism, etc. (see *Rhus Toxicodendron*); and *Arnica Court-Plaster*, for cuts, *Arnicated Corn-plaster*, corns, etc.

CAUTION.—*Arnica* is apt to produce, in some persons, a severe form of erysipelas, when applied externally. Indeed, in some instances, it produces erysipelas by its mere exposure in the room in which susceptible individuals sleep. It should be used with caution, and in a sufficiently diluted form.

ANTIDOTE.—The *erysipelas* produced by *Arnica* may be cured by the application of a lotion composed of forty drops of *Spirits of Camphor* in half-a-pint of water, and by the internal use of the drug at the same time. A too strong *Camphor-lotion* we have often known to produce unpleasant results. *Cantharis* is sometimes used as an antidote.

7.—Arsenicum Album—*White Arsenic—Arsenious Acid.*

Arsenious acid is the ter-oxide of the metal *Arsenicum*, and is usually obtained in Saxony and Bohemia by roasting or smelting cobalt ores, in which arsenic is a considerable ingredient; the metal rises in vapour, takes the oxygen from the air, and so forms arsenious acid. In shops it is generally kept in the form of powder; and being white, is easily adulterated with chalk, carbonate of lead, etc. Taken into the mouth it has no immediate decided taste, but it soon occasions an acrid sensation. It is prepared for use by solution and trituration.

PATHOGENETIC EFFECTS.—Its injudicious or prolonged use occasions a general sinking of the vital powers, with derangement of the digestive and nervous systems, a small, quick, often irregular pulse, sleeplessness, and œdema of the face and extremities. Hence it is admirably adapted to feeble and impoverished constitutions, and to a great number of the maladies of such persons, when administered in appropriate doses. Mr. Hunt states the effects of medicinal doses to be—1, irritation of the conjunctiva; 2, swelling of the face; 3, desquamation of the skin, only observable under a magnifying glass; 4, portions of the skin, protected from light, assume a dirty-brown appearance. Sir Thomas Watson mentions a peculiar silvery whiteness of the tongue as one of the symptoms. The deleterious properties of *Arsenious acid* are widely known, and the foul deeds which have been committed with it have excited prejudices against its employment as a therapeutic agent. Poisonous doses produce violent *vomiting*, *diarrhœa*, burning *pain* in the stomach, *thirst*, *constricted state of the mouth and throat*, *flushed*, *swollen*, *anxious countenance*, *quick pulse*, *extreme debility*, and, usually, convulsions before death.

GENERAL USES.—Affections of persons *debilitated* by excesses, innutritious diet, endemic diseases of *low and marshy districts*, abuse of quinine, etc. It is especially indicated by great, rapid depression of the vital energies, *prostration and emaciation*, irritability of the stomach, relaxed bowels, and a pale, sunken, or bloated countenance, with a hippocratic expression. *Asiatic cholera*, with cold breath, paralysis of the bladder, etc. General *dropsical swellings*, including the swollen feet of aged and feeble persons; many chronic skin-affections, and malignant diseases.

In *cancer* it gives wonderful relief, improves the general

health, and often checks the rapid development of the disease. The pains are of a *burning* character, *worse at night.*

Intermittent fever, the three stages not being well-marked, occurring irregularly, or when one of the phases has predominated or been absent. *Fevers* of a *low type*—putrid, typhoid, etc., with rapid prostration, dry, burning skin, or cold, clammy perspiration; intense thirst; red, irritated tongue; extreme weakness and trembling; rapid, wiry, feeble, intermittent pulse.

Nervous System.—*Intermittent neuralgia*, with burning-pains (some patients compare the pains to a red-hot wire along the nerve); the symptoms are generally worse at night, with mental effort, are not relieved by cold water, and are accompanied by great restlessness and anguish. Persons who have become weakened through long-continued anxiety, over-work, impoverished dietary, etc., are those in whom the *Arsenic* neuralgia is most liable to occur. Depression of spirits; hypochondriac dejection; great weariness and restlessness. Periodic headache; great weight in the head, and stupefaction.

Eyes.—Ophthalmia, with burning-pains and soreness, dread of light, and swelling of the lids.

Circulatory System.—Angina pectoris; some organic affections of the heart; hydrothorax; small, accelerated, and feeble pulse.

Respiratory System.—Swelling, dryness, stoppage, or burning of the nose, with profuse acrid discharge; *influenza;* suffocative paroxysms, especially after lying down at night; chronic *bronchitis*, with oppressive, anxious, and laboured breathing, and great debility; difficult expectoration, the mucus being sometimes streaked with blood; dropsy of the chest; shortness of breath, especially on ascending a hill, with constitutional debility.

Digestive System.—Dryness and bitter taste in the mouth;

disagreeable odour from the mouth; aphthæ, ulcerated; coated, cracked, red, and tremulous tongue; dryness and burning in the throat; throat affections of a serious or gangrenous character. Chronic nausea and vomiting, with heat and burning in the stomach and epigastrium, from ulceration; indigestion, water-brash, and vomiting after food; sensation of weight and anguish, with cold and chilly feeling; great tenderness or violent colic; cancer of the stomach; chronic affections of the liver; diarrhœic stools, with frequent fœtid discharges; tenesmus, and burning at the anus. As, however, the diarrhœa caused by *Arsenic* depends upon "intestinal *inflammation*, this remedy is not called for in merely functional diarrhœa, even if severe. In the various forms of chronic diarrhœa where there is general inflammation, ulceration, or some other kind of disorganization, *Arsenic* is a glorious remedy *(Hughes)*."

GENERATIVE SYSTEM *(Female)*.—Premature, pale, profuse, menstrual discharge, lasting too long; amenorrhœa, with acrid, excoriating leucorrhœa.

SKIN.—Earthy, bluish, cadaverous colour; *burning itching*, not removed by scratching; *malignant variola;* red pimples, which break and form spreading ulcers; pustules, obstinate ulcers, and cancerous affections; fœtid secretions and tendency to run into mortification; *chronic impetigo*, *prurigo*, *urticaria*, and *eczema*.

8.—Aurum Metallicum—*Metallic Gold.*

This metal is found extensively in South America,

constituent particles, by the peculiar process of *trituration*—a process first adopted by Hahnemann, and now generally practised in our school—gold, and any other substance, can be made perfectly soluble. Of late years the opinions of Allopaths have been considerably modified as to the inertia of gold. Our preparations are made from the finest gold-beater's leaf by trituration.

General Uses.—Constitutions broken-down by *syphilis* or mercury; *nightly bone pains;* inflammation and ulceration of bone; exostosis; excessive sensitiveness of the body; palpitation of the heart; faintness, with blueness of the face; susceptibility to pain; etc. *Hypochondria*, tremulous agitation, religious mania, *suicidal tendency*, oppressive anxiety. Our provings of gold show that it causes melancholy and great depression of spirits. *Rush of blood to the head;* hysteric hemicrania; mercurial or syphilitic headache, with severe pain in the bones. *Ozæna*, with caries of the nasal and palatine bones; purulent discharge from the nose; fœtid breath. Induration of the prostate gland; swelling and induration of the testes; chronic *orchitis*, with aching pain; sexual excitement; nocturnal erections and emissions.

9.—Baptisia Tinctoria—*Wild Indigo.*

Baptisia, a medicine of great value, is one of the "New American Remedies," and fills a gap in our previous Materia Medica.

General Uses.—*Gastric or Enteric fever.* *Bry.*, *Rhus.*, etc., more or less used in enteric and other typhoid conditions, are now superseded by *Baptisia*, which antidotes the toxæmic state, at least in the *early stage*. In advanced typhoid cases, *Ars.* is a better remedy. But if given early, the nausea and pains are quickly relieved, and the patient often makes a rapid recovery. It is probably of no value in fevers, not toxæmic; but in scarlet fever, and other diseases with typhoid symptoms, *Bapt.* should be administered as soon as the danger is threatened. Its power in these diseases resembles that which *Acon.* exerts in simple fever. We have repeatedly proved its value. It should be given in a low dilution—the 1st dec., or even the strong tincture. It is also recommended for chronic dyspepsia with *great sinking at the epigastrium*, and a dry brown tongue in the morning.

10.—Baryta Carbonica—*Carbonate of Baryta.*

GENERAL USES.—*Quinsy*—if administered early, the disease may be at once checked; *chronic enlargement of the tonsils;* relaxed and easily-inflamed throat, with hoarseness; facial paralysis; paralytic and other affections of old people (men especially); wens, and steatoma; depression of the sexual functions—nocturnal emissions, and impotence.

Baryta Muriatica is used for *scrofulous affections*—enlargement of the glands, eruptions, etc.

11.—Belladonna—*Deadly Nightshade.*

This is an indigenous plant, of common growth throughout Europe and most temperate latitudes, flourishing upon a dry soil and the slopes of hills. It has a fleshy, creeping root, and herbaceous stem, bearing a beautiful, sweet, but highly poisonous berry, of a violet-black colour, which, when bruised, emits a fœtid, nauseating odour. The plant is readily known by the livid appearance of its flowers, and the character of its leaves, which are ovate-acute, quite entire, and always come off in pairs, of which one is much larger than the other. It flowers in June and July, and its berries are ripe in September. The leaves of the wild plant are considered more valuable than those of the cultivated.

The plant derives its generic name from *Atropos*, one of the Fates, and its specific name, *Belladonna*, from the Italian language, signifying a beautiful lady. This has been said to be owing to its being used as a cosmetic for the face; but more probably from its being employed to dilate the pupils —a practice still adopted by some Parisian women, as it is supposed to confer on them additional charms.

For medicinal uses, the stems, leaves, and flowers are used, from which a tincture is prepared.

POISONOUS EFFECTS.—The following symptoms, produced by a poisonous dose, are most interesting to homœopathists: —Dryness and heat of the mouth and fauces, attended with thirst; difficulty of swallowing and articulation; constrictive spasms of the throat; nausea, sometimes vomiting, and at times swelling and redness of the face; dilatation of the pupils; obscurity of vision, or absolute blindness; optical illusions; suffused eyes; singing noises in the ears; numbness of the face; confusion of the head; giddiness; delirium, simulating intoxication, which may be combined with, or followed by, profound sleep; scarlet eruption on the skin; and if the dose have been very large, complete coma, and death.

GENERAL USES.—*Delirium*, or perverted brain-function, from active congestion; congestive headache, with scarlet flushings of the face; infantile *convulsions*, etc. *Scarlet-fever*, of the *red, smooth, shining* variety (*Bell.* is of little or no use in the other forms of the so-called scarlet-fever, in which the eruption is not smooth or bright-red). As a *prophylactic* against simple scarlet-fever, its application is a striking illustration of the principle of *similia*, and was first announced by Hahnemann, and afterwards confirmed by Hufeland, and since has been largely established by facts. Our own experience both in private families and schools, amply illustrate the value of this appropriation of *Bell.* *Erysipelas*, with

Hydrophobia. *Bell.* is chiefly valuable in affections of a violent character, in which the vessels *(capillaries)* are almost ruptured by the blood. It has a special and powerful action u and its membranes; the mucous lining of the remarkably sensitive to its action. Its chief are—stinging or burning **pains, aggravated** b swelling and shining redness of the affected part

It is especially adapted to persons whose brai of great functional activity, to persons of amiabl inclined to become fat, with light hair, bl delicate, easily-inflamed skin. It is thus spec to women and children.

DIFFERENCE BETWEEN BELLADONNA AND ACO resembles the action of *Acon.* in some point from it in the following respects:—(1.) It p more intense congestion; the inflammations occ attain a higher form and are marked by sympto more dangerous character—delirium, convulsio *Acon.* is adapted to simple fevers, or to the fev of the arterial system *generally*; *Bell.* to fever toms indicating active congestion, or disturb functions, of the *brain*. *Bell.* has also a speci inflammatory affections of delicate organs or tiss the ear, the testicle, etc.—and to individuals refined organism.

NERVOUS SYSTEM.—Giddiness; violent *aching head*, aggravated by stooping and moveme *headache* from cerebral engorgement, **with heat** of the face, and tendency to perversion of (*gastric* headache is better met by *Nux. V.*);

mation of the brain; nightly delirium, or paroxysmal insanity; *acute hydrocephalus; epilepsy*, with active cerebral symptoms, and deep-red colour of the face during the fit; *chorea; squinting* (recent); *infantile convulsions* of true cerebral origin; intermittent *neuralgia*, recurring in the afternoon, with scarlet redness of the face.

Sleep.—Sleeplessness and restlessness, or drowsiness; frequent waking; startings in sleep or when on the point of falling asleep, as in affright, with cerebral excitement; screaming, moaning, or terrifying dreams; sleeping with the eyes open or partially open.

Eyes.—*Dilated pupils:* sensitiveness to light; inflammatory redness and burning pain in the eyes; catarrhal and acute strumous ophthalmia; complete or partial amaurosis; perverted or double vision; *muscæ volitantes.* Dilated pupils, and brilliant or glistening eyes, with scarlet colour of the face, always point to *Bell.*

Ears.—Tingling and roaring noise; catarrhal deafness, with sore throat; deafness following scarlatina or typhus; lacerating pain in the ears; otalgia; swelling of the glands near the ears.

Respiratory System.—*Violent*, dry *cough*, worse at night, excited by a tickling sensation in the throat, with headache and redness of the face; painfulness of the larynx when coughing; spasmodic hooping-cough; *hoarseness.*

Digestive System.—*The Mouth.*—A furred tongue, with red, elongated papillæ appearing through the fur; inflammation of the mouth and tongue; *toothache*, with *red*, *hot* face, *throbbing pains* in hollow teeth, extending to the temples, aggravated by eating and by hot drinks; redness and tenderness of the gums; catarrhal *sore throat*, with sense of rawness, swelling and difficulty of swallowing, (if the swelling be very great, *Apis* should be alternated with *Bell.*); bright-red appearance of the tonsils and uvula, with

toothache, spasms, and colic of pregnant w
fever, with a congested state of the brain.

SKIN.—*Scarlet redness*, with heat and d
redness and burning swelling of the affected
carbuncles, which bear a close resemblance
often strikingly benefited by *Bell.*

12.—Bryonia Alba—(*White B*

There are many varieties of Bryony, but
by Hahnemann, is the *Bryonia alba*, indigen
of Europe, Germany, and some parts of Fra
Bryonia dioica, common in the hedges and
country. This latter variety, *Black Bryoni*
as an external application in *bruises*. P
employ it in the form of a poultice, appl
ecchymosis. It is said to remove all disc
one to two days. The *B. Alba* is, however,
ferred for homœopathic purposes. A deep
bitter tincture is made from the *root*.

GENERAL USES.—Although *Bryonia* occ
rank in our materia medica, it probably
the multiplicity of diseases in which it is
account of their frequent and general occurr

of these diseases are the following:—*Rheumatism*, acute and chronic, worse on movement, and when affecting the joints and muscles; in *rheumatic fever*, it is second only to *Acon.*; lumbago, with acute bruised sensation in the loins; stiff-neck; complaints in which the serous membranes are involved—*pleurisy*, peritonitis, etc.; bronchitis; pneumonia; typhous (not of a low type), bilious-remittent, and relapsing fevers, chilliness being a marked symptom; *dyspepsia*—water-brash, constipation, etc.; some affections of the liver; etc.

Suppressed eruptions are often redeveloped on the surface by a few doses of *Bry.*

Bryonia is well adapted to persons of firm fibre, dark complexion, bilious and irritable temperament; also to affections brought on by exposure to cold, dry weather, and piercing wind; and when *the symptoms are intensified by movement.*

HEAD.—*Congestive headache*—frontal throbbing, with redness of the face, giddiness, sense of weight, fulness, and as if the brain would press through the forehead on stooping. Unlike the *Aconite* headache, it has generally a gastric or rheumatic origin, and the ideas are not disturbed as when *Bell.* is indicated. If bleeding of the nose follow the headache, that is a further indication for *Bry.*

RESPIRATORY SYSTEM.—*Pleuro-pneumonia* and *pleurisy* (after, or in alternation with, *Acon.*); if effusion have taken place, *Bry.* is the best remedy; acute bronchitis, when the disease is not diffused; common "cold on the chest," consequent on a simple catarrhal affection; dry cough, with constant irritation, little expectoration, stitching or catching pains in the chest, sometimes so severe as to induce retching. *Teste* recommends it for croup in alternation with *Ipec.*

DIGESTIVE SYSTEM.—*Water-brash*, heart-burn, *acid eructations*, bitter taste, sense of weight or pressure at the pit of the stomach, as if a stone were lying there; bilious vomiting; *constipation*, from torpor of the bowels, with congestive headache, the fæces being large, and causing pain in passing them; *chronic* constipation, with similar symptoms; congestion of the *liver*, with pain in the right shoulder, dull pain in the right side, and slight jaundiced appearance; red, scanty, and hot urine.

Generative System (*Female*).—Premature and profuse menstruation; milk-fever, and threatened inflammation and abscess of the breast from cold, in nursing women, when the breasts are knotty, swollen, and sore: these symptoms may also be felt when weaning.

13.—Cactus Grandiflorus—*Midnight-blooming Cereus.*

This cactus is indigenous to Mexico and the West Indies. It blooms in the month of July in Naples; and is only found in temperate latitudes, except in conservatories, where, of course, it is not so vigorous as in its natural climate: hence, for medicinal purposes, the plant as it is found in nature only should be used.

General Uses.—*Affections of the heart and large blood-vessels*, in which congestion is dissipated, and irritation removed by the drug; palpitation from nervous or organic disease; heart-complication in rheumatic-fever, with excessive impulse of the heart's action, and intermitting pulse; sense of constriction in the region of the heart, as if the organ "were grasped and compressed by an iron hand," increased by exertion.

Headache, with pressure or weight on the top of the head, especially in women who menstruate too frequently and profusely; faintness and palpitation; acute congestion of the head, with profuse epistaxis.

In some respects it acts similarly to *Acon.*, and is said to have cured chronic bronchitis, pleurisy, pneumonia, hæmatemesis, etc.

14.—Camphora—*Camphor*.

The Laurus Camphora, from which *Camphor* is obtained in great abundance, is a large, handsome evergreen tree, very common in China, Japan, and other parts of Eastern Asia, where it grows to the size of our tall oak. Through all parts of it, the trunk, root, and branches, Camphor is diffused, and is obtained by sublimation. The odour, appearance, and volatility of Camphor are well known.

PATHOGENETIC EFFECTS.—"In doses of gr. ij.–v–x, camphor acts as a stimulant; it increases the action of the heart and arteries, exhilarates the spirits, excites warmth of body and diaphoresis; the pulse is rendered softer and fuller. These effects are transitory, and are followed by depression. In somewhat larger doses, it allays spasm and pain, and induces sleep. In poisonous doses, it produces vomiting, vertigo, delirium, and convulsions. It acts chiefly on the nervous system; and, like sulphur, it transudes through the skin, and is exhaled by the lungs. . . . It exercises a powerful influence on the genito-urinary system; occasionally it causes strangury, yet by some it has been advised to relieve the strangury produced by cantharides" *(Waring)*.

A case of poisoning by Camphor has lately (1869) been reported in the *Journal de Chimie*, of a remarkably small quantity of Camphor, used as an enema, causing most urgent symptoms. "A child of three and a half years, suffering from mild fever, had an enema of five grammes of Camphor, suspended in yolk of egg, administered to it. This was shortly followed by lividity of the face, vomiting, cold sweat, and convulsions, accompanied directly afterwards by insensibility and retention of urine. The child's life was in imminent danger for ten hours. Coffee was given as an antidote, and recovery gradually took place."

GENERAL USES.—*Asiatic Cholera* (see over); *choleraic*

diarrhœa; sudden and extreme prostration of the nervous system, with severe chills, chattering of the teeth, pallor of the countenance, sense of internal heat, cold sweats, cramps, purging, etc. Lassitude, depression, and frequent yawnings; the *primary chill* of catarrh or influenza, when it prevents further development of disease, but only in that stage. *Fainting-fits* from trifling causes, and *hysteric attacks;* in these cases, *Camphor* may be administered by olfaction.

As an antidote to the excess of medicinal action of small doses of a drug, *Camphor* is very useful: a few doses frequently repeated will be sufficient. The erysipelas produced by *Arnica* is readily cured by *Camphor-lotion* (see "Arnica").

The *evanescent action* of *Camphor* requires that it be given in oft-repeated doses; it is only adapted to acute and sudden diseases.

CHOLERA.—A saturated solution, containing equal parts by weight of *Camphor* and of spirits of wine, recommended and successfully used by Dr. Rubini in several hundred cases of cholera, has excited much attention, and was widely used during the outbreak of Cholera in 1866. Dr. Rubini directs that four drops of the saturated tincture of *Camphor* be given *on sugar* (not in water), every five minutes, to patients seized with cholera, or in very severe cases five to twenty drops; and he states that, ordinarily, in two, three, or four hours, reaction will set in. It is gratifying to be able to add that his statements and successes have been abundantly confirmed in this country.*

HEAD.—Congestion and cerebral irritation, amounting even to delirium; giddiness, wakefulness, and nervous irritability. *Sun-stroke* (the remedy being administered by olfaction); head-symptoms from the retrocession of an acute eruption—measles, etc.

* For interesting accounts of Dr. Rubini's treatment, and its successful adoption in this country, see the volume of *The Homœopathic World* for 1866.

Urinary System.—*Sudden stranguary*, with burning and great pain; in infants thus suffering, the remedy may be administered by olfaction for a few seconds, every ten minutes. It is also sometimes useful in sexual weakness and impotence, especially when associated with stranguary or vesical irritability. *Camphor* removes the urinary difficulties consequent on the use of *Cantharides* (blistering-fly).

15.—Cannabis Sativa—*Hemp.*

General Uses.—Affections of the *genito-urinary* organs. *Hemp*, in large doses, causes a difficulty of urinating; paralytic weakness of the bladder; symptoms of stricture; burning and stinging before and after urination; discharge of mucus and pus; chordee; etc. Hence it is homœopathic to the symptoms of *gonorrhœa*, and has proved a most successful remedy, in the hands of Homœopathic practitioners, for that disease. In miscarriage and menorrhagia, and consequent conditions, it is sometimes useful; as also in some eye-affections—opacity of, and specks on, the cornea, etc. The effects of *alcoholic intoxication* have also been remedied by this drug.

16.—Cantharis Vesicatoria—*Blistering-Fly—Spanish-Fly.*

This insect is about eight or ten lines in length, by two or three in breadth, and of a brilliant green colour. During life, the Cantharides have so powerful an odour, that swarms of them can thus be detected, even at a considerable distance. They are abundantly found in the south of Europe, in the early summer months, when they settle upon such trees as the white poplar, ash, privet, elder, and lilac, upon the leaves of which they subsist. We extract their medicinal properties by pulverization and maceration of the entire insect. The "fly-blister," so well known in allopathic practice, is totally repudiated by homœopathic practitioners.

GENERAL USES.—Acute *Inflammatory affections of the urinary organs*—simple nephritis, cystitis, urethritis, etc. Pain in the loins; scanty, high-coloured urine, which is bloody, and sometimes albuminous; burning and scalding pain on passing water; tenderness at the lower part of the abdomen: *stranguary*. Paralysis of the neck of the bladder, especially in females and children. *Hæmaturia*, and *suppression* of urine from acute congestion. The sexual organs are probably only affected through extension of urinary irritations. It may be sometimes useful in dropsy following scarlatina, and in Bright's disease. In hysteric patients, with throat-affection, and partially suppressed urine, followed, after a few hours, by profuse discharge of pale urine, it acts well.

SKIN.—*Burns and Scalds* with small or large *blisters*; vesicular erysipelas; carbunculous and gangrenous sores; shingles *(herpes zoster)*; eczema, with much *burning*. In these affections it is well to apply a graduated *Cantharis-lotion*, besides taking the remedy internally. Burning in the soles of the feet at night in hysteric patients, with profuse and pale urine.

EXTERNAL USE.—*Formula.*—Ten or twelve drops of the strong tincture to a small teacupful of water. If applied promptly to a burn or scald, it will often prevent blistering. *Cantharadine Pomade* is recommended for *recent baldness* and falling off of the hair after fevers and other exhausting diseases (see also *Phos. Ac.*).

ANTIDOTE.—*Camphor-lotion*, as directed for *Arnica*, will correct any unpleasant symptoms from the external use of *Cantharis* (five drops of strong *Camphor-tincture* to one ounce water).

17.—Carbo Vegetabilis—*Vegetable Charcoal.*

Vegetable charcoal is obtained by burning wood in covered-up heaps or in close vessels, with but a limited access of air. For medicinal purposes, the pollard beech of mountainous countries is selected, from the slow combustion of which a black, tasteless, and insoluble substance is obtained, remarkable for its power of counteracting putrefaction, and for combining with, and removing, the odorous and colouring principles of most bodies. From this wood, pulverized, we make triturations, by which the latent, inherent medicinal properties of the crude substance are developed, rendering it a therapeutic agent of great value.

General Uses.—*Chronic derangement of the digestive system*, characterized by *flatulence* and *foulness of the secretions;* diseases marked by *loss of vitality* and *imperfect oxydisation of the blood*, as in intermittent fever in the cold stage, when there is blueness and coldness of the hands and feet; in typhoid, typhus, etc., with similar symptoms, and dry, foul tongue, frequent offensive diarrhœa, and *extreme exhaustion:* it sometimes rouses the sinking nervous energies; *cold extremities*, arising from deficient vitality in the circulation, and associated with general adynamia.

Respiratory System.—*Chronic* catarrhal *hoarseness; chronic bronchitis* in the feeble and aged, when there is scarcely sufficient strength to raise and eject the mucus, which is profuse, and often foul-smelling; threatened gangrene of the lungs.

Digestive System.—*Flatulence* of the stomach, with distension, causing a sense of oppression, palpitation, etc., sometimes felt in the evening and at night; *heart-burn and acidity*, with flatulence, and constipation or diarrhœa; easily-bleeding gums and *foul breath*. It is a valuable remedy in strumous persons, with the above symptoms, and wl

Mercury has been abused. *Diarrhœa*, with offensive motions, especially in scrofulous children; chronic diarrhœa in cachectic persons, with sallow face, acidity of the stomach, flatulence, etc., and without feverishness; chronic constipation, with torpor, heat and fulness in the bowels.

SKIN.—*Foul ulcers* (internal and external use); chronic eruptions, with itching and burning, easily bleeding; inveterate herpes; sores following burns, which do not readily heal, but discharge a foul, ichorous fluid: the *Carbo* should be sprinkled on in very fine powder.

In *poisoning by Arsenic*, charcoal has been found useful; it should be administered in milk or water, and taken in large quantities as quickly as possible.

18.—Causticum—*Caustic.*

GENERAL USES.—*Loss of voice*, from cold, or from over-exertion, as in speaking or singing; cough with involuntary emission of urine; some cases of facial paralysis; pain and weight in the loins with urinary difficulties; neuralgia, or tendinous and muscular pains, with *urging to urinate*, and discharge of pale urine; *enuresis* of children and aged persons; excessive discharges of urine during convalescence from severe disease, with sour perspirations, dejection of spirits, etc.; frequent urging to urinate in hysteric patients; *constipation*, with solid evacuations, expelled with difficulty, and having a shining, greasy appearance *(Bayes)*. In *deep burns*, with formation of scabs, it is sometimes used locally with good results.

19.—Chamomilla Matricaria—*Chamomile-Flower.*

This plant is indigonous to most parts of Europe, and flourishes in corn-fields, waste grounds, and by the roadside, especially on chalky soils. The name of the flower is derived from the Greek word *chama* (low), and from *matrix* (womb), from its supposed specific action on that organ. For homœopathic purposes we gather the plant when in bloom, from which we prepare a tincture.

General Uses.—*Nervous affections* generally, of women and children; derangement of the *nervous and biliary systems* from anger or vexation; chronic abscess has been benefited by *Cham.*, when *Hepar Sulph.* has failed, used internally and externally. Ailments induced by *coffee* and *narcotics*—nervousness, palpitation, etc.—are met by *Cham.* The pains of *Cham.* are worse at night; and after they have somewhat subsided, a sense of numbness remains in the part.

Nervous System.—Extreme sensitiveness to external impressions, without ideal confusion; neuralgia, with the same conditions; face-ache, with swelling; sleeplessness, flushes of heat, and palpitation, with bilious symptoms; spasms and convulsions of women and children; wakefulness, restlessness, and fretfulness, or convulsions of children during dentition, with sour-smelling breath; spasms and convulsions of pregnant women.

Head, Ears, Face, etc.—*Bilious headache*, with stupifying oppressive pain, stitching and burning distress; nervous headache (on one side), with throbbing, flushes of heat, sensitiveness, and irritability of disposition; facial neuralgia with irritable mood. *Ear-ache*, and cracks and soreness of the lips, in infants, from cold.

Respiratory System.—Spasmodic cough, with a sense of tightness in the chest; catarrh of infants; hoarseness and cough of a nervous character in women and children.

Digestive System.—*Toothache* from indigestion, worse soon after eating, and by drinking warm fluids; toothache with swelling, and pain as if the nerve were scraped. Tongue thickly coated with a yellowish-white fur, and red at the edges; sour breath of children, with pinching pains in the abdomen, greenish motions, and flushed cheek; *diarrhœa*, and many other *affections of children during dentition*; dyspepsia, with pressure at the stomach, sudden stitches, sallow complexion, and yellow tongue; aching pain and sourness in the stomach after food, with irritability, and greenish motions: nausea, or vomiting of bile; colic, with extreme soreness of the bowels; affections of the liver from anger, etc.; bilious attack, with heat in the face, thirst, anxiety, and restlessness.

GENERATIVE SYSTEM *(Female)*.—Profuse menstrual discharge,—dark, even blackish, and coagulated, with griping or labour-like pains, sickness, frequent urging to urinate, and nervous irritability; pains in the veins of the leg; cramps of pregnant women, with nervous sensitiveness; false labour-pains, with cramps and twitches; uterine disturbance from mental excitement, anger, vexation, etc.

SKIN.—*Rash in children*, alternating with diarrhœa; simple intertrigo; ulcers, with burning-pains, and great sensitiveness; scrofulous ulcers, and ulcers of the breast, secreting unhealthy pus; ulcers occurring in connection with bilious derangement, sallow complexion, etc.; in these cases *Cham.* should be used both internally and externally.

20.*—Calcarea Carbonica—*Carbonate of Lime.*

Calcarea Carbonica is found abundantly in the form of chalk, marble, eggshells, oyster-shells, etc. The insolubility of the salts of lime formed an obstacle to their general use by Allopathic medical men; notwithstanding this they use them occasionally for their antacid and astringent properties. For Homœopathic purposes we employ *oyster-shells*, from which, after washing, boiling, exposing to a charcoal fire, sifting, and reducing to a powder, we first make triturations.

* By an inadvertence, *Calc. Carb.* and *Calendula* were omitted from their proper alphabetical arrangement.

GENERAL USES.—*Scrofulous, rachitic,* and *tuberculous* affections, and others depending on defective assimilation and nutrition; debility, loss of flesh, etc.; difficult teething; soft condition of the bones (rickets), on account of which the child is late in walking. Scrofulous consumption, with tight cough, oppression, expectoration of yellow or green fœtid *pus*, hæmoptysis, hectic-fever, night-sweats, etc. Chronic urticaria, porrigo capitis, and other chronic eruptions. Warts and polypi, as results of disordered nutrition and growth, are curable by *Calc.* "It may be laid down that *Calcarea* is best adapted to the disorders of women and children, to persons of leuco-phlegmatic temperament, with tendency to obesity" *(Hughes).* The flesh is pale, soft, and flabby.

HEAD.—Chronic nervous headache, with eructations, and sense of *coldness in the head;* dull headache, worse in the morning, as from brain-fag.

EYES, EARS, THROAT, ETC.—Ophthalmia and conjunctivitis: otorrhœa and chronic otitis; chronic yellow or greenish purulent discharge from the nose *(ozæna):* chronic sore-throat, with dryness, and swollen tonsils; glandular enlargements. In these local affections, *Calc.* probably acts chiefly by improving the constitutional condition: it is not adapted to acute manifestations of the dyscrasia. Its external use, in the form of diluted lime-water, is sometimes very serviceable in connection with the internal use of the drug.

DIGESTIVE SYSTEM.—Anorexia; *chronic acid eructations,* with burning sensation in the stomach; chronic diarrhœa, with slimy, foul-smelling stools; diarrhœa of children during dentition, offensive motions, part being light and part dark-coloured; colliquative diarrhœa of consumption; chronic constipation with swelling of the bowels; mesenteric disease in scrofulus children.

GENERATIVE SYSTEM *(Female).—Premature and profuse catamenia;* itching and burning leucorrhœa; chlorosis in *scrofulus girls.*

CALCARIA PHOSPHORATA—*Phosphate of Lime*—is used especially in diseases of the osseous system—curvature of the spine, spina bifida, hip-joint disease, psoas abscess, scrofulous ulcers, etc.

21.—Calendula Officinalis (*Marigold*).

The marigold is a native of France, but is now found in cultivated grounds in nearly all parts of Europe. The leaves and flowers are the parts used in medicine.

GENERAL USES.—This remedy is almost exclusively used as an external application, and in this way exerts a most favourable influence in promoting the union of wounds with the least resulting scars, and with the smallest amount of suppuration. *Cuts*, whether accidental, or inflicted in operations, or injuries, in which *the flesh is much torn*, and which do not heal without the formation of matter; wounds penetrating the joints, etc. In all such cases it is much preferable to *Arnica*, especially in constitutions having a tendency to erysipelas. It controls hæmorrhage (but to a less extent than *Hamamelis*), and relieves the severest pains attending various accidents. In the late civil war, it was largely used by our American colleagues in the treatment of injuries, and with the most beneficial results. It is an invaluable remedy in *ulcers* of the lower extremities—bad legs as they are called—such as often occur in broken-down constitutions, especially in the decline of life. Mr. Nankivell informs us that *Calendula-lotion*—20 drops to a teacupful of water—is very useful in many chronic affections of the eye-lids: he has never known it to have any repellent or inconvenient effect.

FORMULA.—A *lotion* may be made by adding a teaspoonful of the pure tincture to half or three-quarters of a teacupful of water. If the bleeding be considerable, the lotion may be made much stronger.

22.—China—Cinchona Officinalis—*Peruvian Bark.*

The Cinchona-tree is a native of Peru and the adjacent provinces of South America, and is of great beauty, with evergreen laurel-like leaves, which diffuse a delicious fragrance around. It is not found at an elevation of less than 2,500 feet above the sea, and sometimes extends as far up as from 9,000 to nearly 12,000 feet.

We make an alcoholic tincture from the bark, or triturations of its alkaloid *Quina* (Quinine).

General Uses.— *Debility caused by loss of animal fluids*—hæmorrhage, diarrhœa, spermatorrhœa, profuse sweating, expectoration, or suppuration, excessive lactation, etc. *Simple intermittent fever; simple remittent fever* with much prostration and variable pulse; *hectic-fever*, from abscess or prolonged suppuration in any part; *periodically-recurring neuralgias*, and other affections marked by periodicity; sensitiveness of the nervous system to physical impressions; *anasarca* when associated with ague or disease of the spleen; *sweating*, in cases of extreme debility, especially after severe fevers, the patient waking up every night with his linen soaked with sweat. Disturbing dreams causing anxiety and starting, the anxiety or confusion remaining some time after waking. "*Irritation of the spine*, and spinal pain, with imperfect circulation, shown by blueness of the nails, coldness of the extremities, with numbness, etc., is well met by *China*" *(Bayes)*.

Debility, however, is little benefited by *China* so long as its cause remains in operation.

The pains indicating *China* are *increased by movement*, by *contact*, and by *currents of air;* and perspiration is easily induced by exertion.

Nervous System.—*Intermittent neuralgia; vertigo*, with dimness of sight, humming in the ears, and flushed face, succeeded by depression, yawning, etc.; tremblings, debility caused by excessive mental labour.

HEAD, EARS, ETC.—Neuralgic and congestive headache and face-ache, occurring *periodically*; headache, with sense of *constriction*, as if a band were passed over the top of the head from side to side, with noises in the head and ears,—buzzing, singing, humming, roaring,—or congestion—weight, fulness, and tension in the head, flushing of the face, etc.—the symptoms being aggravated by movement, currents of air, or contact; pains in the head, relieved by eating; *brow-ague* (malarial); nervous *deafness*, with hissing or other noises in the ears.

DIGESTIVE SYSTEM.—*Diarrhœa* (chronic), or diarrhœa occurring early in a morning or after a meal, without pain; simple summer diarrhœa with severe griping, or absence of pain; passage of undigested food; periodic (malarial) *dysentery*, with debility—cold extremities, feeble pulse, etc.; *sinking at the stomach*, relieved by eating, but soon recurring; sensation of emptiness with or without hunger; *jaundice*, in feeble persons, with sallow, dirty-yellow complexion, stitches in the liver, slimy-bilious taste, and loss of appetite; drowsiness and oppression after eating, and qualmishness in the stomach; congestion and enlargement of the spleen; ascarides, especially if occurring in scrofulous children with large abdomens, and subject to diarrhœa.

URINARY SYSTEM.—Scanty and turbid urine, with whitish or brick-dust sediment; periodic paroxysms of *hæmaturia*.

GENERATIVE SYSTEM.—Nocturnal emissions and spermatorrhœa, with debility, depression of spirits, indigestion. Menstruation continuing too long, or being *profuse*, the discharge consisting of *lumps of dark coagula; irregular* menses; irregularity of labour pains; debility from excessive menstruation, leucorrhœa, or lactation.

SKIN.—Unhealthy *ulcers* in cachectic patients of a sallow appearance, with cold and dry or clammy skin; ulcers connected with ague; dropsy; moist gangrene.

ANTIDOTES.—The ill-effects resulting from the too free use of *Bark* or *Quinine* are best met by *Arsenic*, *Ferrum*, *Veratrum*, *Belladonna*, or *Ipecacuanha*, according to the existing symptoms.

23.—Cimicifuga Racemosa—Actæa Racemosa—
Black Cohosh—Squaw-Root.

This plant grows abundantly in shady and rocky woods, on rich grounds, from Maine to Michigan, and in some other parts of America. It is very stately in appearance, being from four to eight feet high, and gives off its flowers in bunches or racemes, as its name indicates. In late autumn and winter, any motion of the plant causes a rattling of the seeds so much resembling the alarm of the rattle-snake as to cause the hunter to start involuntarily; hence its name of *Rattle-weed*, given to it by the country people. The term *Squaw-root* is given to it in consequence of its use by the Indians and settlers who, for centuries, have employed it for many uterine diseases, in labour to assist the expulsive efforts of the womb, and for chorea.

In common with most English Homœopathic physicians, we have derived our knowledge of this drug chiefly from Dr. Hale's admirable work on the "New Remedies." Since our first experience with it, many years ago, we have used it largely, and can abundantly confirm the greater part of Dr. Hale's recommendations.

GENERAL USES.—Its special sphere of action is in *rheumatic*, *muscular*, *nervous*, and *uterine* affections. The *left* side of the body is chiefly involved. It will be seen from the following remarks that those maladies which can be traced to, or are associated with, the uterine system, or rheumatism, are most amenable to its action. Dr. Ringer states that its action on the uterus is very similar to that of *ergot*, but that it

ployment endangers the life of the child, a
tures of the mother, much less than ergot.

Nervous System.—Restlessness; "fidgeti
ness;" nervous weakness and prostrati
followed by irritation, and consequent exh
neuralgia; *pains in the left side, under the b*
and lumbar region. Nervous tremors—al
or connected with deranged menstruatio
depression of spirits, from over-nursing, or
Weariness, sense of confusion, and the pecul
dulness arising from mental labour or want
irritation, not from organic disease, but fr
uterine causes.

Head.—*Rheumatic, nervous*, and menstr
severe *aching-pain in the eye-balls*, and over th
by movement of the head or eyes; dull pai
region, *from within outwards*, with shooting
back of the neck; fulness, heat, and throbb
and sense as if the top of the head would
up stairs; neuralgia in the forehead and
ague). Throbbing, aching pain in the top
head, extending to the shoulders and down
strange and wild appearance, dilated pupils, d
illusions of visions,—rats, mice, insects, etc.-
the eye-balls, sense of soreness in the eye
diplopia, roaring in the head, etc.; *hyste*
pains, sensations, and illusions. *Cimicifuga*
to the "nervous sick-headaches," and headac
delicate, nervous, and hysteric females, especi
with menstruation, pregnancy, or the critic
the headaches of hard students, and the c
and distress of drunkards after alcoholic
these conditions, the latter especially, the al
disturbance would be a further indication for

CIRCULATORY SYSTEM.—Recent affections of the heart following, or due to, rheumatism, with *irregular pulse*, palpitation, pain, etc.; paroxysms of pain and distress,—the heart's action seeming to cease suddenly, with a feeling as of impending suffocation,—similar to those of angina pectoris, chiefly felt after lying down at night,* especially from rheumatic or uterine irritation; pain or anxiety about the heart, down the left arm to the hand, with palpitation, numbness of the left arm, and exhaustion. Pain in left side, under the left breast, in females (see "Nervous System".)

RESPIRATORY SYSTEM.—The reputed virtues of this remedy in lung-disease are not sufficiently verified to warrant us in recommending it; but we have had ample experience of its uses in some secondary affections of the respiratory system. Nervous cough, and dryness of the throat, or sense as of a dry spot in the larynx, inducing cough, in girls and women, from uterine disorder, pregnancy, hysteria, etc.; spasmodic action of the larynx in hysteric patients, with hoarseness, sense of fulness or choking. Pleurodynia, *stitch-in-the-side* (not to be confounded with pleurisy), worse on exertion, and when taking a full breath. It has also cured a true pleurisy. In the catarrhs of women and children, with acute pains in the limbs, aching in the eye-balls, watery coryza, head-, face-, and tooth-ache, dry, tickling cough, worse at night, *Cimicifuga* is very useful.

DIGESTIVE SYSTEM.—The *vomiting* and *sinking at the*

* While these pages were passing through the press, we prescribed the 1st dec. dil. of *Cimicifuga* for a patient suffering from cardiac disease. The first dose was taken a short time before going to bed, and on lying down she experienced the distressing sensation in the region of the heart described in the text, and exclaimed, in great anguish, "I am dying!" In a short time the sensation subsided, and she took another dose of the medicine. After the second dose the distress quickly returned, and in a more intense form. It was clearly the effect of the medicine, and an antidote was administered. She was afterwards put on the 3rd dil. of this drug and rapidly improved.

stomach, caused by *Cimicifuga*, are sy uterine disturbance, and not gastric. are not within its sphere.

URINARY SYSTEM.—Pale, profuse ur pression,—as in hysteria, some uterine etc.

GENERATIVE SYSTEM (*Female*).—A cient nervous energy in the ovaries, organs, manifested by chorea, hysteria, cold, with intense headache, pain in th limbs; uterine cramps, etc. *Delayed* heavy headache, palpitation, and melanc —with severe headache before menstru discharge, aching in the limbs, pain region, hips, and thighs, with pressi pains in the abdomen, tenderness in t depression, nervousness, etc., the disch coagulated; after the menses, the patie neuralgic pains, with lowness of spirits *atony of the uterus*—with dark, coagul *orrhœa*, also associated with uterine rheumatic, and congestive affections of may require the aid of *Bell.* or *Vera* *miscarriage*, even when habitual, is som trol of *Cimicifuga*, if administered early i or for some time before the usual perio the general symptoms correspond. *Dis* nervousness, depression, sleeplessness, disturbance, cramps, and other neuralg *Sinking at the stomach*, occurring at the nection with other uterine troubles; ch ache, aching in the eye-balls and limbs, d *labour-pains*, and other difficulties atte best as a *preventive*, administered for se before labour. *After-pains*, with nervous irritability, sleeplessness, and melancholy, especially when arising from exhaustion of the uterus after prolonged or frequent labours; *prolapsus uteri* from the same causes. *Suppressed lochia*, with uterine spasms, cramps in the limbs, headache, and even delirium; *puerperal mania*—great despondency, etc., especially in rheumatic patients.

ORGANS OF LOCOMOTION.—*Stiff-neck*, *crick-in-the-back*, and *lumbago*, of rheumatic origin; the lumbago is worse when the patient is standing or sitting still, and in cold and stormy weather, but better when laid down; *stitches in the side;* sciatica; articular rheumatism of the lower extremities, with heat and swelling. Muscular cramps and pains from rheumatism.

SKIN.—Urticaria and other irritations of the skin, due to reflex uterine action.

24.—Cina Anthelmintica—*Worm-seed*.

This plant is a hardy perennial shrub of Asia Minor, Judæa, etc. We use the seed, from which we make a tincture or trituration.

GENERAL USES.—Affections characterised by some of the following symptoms:—*voracious* or *variable appetite; grinding of the teeth;* pinching in the abdomen; *itching of the anus;* diarrhœa; wetting the bed; white and thick urine; spasmodic cough, sometimes inducing vomiting; emaciation; large abdomen; starting, restless sleep; pale face; semicircles under the eyes; picking of the nose; frequent feverishness; twitching of the eyelids; dilated pupils, with dimness of sight; twitchings in various parts of the body; convulsions; epileptic spasms.

Since the presence of *worms* (especially round-worms) in the intestinal canal gives rise to more or less of the foregoing symptoms, it is clear that *Cina* is homœopathic to *helminthiasis* with similar symptoms: hence it is found curative in nearly all affections arising from, or coinciding with, the existence of worms; it does not simply expel them but corrects the condition on which the growth of the parasites depends. *Whenever the above symptoms occur*, whether worms can be detected or not, *Cina* will be curative.

Hooping-cough associated with worms; some amaurotic conditions, with illusions of colour; pain below the stomach worse on first waking in the morning and before meals, and relieved by eating; etc.

25.—Cocculus Indicus—*Indian Berries.*

The fruit of a parasitic shrub, growing on the mountainous parts of Malabar, Ceylon, and the Indian Archipelago. Although poisonous, it is, nevertheless, used in considerable quantities for imparting an intoxicating property to malt liquors: by two writers "On Brewing" (Childe, and Morrice), it is openly recommended. It is also used to poison fish and game. We make a brownish straw-coloured tincture from the seeds.

GENERAL USES.—*Functional* disease of the nervous system; especially if the voluntary muscles be involved—*paralytic rigidity* of the lower extremities; paralysis following diphtheria, and *hemiplegia*, with painful stiffness and cracking of the joints; *confused* heavy sensation in the head, with *giddiness*, especially after eating or drinking; giddiness with hot, flushed face, and *sick-headache*, like that occurring in sensitive persons from riding in a carriage, etc.; sea-sickness, in which *Cocculus* is often very useful. Spasms in the abdomen, of a nervous origin, especially after eating; spasms of the uterus *(menstrual colic)*, with dull, indescribable headache, and sickness; disordered digestion, flatulent colic, or spasms of pregnant women, or during menstruation, with *nervous* symptoms; serous and purulent leucorrhœa, with great soreness, and flatulent distension of the bowels.

Antidote.—*Camphor*, in a strong form, frequently administered, will antidote the effects of large medicinal doses of *Cocculus*.

26.—Coffæa Cruda (*Raw Coffee*).

We use the berries of the *Coffee-shrub* indigenous to the elevated regions of Arabia Felix, from which we make a tincture.

General Uses.—"*Excitation* of all the organic functions; increased *irritability of the organs of sense*—sight more acute, hearing more sensitive, taste finer, and sensorium more vivid; mobility of the muscles is increased, sexual desire is more excited, and even the nervous activity of the digestive and secretive organs is increased: hence a *morbid sensation* of excessive *hunger*, increased desire and facility of the alvine evacuations and of the emissions of urine" (from *Stapf*). *Increased susceptibility to pain; sleeplessness*, either from simple nervous wakefulness, or from agitation of mind or body, extreme anxiety, or mental labour; the *wakefulness of children and old people* is especially under its control, it being, in the 3rd or 6th dilution, so effectual in producing calm sleep, that we have sometimes been asked, "Is it an opiate you have been giving?" *Headache* and *hemicrania* commencing in the morning, with *excessive sensitiveness*, chilliness, nausea, and feeling as if a nail were driven into the parietal bone (at the side of the head); *neuralgia* of the right side of the head and face; *toothache*, with great restlessness, flushed face, relieved by cold water, sometimes recurring every night; nervous *palpitation*, with irregular, intermittent pulse; oppression of the chest, as during an attack of asthma; pyrosis;

vomiting of pregnancy; difficulty in passing urine; strangury; extreme sensitiveness and pain during menstruation and labour; irregular, spasmodic labour-pains, with irritability; hysteria, with alternate fits of liveliness and depression; flushes of heat, etc. In the sleeplessness, restlessness, and nervous disorders of children and females, it is a sovereign remedy, second only to *Cham.*

A spoonful or two of a strong decoction of *Coffee* will often immediately relieve an *acute indigestion from over-eating*, especially if the stomach remain inactive, and the food cause a painful sense of distension or cramp.

Coffee is also useful as *an antidote* to over-doses of *Opium*, *Aconite*, *Belladonna*, and many other vegetable poisons: for this purpose it may be given in frequently-repeated doses of a strong infusion. Strong coffee helps to keep awake persons poisoned with *Opium*.

As a *beverage*, *Coffee* should not be used more than once a day. In some, it occasions palpitation of the heart, sleeplessness, and mental excitement, and by such should not be taken at all as a beverage.

27.—Colchicum Autumnale—*Meadow Saffron.*

General Uses.—*Gouty* and *rheumatic affections*, characterized by paroxysms of acute tearing or lacerating pains, with irritated pulse, rose-colour of the skin of the affected part, becoming white on pressure, nodosities; *inflammatory irritation* of the stomach, bowels, heart, or urinary organs *of gouty persons*; asthma, palpitation and tearing pains in the heart, cutting pains in the bowels, etc., alternating with paroxysms of gout; swelling, pain, heat, redness, and lameness in the extremities; *neuralgic pains*, tearing or lacerating, in the chest, abdomen, bowels, or anus, in persons having an arthritic diathesis: there may also be general debility, dropsy, heat and dryness, or perspiration. *Colchicum*, in drop-doses of the strong tincture, is one of the best remedies in preventing an immediately-threatened, or recently-developed *attack* of gout, especially if alternated with *Aconitum* to quell circulatory excitement; but it has little or no curative power over the gouty *diathesis*. In its effect on the bowels it somewhat resembles *Veratrum*.

28.—Collinsonia Canadensis—*Stone-root.*

This plant is indigenous to the Northern American States, and is one of the "new American remedies" with which our Materia Medica has been enriched.

General Uses.—*Constipation*, and *piles* (blind or bleeding); indigestion from want of tone in the stomach: especially if these diseases be associated with *flatulence*, colic, and spasms in the bowels; throbbing headache and fulness in the head, and many other disorders from constipation or hæmorrhoids; much straining and dull pain at stool; heat, and *itching of the anus*; "hæmorrhoidal dysentery;" diarrhœa of children, and *cholera infantum*, with colic, spasms, flatulence, and mucous, papescent, or watery discharges; *dysmenorrhœa menorrhagia*, *prolapsus uteri*, and *leucorrhœa*, when depending on hæmorrhoidal or rectal troubles; and even amenorrhœa, when the hæmorrhoidal discharge is vicarious of menstruation; *pruritus vulvæ*, *constipation*, or *piles*, from pelvic congestion or *during pregnancy*; frequently with the various affections there is considerable concurrent exhaustion. In some rheumatic and cardiac affections, *Collinsonia* is also of service. The Indians use it for the healing of sores and wounds; it is also domestically used in America as a poultice and wash, much as we use *Arnica*.

29.—Colocynthis—*Bitter Cucumber.*

This plant is a native of Turkey, Egypt, North of Africa, the islands of the Archipelago, etc. It is an annual, much resembling the common cucumber, but is distinguished from it by the fruit, which is of a *globular* shape, smooth, and of a yellow colour when ripe. *Colocynth* has been used in medicine from a remote period, and is one of the plants supposed to be the Pakysth or *wild gourd* of Scripture. The seeds, and the pulpy or medullary matter, yield the medicinal product: we make a straw-coloured tincture, or a trituration.

General Uses.—*Colic with diarrhœa;* and *neuralgia.* Severe griping or *cutting-pains* as from knives, in the abdomen and about the navel, increased by taking food, with sensation as if the bowels were about to act, followed by copious diarrhœa, with *straining*, after which there is relief: but the symptoms may speedily recur; dysenteric diarrhœa, with severe colic; peritonitis involving the ovaries; colicky and stitching-pains in the ovaries and liver. *Neuralgic hemicrania*, with sensation as if the head were in a vice, and pressive, or burning-cutting pain in the eye-ball; violent stitches in the forehead and eyes, from within outwards; *facial neuralgia*, chiefly on the left side, with *headache and toothache*—the pains being tearing-stitching, aggravated by warmth and motion, and occurring periodically. *Sciatica*—the pain being lancinating, and darting down the leg from the hip to the foot, worse when raising the limb, but better with continued exercise: and especially when diarrhœa and colicky pain also exist.

30.—Conium Maculatum—*Spotted Hemlock.*

The spotted hemlock is the plant with which, it is believed, the great Socrates was poisoned. It grows abundantly along hedges and in waste places. From its resemblance to fool's parsley and common parsley it has been mistaken for those plants and eaten.

General Uses.—Paraplegia, when the affection commences in the feet, and gradually extends upwards. Inflammation of the eye-lids, with suppuration, ulceration, excessive sensitiveness to light, and violent burning and itching, in scrofulous patients; photophobia and discharge of scalding tears without inflammation; presbyopia, especially the far-sightedness of old people when it comes on prematurely; scrofulous ozœna. Dry, hacking cough, with constant irritation, scraping in the larynx, worse on lying down and at night. "Engorgements of the mammary and other glands resulting from mechanical causes;" atrophy of the breasts and testicles; amenorrhœa; swelling of the testes from a blow; impotence and sterility. Scaly and tubercular eruptions on the skin; hard, *schirrous* tumours, which form in consequence of mechanical injury. In many of the ailments of old persons, especially females, it is a valuable remedy.

31.—Cuprum Metallicum—*Metallic Copper.*

This metal occurs pure, in a native mineral state, and in different forms, chiefly in England, Sweden, North America, etc. It derives its name from having been first found in the island of Cyprus. When combined with acids it is a violent irritant poison: even food cooked in untinned copper vessels, by dissolving a portion of the metal, becomes highly poisonous.* For homœopathic uses, it is prepared in the first instance as a trituration.

General Uses.—Derangements of the nervous system characterized by *cramps*, *convulsive movements*, and *spasm*.

* An instance of the poisonous effects, on a whole family, of this drug, through drinking water from a well in which a copper-kettle had been immersed for some time, is cited in *The Homœopathic World*, Vol. II. p. 207.

Chorea, especially of the upper extremities or of one side of the body, with neuralgic pains previous to or during the attack, and followed by paralysis of the affected parts; *epilepsy*, which began and is characterized by the violence of the convulsions, and, usually, paleness of the face, vertigo and headache, and muscular tremors; melancholy, debility, very slow pulse, languor, muscular tremors, loathing of food sallow complexion, and emaciation of nervous affections, hysteria, etc.; chronic vomiting and diarrhœa; the cramps and *vomiting* of *choleraic diarrhœa* and *Asiatic cholera;* some forms of *enteralgia*, gastritis, and dysphagia. *Spasmodic* asthma, croup, and hooping-cough, and angina pectoris. Some cases of itch are curable by *Cuprum*.*

Cuprum Aceticum is also used by homœopaths; but there is no difference in the sphere of action of the two preparations.

32.—Digitalis Purpurea—*Purple Fox-glove.*

Fox-glove is a native of England and Western Europe. Fuchsius first described it, and named it *digitalis*, from *digitus*, a finger, in consequence of the resemblance of its flowers to the fingers of a glove. It grows on pastures and exposed hill-sides, and in plantations. This drug is much used by quacks and old women for dropsy and other diseases, often with mischievous results. Mr. Nankivell informs the Author that two of his patients recently were thus killed. For homœopathic uses we employ the *leaves* only.

General Uses.—Disease of the *heart*, with dizziness, tendency to faint, shortness of breath on exercise, palpitation,

† "Copper pennies have gone out of circulation, hard bronze coins have taken their place, and *itch* has increased wonderfully, all within two or three years. Is this a mere coincidence? Next to *Sulphur*—and in some cases beyond *Sulphur*—*Cuprum* is curative in itch."—*Dr. Bayes in the Monthly Homœopathic Review*, March, 1867.

slow, *irregular, and intermittent pulse*, or *quickened and feeble* action of the heart; frontal headache, with heaviness and throbbing, dimness of sight, sparks and colours before the eyes, and buzzing in the ears, also nausea and vomiting, associated with heart-disease; hypertrophy, dilatation, and enfeeblement of the heart, leading to dropsy; dropsy of the kidneys, and suppression of urine; *cyanosis, ascites*, and even *anasarca*, depending upon, or associated with, vascular derangements—heart-disease, menstrual irregularities, etc.; white or ash-coloured stools, either dry or papescent, with white-coated tongue.

33.—Drosera Rotundifolia—*Round-leaved Sundew.*

This plant is indigenous to elevated situations in Great Britain, and flourishes in mossy, turfy bogs. It is called Drosera *(dewy)*, in consequence of its having an appearance as if covered with dew. We express the juice from the whole plant.

General Uses.—*Spasmodic cough; hooping-cough* (the *best* remedy after *Acon.* in uncomplicated cases); *phthisis pulmonalis*, with spasmodic cough, profuse expectoration, hæmoptysis, and gastric irritation, the cough inducing vomiting; coughs, generally, of a *spasmodic* character, coming on suddenly, producing a *fit of coughing*, especially if accompanied with retching or vomiting; nervous and sympathetic cough.

34.—Dulcamara—*Bitter-Sweet—Woody Nightshade.*

This plant flourishes in moist shady hedges and thickets, or on the banks of ditches or streams, bears clusters of bright-red berries, and attains, when supported, to the height of from eight to ten feet. It has acquired its name from *dulcis* (sweet), and *mara* (bitter), owing to the transition of tastes which it yields. We employ the young branches and leaves of the plant when it commences flowering.

General Uses.—Various affections resulting from damp, *or a thorough wetting*, such as cold in the head, short hacking cough, nausea, *diarrhœa*, catarrh of the bladder, itching or stinging *eruptions on the skin*, glandular enlargements about the neck, mild *rheumatism*, with pains worse during rest, and relieved by movement, and other conditions following a *cold*. If this medicine be taken immediately after exposure to damp, it will often prevent the ordinary consequences of a cold. "Threatened paralysis of the lungs which we meet with in old persons at the first setting in of cold weather. It may also be helpful to the same patients when, from weakness, they have to cough a long time to expel phlegm" *(Hughes)*. The alkaloid of *Dulcamara* — *Solania* — is suggested in these affections. Altschul, Hempel, Hughes, and others mention *Dulcamara* for the first stage of Bright's disease.

35.—Euphrasia Officinalis*—*Common Eye-bright.*

This pretty unassuming plant grows on heaths, over the sides of chalky cliffs, and on mountainous meadows, in all parts of Europe. The names given to it in different countries, and during several centuries,—"eye-bright," as in England; "eye-comfort," or "spectacle-breaker," as on the continent; etc.,—all indicate its specific uses in restoring and strengthening the vision.

General Uses.—*Catarrhal inflammation*, with *abundant watery secretion*, sensitiveness to light, and irritation of the frontal sinuses and of the lining of the nose, with sneezing, and copious mucous discharge; smarting or stinging in the

* Abridged from an article in *The Homœopathic World*, Vol. iv, p. 30 *et seq.*, in which cases are given illustrative of its power.

eyes—the effects of light or of cold air; catarrhal inflammation in the first stage of measles; simple *acute inflammation* of the eyes; chronic sore eyes; *amaurotic* conditions from suppressed nasal catarrh; strumous ophthalmia (with *Sulph.*); specks on the cornea. The remedy may also be topically applied as a lotion—six to ten drops in a wine-glassful of water.

36.—Ferrum—*Iron*.

Iron is a metal which is more generally diffused over the globe than any other, and has been known from time immemorial. It occurs native in small quantities, seldom pure, generally oxidized, and united with acids; such as the carbonic, phosphoric, etc. Iron is distinguishable in the residue of the combustion of many plants, and it forms an important constituent of the blood, and other parts of the animal organism. For homœopathic purposes, either the filings of pure metallic iron, prepared by trituration, are used, or the Acetate of Iron—*Ferrum Aceticum*—which is a convenient solution. Other supplementary preparations are also sometimes used—*F. Iodatum*, *F. Muriaticum*, *F. Redactum*, etc.

Pathogenetic Effects.—"According to allopathic physicians, iron is a nervine tonic. This is one of those superficial statements of which old-school treatises on materia medica abound. So far from iron being a tonic, it has, on the contrary, a debilitating and disintegrating effect upon the system. It is no more a tonic than *Arsenic* or *China*. The first effect of iron may be to cause an apparent stimulation of the vital functions, but the physical condition of those who live near iron springs might have sufficed to enlighten physicians concerning the ultimate debilitating effect of iron. We find these people tainted with chronic diseases more than almost any other class of men, even when their mode of life is otherwise unexceptionable. A general or partial debility, bordering upon paralysis, certain violent pains in the extremities, various affections of the abdominal viscera, vomiting of food day and night, pulmonary phthisis, bloody cough, want of animal heat, menstrual suppression, miscarriage, impotence, sterility, jaundice, and other symptoms of cachexia prevail among them" *(Hempel)*.

General Uses.—*Anæmia* and *chlorosis*; *anæmic*, *chlorotic*, and *debilitated conditions*, and other ailments *contingent* upon, or associated with, them; congestive headache; languor; neuralgia; chorea; phthisis; pneumorrhagia; dyspepsia—loss of appetite, coated tongue (white or yellow), oppression and fulness of the stomach and bowels after eating, frequent vomiting of food, constipation with ineffectual urging, or chronic diarrhœa with slimy, and even bloody stools, straining; colliquative diarrhœa; lienteria; ascarides; catarrh of the bladder; involuntary urination of children during the day; impotence; sterility; spermatorrhœa; amenorrhœa; leucorrhœa; dropsy; cold hands and feet, chilblains, and sores in leuco-phlegmatic constitutions; etc.

37.—Gelseminum Sempervirens—*Yellow Jessamine—Woodbine.*

"This is one of the most beautiful climbing plants of the Southern States (America), ascending lofty trees, and forming festoons from one tree to another, and, in its flowering season, in the early Spring, scenting the atmosphere with its delicious odour. On account of its gorgeous yellow flowers, and the rich perfume which they impart, as well as the deep shade it affords, it is extensively cultivated in the gardens of the South, as an ornamental vine" *(Hale)*. We make a tincture from the root.

General Uses.—Affections of the *nervous* and *muscular*

systems. Its action seems to come between that of *Acon.* and *Bell.*; and in some respects it is very similar to *Chloroform.* It is useful in acute pain in the muscles, as from long-continued exertion; the head-symptoms arising from heart-disease; cerebro-spinal meningitis; scarlatina simplex, especially in young children, when there is great restlessness, tendency to remittency, and *Acon.* and *Bell.* fail to bring out the eruption fully and bright; simple fevers of women and children when *Acon.* is not sufficient, or when there is a condition of the brain beyond the reach of *Acon.*, yet not demanding *Bell.*; *infantile remittent fever*, and other fevers having a *remittent* character—evening exacerbations passing off without perspiration,—and without dyspeptic symptoms; nervous fever, "inward fever," etc., without intestinal lesion; measles—in the forming-stage, with chilliness, thin watery discharge from the nose, hoarseness, etc.; tendency to convulsions in children about the time of the eruption in fevers; feverish conditions with great restlessness.

NERVOUS SYSTEM.—Nervous rigors with chattering of the teeth, and shivering, *without chilliness*, from fright, mental emotion, or hysteria; feeling of lightness in the body; aches and pains in the back, shoulders, neck, etc., from spinal irritation; excessive irritability of body and mind; causeless nervous excitement of hysteric patients; semi-stupor, languor, and physical prostration, from night-watching, etc.; sleeplessness and mental apathy of drunkards; hysterical insensibility and lock-jaw; catalepsy; spasm of the glottis; spasmodic croup, when *Acon.* fails, or the brain is involved; coma, and apoplexy from intense passive congestion; sleeplessness from mental excitement; drowsiness in hot weather, when not arising from deranged stomach or liver. In large doses, *Gels.* so paralyses the muscular system, that while the patient is fully conscious, he lies utterly powerless to open his eyes to see, or his mouth to speak; hence it is very useful in some local paralyses.

HEAD.—Passive, venous cerebral congestion, with dull headache and vertigo; hemicrania—dim sight, double vision —and great sensitiveness to all sounds; nervous headache—the pain commencing in the neck and spreading thence over the whole head; sudden headache, with dizziness, heaviness, dulness, and a state of semi-stupor; sunstroke with similar symptoms; brain-fever.

EYES.—Heaviness of the eye-lids; *ptosis*, caused by congestion of the brain; weakness of sight from over-exertion, with *dimness, dryness, and double vision;* heaviness in the head; paralytic squinting; amaurosis, from congestion of the brain, with dilated pupils, or from worms, or from over-doses of *Quinine*, with black spots before the eyes; "thirst for light."

FACE, ETC.—Neuralgia, with twitching of the muscles near the affected part; erythema; papulous eruption, having an evanescent character. Roaring in the ears, with sudden deafness.

CIRCULATORY SYSTEM.—Excessive action of the heart from functional causes, and palpitation, with heavy throbbing; affections of the head and eyes from heart-disease.

RESPIRATORY SYSTEM.—Nasal catarrh—discharge of watery fluid from the nose, with hoarseness, cough, soreness in throat and chest; aphonia, from catarrhal paralysis; affections "from relaxation from the return of hot weather after winter;" acute bronchitis and pneumonia in the first stage, when there is not the excitement calling for *Acon.*

DIGESTIVE SYSTEM.—Pure nervous toothache from cold—a drop of the tincture may be applied to the tooth; "painful dentition, with sudden loud outcries, pulsating fontanelles, and feverishness;" spasmodic affections of the throat, as in hysteria; paralysis of the glottis and other organs of swallowing, whether or not after diphtheria; sore throat, with pain shooting up to the ears, and deafness; cramps and spasmodic conditions of the stomach; congestion of the stomach—sense of a heavy load, with tension, and dull pain; emptiness, "goneness," or false hunger—a gnawing sensation. Diarrhœa, with bilious, papescent stools, much flatulence, and excess of nervous prostration; dysentery, with inflammatory symptoms, creamy or tea-coloured stools, from passive congestion of the liver, inducing languor, drowsiness, dulness or depression, with dull headache, dimness of sight, etc.; jaundice.

Urinary System.—Enuresis in children and old people, from paralysis of the sphincter; spasm of the bladder; spasm of the ureter from the passage of a calculus.

Generative System.—Involuntary emissions *without* erections; flaccidity and coldness of the genitals; seminal weakness from emotional, or local congestive, causes; some cases of spermatorrhœa and spinal exhaustion, from self-abuse. Congestive amenorrhœa from cold; neuralgic or spasmodic dysmenorrhœa and after-pains; simple menorrhagia, without other symptoms; spasmodic gastrodynia of pregnant women; rigidity of the os uteri; puerperal convulsions.

Skin.—Simple erythema and erysipelas, with slight fever; eruptions resembling measles, with pain or irritation.

38.—Glonoine—*Nitro-Glycerine.*

This is a preparation of Glycerine, and Nitric and Sulphuric Acids. While of great service in excavating, its great explosive properties render it extremely perilous; many serious accidents having occurred through the least mismanagement in the transit or storage of the drug. In the human body it acts as quickly as Prussic Acid.

General Uses.—*Congestive headache, fulness, tightness,* and *vertigo; sunstroke,* with sudden falling down, violent dizziness and distress; effects following sun-stroke; congestive headache at the climacteric period and in amenorrhœa from suppression; neuralgia, and puerperal convulsions, with violent cerebral congestion; *nervous palpitation*, etc., from fright, hysteria, etc.; *rush of blood*, with throbbing in the arteries and neck, quickened pulse, etc.

39.—Graphites—*Black-lead—Plumbago.*

The name of this substance is derived from the Greek word *grapheo* (to write), because it is used for writing with. We first make triturations.

General Uses.—Unhealthy condition of the *skin*—chronic eruptions, ulcers, and erysipelas; cracks, and excoriations; tetter. *Constipation*, with large and knotty stools; delayed and scanty menses, especially when co-existing with unhealthy states of the skin, and constipation; swelling and indurations of the testicles; etc.

40.—Hamamelis Virginica—*Witch-hazel.*

An American plant, growing from ten to twenty feet high, somewhat resembling the hazelnut-bush, and bearing fruit which ripens every second year. It derives its English name from its supposed virtue of divination, being relied upon for the discovery of hidden treasures, etc. We use the bark and leaves.

General Uses.—*Varicosis, phlebitis,* and *hæmorrhage.* Varicose veins, not ulcerated (internal and external use); varicose condition of the throat, the veins looking blue, with uneasy sensation in the parts, pain, and hawking up of mucus and blood; painful and *bleeding piles*, with sensation as if the back would break off, for which it is one of the best remedies; *inflammation of the veins*, especially if associated with a varicose condition; hæmorrhage from the *nose*, mouth, cavity of an extracted tooth, *stomach, lungs, bowels,* bladder, *uterus*, or *anus*, when the blood is *venous*, steadily flowing in a dark stream; "hæmorrhage with asthenia or anæmia, or from asthenic tendency, is of itself an indication for the use of *Hamamelis*" *(Belcher)*; headache—fulness, dull pain, and crowding pressure in forehead and between the eyes from venous congestion, especially when leading to expistaxis; blood-shot eyes from hooping-cough; burns of the tongue and lips from hot drinks; intestinal hæmorrhage; dysentery, when the quantity of dark blood is a more prominent symptom than the straining; *ardor urinæ*; vaginal leucorrhœa, with relaxation of the mucous lining, etc.; *vicarious menstruation*—hæmatemesis, etc., or varicosis, with constipation; varicocele; purpura; neuralgia of the testes and ovaries; etc. *Ecchymosis* from a bruise.

External Use.—*Formula.*—One part of the strong tincture to four of water. Besides its external use in nearly

42.—Hepar Sulphuris Calcareum—*Hepar Sulphur—Liver of Sulphur.*

A combination of *Calcarea Carbonica* and *Sulphur*, effected by heat in a hermetically-closed crucible, and forming *Sulphuret of Lime.*

General Uses.—Affections of the *glands, respiratory system*, and *skin;* the *scrofulous* and *syphilitic dyscrasia;* and the evil effects of *Mercury*. Chronic glandular swellings, especially when abscesses form; scrofulous disease of joints; ulcers, and scaly eruptions due to syphilitic infection; suppuration from any part, in scrofulous persons. It promotes and regulates suppuration in a remarkable manner (second only to *Silicea*).

Head, Eyes, etc.—Headache at the root of the nose; chronic periodical hemicrania, with boring pain; "shudderings extending to the top of the head, the hair being painful to the touch;" ulcers of the conjunctiva which are apt to return; sore eyes, chronic, with frequent inflammation and free discharge, in scrofulous children; scrofulous ozœna and otorrhœa.

Respiratory System.—Hoarseness, with wheezing breathing; hoarse cough following measles; membranous croup; catarrh of the larynx and trachea, with roughness and hoarseness, severe, deep, dry cough, particularly in the evening, and easily excited by exposure, "sensation as of a clot of mucus, or of internal swelling, when swallowing," and titillation in the throat; cough with those symptoms, at first dry, afterwards moist, and yielding tenacious mucus; chronic bronchitis; phthisis pulmonalis in the scrofulous.

Skin.—Unhealthy, and chapped or cracked skin; fissures in the palms of the hands; *abscesses, whitlow, boils*, and threatened *carbuncles;* chronic erysipelas; chronic herpes.

Digestive System.—Acute quinsy; swollen tonsils; salivation, spongy gums, and other conditions of the mouth, from Allopathic doses of *Mercury*; chronic dyspepsia, with frequently and easily deranged stomach; chronic congestion of the liver, with abdominal distress, impeding free respiration, and causing a sense of oppression; "obstinate constipation, from a congested condition of the rectum" *(Bayes)*, and piles, from the same cause.

43.—Hydrastis Canadensis—*Golden Seal.*

We are indebted to America for this valuable remedy. The plant is indigenous to North America, flowers in May and June, and is used by the Indians to colour their clothing yellow; combined with Indigo, it forms a fine green.

General Uses.—*Cancerous affections*, especially when involving *glandular* structures, and their associated *debility*: in

44.—Hyoscyamus Niger—*Black Henbane.*

This plant is indigenous throughout Europe, growing in uncultivated places in the neighbourhood of farms, villages, etc. The shrub may be recognised by its fœtid odour when pressed. We use the whole plant.

General Uses.—Functional diseases of the *brain and nervous system*, characterised by great nervous irritability and a too-active condition of the sensorial functions.

Nervous System.—Delirium, without the congestion indicating *Bell.*, or the fury calling for *Stram.*; "complete loss of sense, urine being passed unconsciously, delirium coming on with occasional fits of excitement, in which the patient tears at the bed-clothes, attempts to fling off everything, or makes motions as if he were at his employment; afterwards he falls asleep for some hours, waking at intervals with fits of excitement" *(Bayes)*; delirium tremens; brain-troubles of children, not requiring *Bell.*; excitement preventing sleep; mild delirium of typhus, typhoid, and puerperal fevers; phrenitis; epileptic and hysteric convulsions, and eclampsia. Fainting fits of hysteria.

Head, etc.—Squinting, stammering, twitching in the face, and other choreaic movements in children; giddiness and stupefaction, dull and haggard expression, excessive dilatation of the pupils, and loss of speech; disturbance of the visual function—a tailor, under the influence of this plant, could not thread his needle, it seemed to have three points.

Respiratory System.—Nervous dry cough, *commencing on lying down*, relieved by sitting up, and coming on at night; spasmodic, nervous coughs of children, old people, and hysteric persons.

Digestive System, etc.—Vomiting from brain-disturbance; hysterical vomiting; painless diarrhœa, especially in females; involuntary nocturnal urination.

45.—Ignatia Amara—*St. Ignatius' Bean.*

The *Strychnos St. Ignatii* is a climbing bush, which, like the *Strychnos Nux Vomica*, grows on the islands of the east and south-east coasts of Asia. Although the two plants are of one family, the seeds of the former contain more strychnia than the latter, and there is a considerable difference in their respective therapeutic effects. "There is a great correspondence between *Ignatia* and *Phosphoric Acid* in their general sphere" *(Bayes)*.

General Uses.—*Hysteria*, and other *nervous disorders*; sensation in the throat as of a lump there; globus hystericus; epileptiform convulsions, and other convulsive affections of children, especially if from fright or worms; hypochondriasis; alternate sadness and gaiety; very acute sensibility of the body; sleeplessness, and the consequences of *fright or grief* in persons of an exalted impressionability, especially women and children; excessive convulsive yawning; great perspirations during meals; stiffness of the back from irritation of the spine.

Head, etc.—Paroxysms of headache, with sensation as if a nail were pressed into the brain; weight at the back of the head, the patient being continually inclined to lean it back upon something for support; face-ache and tooth-ache, with crushing pain, or digging and soreness in the teeth.

Respiratory System.—Sensation as if a cold in the head were coming on, with aching in the forehead; nervous cough, with irritation in the throat-pit, in females; bronchial catarrh of old people where *spasm* is a prominent symptom; constriction of the chest; dyspnœa.

Digestive System, etc.—Indigestion, with great n depression; distress in the stomach, and periodica hysteric persons; feeling of weakness at the acute pain in the anus; constipation, with free ful desire for stool, and prolapsus ani, in *children; premature menses, etc.*

46.—Iodium—*Iodine.*

This is an elementary substance, named from *Iodes* (violet colour), on account of the beautiful and characteristic colour of its vapour. It exists in the mineral and vegetable kingdoms, and largely in marine plants. It is chiefly obtained from incinerated sea-weed or kelp. Coindet, who first instituted inquries concerning the curative properties of *Iodine*, found that the therapeutic virtues of *Spongia* were due to the presence of *Iodine* in that substance; nevertheless, *Spongia* has a sphere of its own apart from that of *Iodine*.

General Uses.—Scrofulous affections of the glands; scrofulous inflammation of the joints; *goitre;* inflammation of the lymphatic glands; general emaciation, with colliquative sweats and diarrhœa, like as in hectic fever; wasting of the body from non-assimilation of the fatty elements of food, with a tendency to consumption of the lungs, or, in children, of the bowels; fainting-turns; thin, watery condition of the blood and secretions; scrofulous ulcers and caries; great and lasting anxiety of a peculiar character, referring to the present rather than the future—a sense of "discouragement and dispiritedness, which is particularly depressing."

Nervous System.—Tremblings, with emaciation; chorea, in scrofulous subjects, with exhaustion, wasting, etc.; marasmus of children and females; mercurial wasting, and tremor; paralysis from deficient innervation, with atrophy and sinking of vitality, from care, want, etc.; despondency.

Head.—Pressure in the forehead and back of the head, with confusion, sense of gnawing hunger, followed by thin diarrhœic discharges; chronic nervous headaches from stomachic derangement; congestive headache, with fulness, giddiness, drowsiness, etc., especially in old people.

Eyes, Ears, and Nose.—Scrofulous ophthalmia, with photophobia, obscuration of vision, etc.; chronic catarrhal deafness with, or following, glandular or throat affection; scrofulous or syphilitic ozœna, with fetor, loss of smell, etc.

Circulatory System.—Palpitation, with quickened pulse, and weakness, leading to fainting; intermittent pulse; constriction about the heart and chest.

Respiratory System.—Inflammatory croup (when membrane forms, *Iod.* should be administered internally and by inhalation); chronic laryngitis, with hoarseness, aching and sore pains; paroxysms of cough with discharge of lumps of hardened mucus; laryngeal phthisis; hoarseness, with fits of deep, dry cough; dry, hard, barking cough; chronic bronchitis, with tearing and suffocative cough, tickling in the throat, constriction, burning sensation, wheezing, and expectoration of blood-streaked, or even purulent, mucus; chronic pneumonia, with abscesses; tightness of the chest, with pressing, burning, and palpitation; cough with hæmoptysis, wasting, and night-sweats; cough and phthisical symptoms following the disappearance of glandular swellings; phthisis pulmonalis, with the general symptoms indicative of this remedy.

Digestive System.—Salivation, especially mercurial, with disorganization of the gums, paleness of the face, emaciation, and small quick pulse; salivation from pregnancy; unnatural hunger with emaciation; bad digestion, with morbid hunger, diarrhœic stools, and wasting, the food not being assimilated; diarrhœa of scrofulous children, the discharges being thin and fœtid, and accompanied by distension of the bowels, pinching and cutting pains, etc.; tabes mesenterica, with cough, and hectic symptoms; disease of the pancreas; enlargement of the liver, chronic jaundice, etc., in the scrofulous, with wasting, especially when dependent on organic disease.

Generative System.—Atrophy or induration of the testes, with impotence; hydrocele. Amenorrhœa in girls having a phthisical tendency, emaciation, etc.; falling away of the

breasts; amenorrhœa of scrofulous subjects, wit
loss of appetite, costiveness, distension of the bow
breathing, palpitation, etc.; premature and pr
or profuse discharge of thin, watery fluid, with
dizziness, frontal headache, etc.; dysmenorrhœa
symptoms; sterility, metritis, and chronic vag
scrofulous; fœtid leucorrhœa, with emaciation
flow of milk, continuing after ceasing suckling, v
ovarian cysts, atrophy, etc.

SKIN.—Chronic erythematous, papular, and p
tions of scrofulous children; "a remarkable im
the beauty of the hair and cleanliness of the sc
observed to follow its use in these subjects" (H

47.—Ipecacuanha—*Ipecacuanha.*

This is a creeping herbaceous perennial pla
plentifully in the wooded tracts of Central Sou
particularly in Brazil. Its root is the *Ipecacu*
merce.

GENERAL USES.—*Spasmodic* affections of th
system and *stomach*, of an intermittent or paroxy
ter, especially occurring at night; intermittent
predominence of gastric symptoms. *Ipec.* best s
who are feeble and slender, with sensitive temper
fretful, impatient, or apathetic disposition.

HEAD.—Hemicrania, paroxysmal, with fine sti
and soreness.

RESPIRATORY SYSTEM.—Spasmodic sneezing,
bleed, or running of watery fluid from the nose, an
redness, and smarting of the eyes; spasmodic cou
with tickling in the larynx, retching, and vomitin
cough with pain in the umbilical region, as i

would be ruptured; hooping-cough, during the early stage, with great accumulation of mucus, and vomiting; paroxysmal cough with *hæmoptysis;* bronchial catarrh, with excessive quantities of mucus, causing vomiting in the effort to expel it. *Ipec.* is a good expectorant. Sudden hæmorrhage from the lungs in phthisis; hay-fever; spasmodic asthma, with anguish, deathly paleness, dread of death; nocturnal asthma, coming on suddenly, with similar symptoms, cold extremities, ending in profuse expectoration of mucus.

Digestive System.—*Nausea and vomiting,* with abundant flow of watery saliva, qualmishness, sense of emptiness of the stomach, and *moist, yellowish* or *white-coated tongue;* vomiting of pregnancy, with similar symptoms; *hæmatemesis* (see also "Generative System"), with moist tongue and flow of saliva; vomiting of blood, mucus, or bile, of a greenish or blackish colour, with straining and retching; loss of appetite; oppression after food, want of tone in the stomach, flow of saliva, frequent retching and vomiting; spasmodic cardialgia, neuralgic and bilious colic, with pinching and cutting pains about the navel; diarrhœa, with nausea, vomiting, and bloody, or foul-smelling stools; dysentery, with moist furred tongue, profuse discharge of mucous and greenish matter, and blood; autumnal diarrhœa, with griping, straining, nausea, and vomiting.

Urinary, and Female Generative Systems.—Hæmaturia, with qualmishness and nausea in the stomach and bowels; thick, reddish urine. Sudden discharge of bright-red blood from the uterus, after labour, with sickness at the stomach, dizziness, headache, cold, pale face; menorrhag with similar symptoms; *hæmatemesis* associated with *irr menstruation* or the critical age.

48.—Iris Versicolor—*Blue-flag.*

Blue-flag is an aquatic plant common throughout the United States, presenting blue or purple flowers from May to July. "It is probable that its employment as a remedial agent was first suggested to the profession by the Indians, who, it is said, value it as one of their most powerful medicines. A traveller among the tribes in Georgia and Florida mentions having seen an artificial pond in almost every village, covered with a luxuriant growth of the *Iris*, and which was constructed for its especial cultivation. In times of prevailing sickness, they would partake freely of a decoction of the root, which, together with prayer and fasting, they consider an efficient guard against an attack of the epidemic" *(Hale's "New Remedies")*.

General Uses.—Affections of the mucous membrane, stomach, and alimentary canal, and the pancreas and other glands, associated with abnormal secretion, salivation, vomiting, and purging; some scrofulous, mercurial, and syphilitic conditions; vesiculo-pustular eruptions on the skin and scalp; mercurial salivation; etc. *Iris* similates Mercury to a remarkable degree, stopping short of the great disorganizing effects of that drug.

"Nearly all the conditions for which *Iris* is applicable are characterized by unusual lassitude, prostration, and lowness of spirits, these conditions being probably due to the disturbing action which the drug exercises upon the liver and gastric mucous membrane. It is most useful in persons of bilious temperament, subject to gastric and bilious disorders."

Head.—*Sick-headache*, gastric or hepatic: in this affection, *Iris* is considered to be the best remedy; the pain is generally in the forehead and right side of the head, is aggravated by rest and on first moving the head, but relieved by continual motion, and is often accompanied by vomiting or diarrhœa; neuralgia of the right side of the face.

EYES.—Simple inflammation of the eye-lids from cold, especially when associated with diarrhœa.

DIGESTIVE SYSTEM.—Inflammation of the mouth and fauces, with or without ulceration, with painful burning, and salivation, but without fetor; salivation, etc., after diphtheria; burning distress in the region of the stomach and pancreas; "pancreatic salivation;" sour *vomiting*, with headache; acidity, and eructations of food; indigestion dependent on defective secretion of the pancreas, rendering the digestion of starchy and fatty foods imperfect; simple affections of the liver; *diarrhœa*, with burning in the rectum and anus; diarrhœa not followed by constipation; looseness of the bowels, with almost constant uneasiness and grinding in the bowels—"a grumbling belly-ache"—discharge of fetid flatulence and fæces, or the evacuations may be green; periodical diarrhœa occurring at night; cholera infantum, especially when vomiting is very prominent; cholera, with great pain in the pit of the stomach, around the navel, or low down in the bowels, with every fit of vomiting or purging; English cholera; involuntary diarrhœa, rice-water evacuations, cramps, and choleraic expression of countenance; summer and autumnal diarrhœa with watery or bilious evacuations, and when *vomiting* is frequent.

GENERATIVE SYSTEM *(Male)*.—Seminal emissions with amorous dreams; spermatorrhœa, with lowness of spirits.

49.—Kali Bichromicum—*Bichromate of Potash.*

We are indebted to Dr. Drysdale of Liverpool for the introduction of this drug into our Materia Medica. by the symptoms which have been observed in the employed in the bichromate-of-potash factories, now recommended, and has been used with suc important affections. It is prepared for use ei *or trituration.*

General Uses.—Affections of the [illegible] skin, fibrous tissues, liver, and kidneys; ophthalmia; *rheumatism*, with coldness of the affected parts, esp there are, at the same time, papular eruptions on syphilis; etc. It is probably seldom indicated nervous system is involved, or in toxæmic conditions

Eyes and Nose.—Ophthalmia, catarrhal or with redness of the conjunctiva, agglutination of the discharge of yellow matter. Inflammation and of the nose, with serous, purulent, and bloody sometimes coming away in tough, elastic plugs; p the nose.

Respiratory System.—Acute coryza; chronic c head; influenza, without much nervous prostratio and *chronic bronchitis*, with *tough and stringy*, or *expectoration*, and dyspnœa, especially when there i tion at the same time; membranous croup; burn in the middle of the sternum; cough, followed b dizziness, and *difficult expectoration* of *tough*, blood mucous.

Digestive System.—Ulcerated sore throat, with of a yellow, *tenacious* matter, and syphilitic sore thr the ulceration is not deep; indigestion, "from chron catarrh, with *yellowish* coated tongue;" nausea and with sense of coldness in the stomach; ulceratio stomach, with soreness and tenderness, dryness of th etc.; ulceration of the intestines; dull pain in hypochondrium, and whitish stools; suppression following Asiatic cholera.

Skin.—Pustular eruptions; ulcers of the legs; ul dark centres and over-hanging edges, especially of a character; pimples on the face, nose, forehead, and s

---

50.—Kali Hydriodicum—*Kali Iodidum—Iodide of Potash.*

This remedy is very largely used by Allopathic practitioners, and has a similar general sphere of action to that of *Iodium*.

General Uses.—Secondary and tertiary syphilis; chronic rheumatism; coryza, the nose being red and swollen, and the discharge not causing soreness; ozœna; swelling and cracking of the tongue; sore eyes; chronic sore throat; acute and chronic hydrocephalus; epilepsy and paralysis of a syphilitic origin; some forms of cutaneous disease—psoriasis, lupus, etc. "The pains which *iodide of potassium* removes are almost always worse at night, and such a character of the disease may be accepted as a strong indication for the medicine" *(Ringer).*

51.—Kreasotum—*Kreasote.*

This substance is obtained by the destructive distillation of organic substances, contained in tar, the smoke of wood, etc. The word is derived from *Kreas* (flesh) and *sodso* (I preserve), on account of its antiseptic properties. The word is frequently spelt *Creosote*, which is incorrect. M. Teste declares that the continued use of *smoked meat* produces destructive effects in the mouth, carrying off the teeth, inducing foul breath, costiveness, and a bad state of the body generally.

General Uses.—*Decay of the teeth*, and *toothache* from that cause (compare *Mercurius); morbid dentition*, especially when the teeth decay as they appear, and the patient is cachectic and troubled with constipation (compare *Chamomilla*); *vomiting*, sympathetic of disease not in the stomach, as in phthisis, cancer of the liver, kidney-disease, etc; vomiting of pregnancy and hysterical vomiting; constant nausea and inclination to vomit, without actual vomiting, but with a sense of coldness in the stomach; diarrhœa and dysentery, when the discharges are putrid; gastro-intestinal inflammation; diabetes mellitus. Foul vaginal discharges, malignant uterine ulcerations, premature menstruation with discharge of fœtid blood, nervousness, etc.; *foul, corrosive leucorrhœa;* putrid-smelling lochial discharge. Syphilitic eruptions. In burns, scalds, chilblains, and foul ulcers a lotion may be applied externally—one drop of pure *Kreasote* to sixty or eighty of water. M. Teste thinks that *Kreas.* is most suitable to delicate or cachectic children. In affections of the teeth the higher potencies should be used—12th to 30th; in vomiting, the lower—2nd or 3rd.

52.—Lachesis—*Lachesis.*

The substance known in Homœopathic therapeutics by this name is the poison of the lance-headed viper *(Trigonocephalus lachesis).* The bite of this serpent is generally fatal. Our use of its virus is chiefly founded on the symptoms presented by those who have been bitten. We have very little personal experience of this medicine.

General Uses.—Putrid sore-throat (not diphtheritic); irritable throat, inducing cough; globus hystericus; suffocative fits of cough; excessive vomiting during hooping-cough; spasmodic stricture of the œsophagus; nervous palpitation from heart-disease, accompanied by anxious, wheezing respiration, asthmatic cough, tendency to vomit, etc.; some cases of chronic constipation in females, and when there is alternate relaxation and constipation; nervous affections of women at the climacteric period—flushes, with headache and sleeplessness; burning pains in the top of the head; pains in the back; melancholy; etc. Traumatic, gangrene, and skin and other diseases, in which, as in cases of the serpent's bite, the blood becomes tainted by the local affection—carbuncle, pyæmia from phlebitis, putrid sore throat—with prostration of the nervous energies.

53.—Lycopodium Clavatum—*Wolf's-foot, Club-moss.*

This plant is found throughout Europe, in stony and hilly places. We use the pollen or powder (Sporulæ Lycopodii); it will not sink in, or absorb, water, and adheres to the fingers when touched. In its crude state it is all but inert; but Hahnemann's process of trituration renders it a potent remedy in many diseases.

General Uses.—Affections of the digestive, urinary, and respiratory mucous membrane, and the skin.

In the following conditions, if there be consentaneous mental and physical weakness, sallow complexion, loss of appetite, slow and depraved digestion, flatulence, and constipation, *Lycopodium* will almost certainly prove curative.

Respiratory System.—*Chronic* catarrh, and, perhaps, bronchitis, with *much general weakness;* "chronic superficial ulcerations, having a tendency to spread, in the throat, soft-palate, tonsils, and pharynx" *(Bayes).* "Chronic pneumonia, with purulent, foul-smelling expectoration; early stages of phthisis pulmonalis, when supervening on bronchial catarrh, with much free mucous expectoration."

Digestive System.—*Dyspepsia—water-brash, acidity, heart-burn, flatulence* in the intestines, *constipation* with torpor, sense of warmth and dryness of the bowels, and *gravel* in the urine; enteritis of infants, from indigestible food; chronic congestion of the liver, with pain in the right side and back; "unconquerable sleep after dinner, followed by great exhaustion."

Urinary System.—Frequent or painful urination, the urine being cloudy, depositing a sediment, and sometimes mixed with mucous and blood; catarrh of the bladder; spasmodic retention of urine or incontinence of urine, of children; stranguary dependent on the presence of gravel or pus in the urine, or atony of the mucous membrane; *gravel* (lithic acid deposits).

SKIN.—Intertrigo; porrigo favosa; plica polonica; chronic inflammation of the skin; sallowness; cold extremities.

54.—Mercurius—*Mercury*.

There are several preparations of *Mercury* used by Homœopathic physicians, the principal of which are—*M. Solubilis Hahnemanni*, the black oxide of Mercury, first prepared by Hahnemann; *M. Vivus*, quicksilver; *M. Corrosivus*, corrosive sublimate or bichloride of Mercury; *M. Iodatus*, or *Bin-iodatus*, iodide, or bin-iodide of Mercury; and *Cinnabaris*, red sulphuret of Mercury. The general effects of all are so similar, that we have thought it best, in this edition, to speak of them under one signature—MERCURIUS—pointing out at the end of the section the main distinctions between different forms or combinations of the drug.

GENERAL USES.—*Unhealthy and liquefied state of the blood*, the secretions being fœtid, the complexion sallow, the skin generally pale and dull, and the system liable to ecchymosis passive hæmorrhages and effusions—purpura hæmorrhagica, anæmia, anasarca, etc.; *cachectic conditions of the whole nervous system*, the mind losing its power, the patient becoming irritable, the limbs trembling, and the body wasting or appearing to be ill-nourished and unhealthy; the glands enlarge and tend to suppuration or disorganization, the mucous membranes and the skin are disposed to ulceration generally unhealthy, and the secretions from the former are abnormal and excessive, and the perspirations from the latter copious, and sour or fœtid.

Congestions of the head, lungs, liver, bowels, etc., accompanied by chills, and followed by *slight* fever, heat, dryness of the mouth and throat, restlessness, etc., aggravated in the evening and night. *Dropsy* of the extremities, and ascites, when due to jaundice, liver-disease, or general cachexia, with sallow, yellowish-greenish and cold skin, feeble and slightly hurried pulse, thick and foul-smelling urine, constipation, and dry, light-coloured fæces. *Rheumatism*, the pains being hard aching, or crushing pains in the bones, with coldness or chilliness, followed by slight fever; local rheumatism, chronic, or during rheumatic fever, the parts perspiring freely without relief of the pain; rheumatism, with profuse, sour sweats, not relieving the symptoms; sub-acute periostitis, in cachectic patients; *scurvy*.

The following are the general indications for the employment of *Mercurius*. *Impoverished, pale, sallow,* or *unhealthy appearance;* symptoms of *bilious or liver derangement; offensive breath;* impaired appetite; *liability to derangements of the mucous membrane*—cold in the head, inflammation of the eyes, sore throat, dyspepsia, diarrhœa, etc.—*from a draught of air, unfavourable change of weather, etc.;* increased susceptibility to impressions; *sensitiveness of the skin* to cold and damp, with *chilliness;* in febrile conditions, the *fever* is slight, with somewhat quickened, soft, full, and easily compressed pulse, and the precursory chills, though very uncomfortable, are slight; the pains and symptoms generally are *worse* in the evening and at *night;* there is *chronic perspiration*, especially at night, or clammy sweat on the least exertion; and there is weariness, coldness of the extremities, *depression of spirits* or enfeebled mental power, irritability, restlessness, etc.

Mercurius, however, is not adapted to patients who have been previously drugged with large and long-continued doses of Mercury; *Hepar Sulph.*, *Nit. Ac.*, or some other remedy, is then more suitable.

Nervous System.—Trembling of the hands and the body generally, in cachectic individuals, from want, etc.; imbecility, softening of the brain, chorea, and hydrocephalus, from previous impoveri the nervous system; syphilitic paralysis; wakef night, and disturbing dreams, with drowsiness by da lessness with beating at the pit of the stomach, profus and depression of spirits.

Head.—*Headache from cold*, as in cold in the h sense of *tightness* round the head, irritation of the ey ness over the nose and in the jaw-bones, running from the eyes and nose, chilliness; *rheumatic heada* pains in the bones of the skull, tearing in the sensation as if the skin were tightly drawn over pains in the forehead, and general chilliness, cold h face; *bilious headache*, the head feeling full, as if ti with sensitiveness, flushed, swollen, and hot face, flow of saliva, vomiting of bile, etc.

Eyes.—Inflammation of the eyes from cold, with and burning, agglutination of the lids, sensation as in the eyes; chronic sore eyes in unhealthy subjec fulous and syphilitic ophthalmia; conjunctivitis, i retinitis; chronic inflammation and swelling of the m glands.

Ears.—Otitis, with severe pain, discharge of fœti pus and blood, buzzing and fluttering noises, worse earache, and partial deafness, from cold, with much and muco-purulent discharge from, the ears, swellin glands, offensive breath, etc.

Nose.—Swelling and inflammation of the nose, g to suppuration or ulceration, and discharging foul p mation of crusts in the nostrils; muco-purulent runn the nose; syphilitic ozœna.

Respiratory System.—Cold in the head—runnin

coryza, sneezing, watering of the eyes, tightness of the head, and chilliness; hoarseness, with dryness of the throat; cough, with yellow expectoration consisting of mucus or mucus and pus of a sweetish or saltish taste; dry, hacking cough, which shakes the chest, with dryness and tightness in the chest, worse at night, relieved for a time by drinking cold water, and a sense as though the cough would be altogether relieved if the parts could be lubricated; cough in chronic bronchitis and consumption, with similar symptoms, or expectoration of muco-purulent matter and blood, when occurring in cachectic patients, and following scarlet fever.

Digestive System.—*Mouth, etc.*—Inflammation and ulceration of the mouth, tongue, fauces, and tonsils, with swelling of the glands, and slight fever; sore mouth of nursing women; thrush, even with ulceration, and especially when the affection extends down the alimentary canal; cancrum oris; low inflammation and swelling of the tongue; scurvy, sponginess and bleeding of the gums; cracks at the corners of the mouth; coppery or brassy taste, or foul taste, whitish or yellowish coating on the tongue, slimy state of the mouth, and offensive breath; salivation, simple, or in pregnant women; mumps; swelling of glands after scarlet fever. *Teeth.*—*Toothache*—the teeth are *loose* and feel *sore*, the gums swell and are sensitive, the pains are throbbing or jerking, *worse at night*, accompanied by *salivation*, and often make the patient perspire, though there is a general sense of *chilliness;* gum-boils, with similar symptoms. *Throat.*—Sore throat, with *aching* pain which makes swallowing difficult, or with pain as if a sharp body were sticking in the throat, with dryness, and, occasionally, a sense as of hot vapour rising in the throat; low form of, or chronic, sore throat, with pale or *bluish-red swelling*, great sense of dryness, hawking of tenacious glassy mucus, and tendency to ulceration; syphilitic sore throat, with similar symptoms; sore, ulcerated, putrid, gangrenous throat of scarlatina anginosa, with *swelling* of the glands. *Glands.*—Inflammation, swelling, and induration or suppuration of the parotid, submaxillary, or sublingual glands, from cold, with soreness and heat, and, perhaps, salivation; mumps. *Stomach.*—Burning in the pit of the stomach, with soreness, oppression after food; dyspepsia, from torpor of the liver, with bilious vomiting, constipation, offensive urine, depositing brownish sediment; acute gastritis. *Pancreas.*—Fulness in the left hypochondrium, with burning pain and tenderness in the region of the pancreas, and increased secretion from the organ—frothy and watery diarrhœa, or whitish, tough, and greenish evacuations. *Liver.*—Chronic congestion, enlargement, and induration of the liver, with aching, dull pain, oppression, soreness, uncomfortable heat, oppressed breathing, the patient being unable to lie on the right side, and general bilious symptoms; torpid liver, deficient secretion of bile, pale, costive, and offensive motions, loss of appetite, depression of spirits; cirrhosis; chronic jaundice, with constipation, pale and dry fæces, deep-yellow urine, soft and feeble pulse; *simple jaundice, especially in children. Bowels.*—Diarrhœa—vitiated, coloured, slimy, offensive, excoriating the anus, especially in children; diarrhœa from cold—watery, with heat and flatulence, and sensation as if the bowels were loose in the abdomen, shaking when walking, chilliness, headache, foul taste, salivation, debility; bilious diarrhœa, with green, dark-brown, or excoriating evacuations, distension and soreness of the bowels; watery diarrhœa, and emaciation; diarrhœa of infants, with green motions, or like stirred eggs, flatulence, etc.; dysentery—passage of bloody mucus, tenesmus or involuntary pressing down, chilliness or slight fever, with chalky sediment in urine; inflammation of the cæcum, colon, and rectum, with ulceration; pains in the hip and sacrum from disease in the rectum—hæmorrhoids, dysentery, etc.

Constipation, following bilious diarrhœa, the fæces being dark-brown or green, lumpy, and covered with mucus; or constipation, with an occasional attack of bilious diarrhœa. *Anus.*—Soreness of the anus, sharp, sticking pains, with oozing of serous fluid, foul smelling; white piles. Ascarides and lumbrici in patients having the characteristic cachexia indicating *Mercurius*. Peritonitis, with effusion.

URINARY SYSTEM.—Nephritis, non-desquamative; catarrh of the bladder; albuminuria; suppression of urine from acute inflammation or congestion; frequent and painful urination.

GENERATIVE SYSTEM.—Inflammation of the mucous membrane of the glans penis; swelling of scrotum, with erection of penis; coldness and shrinking of the genitals; spermatorrhœa, and gleet, in cachectic subjects; gonorrhœa; chancre; syphilitic sores. Mr. Nankivell informs the author that *Mercurius* will resolve incipient buboes, and even when these are on the point of suppuration. Purulent and corrosive leucorrhœa, and prolapsus of the vagina, with heat, pain, and soreness; profuse menstruation from liquefaction of the blood, in patients presenting the *Mercurius* cachexia—general weakness and wasting, œdema, coldness, paleness, short breath, etc.; sore breasts in similar patients.

SKIN.—Chronic *sweating*, sour or fœtid; perspiration on the least exertion; vesicular and pustular eruptions; cracking of the hands; porrigo of the scalp; scrofulous and syphilitic eruptions and ulcers; impetigo, rupia, and other destructive conditions; nightly itching or fine biting sensations without eruption (from approaching jaundice). "The only practical rule for the administration of *Mercurius* in vesicular, pustular, and papular rashes, in the absence of general indications is, that on pressure over the reddish blush which surrounds these, the colour of the skin remains coppery or yellowish-brown until the blood returns to the surface. In very unhealthy subjects these vesicular and pustular rashes have a tendency to run into sores" (*Bayes*).

Different Forms of Mercurius, and the Diseases to which they are specially adapted.

Merc. Bin-iodatus.—Goitre; glandular swellings; also when such swellings occur during, or follow, scarlet fever; chronic bronchitis in the strumous; polypus of the nose; chronic catarrh.

Merc. Corrosivus.—Ophthalmia, gastritis, enteritis, dysentery, liver-disease, peritonitis, urinary affections, gonorrhœa; impetigo capitis; some of the syphilitic eruptions.

Merc. Sulphuratus Ruber—Cinnabaris.—Chronic gonorrhœa, gleet, chancre, and enlargement of the inguinal glands.

Merc. Solubilis and *Merc. Vivus* are prescribed by many Homœopathic physicians indifferently, as the effects of both are nearly identical throughout. It was the *Merc. Sol.*, however, which was proved by Hahnemann.

55.—Muriatis Acidum—*Muriatic Acid—Hydrochloric Acid.*

General Uses.—*Low forms of toxæmic fevers*—typhus, etc.; aphthous, ulcerative, and malignant affections of the mouth, tongue, and throat; scarlatina anginosa in the putrid stage; diphtheria (as a local application); blackish or brownish sordes on the teeth; etc. In the above conditions it rivals *Arsenicum*. Hempel suggests *Muriatic Ac.* for chronic catarrh following scarlatina, and we have found it very useful in several affections during, or consequent on, scarlatina, typhoid, etc., especially deafness, offensive purulent running from the ears, nose, etc., more particularly in scrofulous patients; burning itching eruptions, ulcers secreting a fœtid ichor, eczema

56.—Nitri Acidum—*Nitric Acid.*

General Uses.—Chronic *scrofulous*, *syphilitic*, and *mercurial*, affections:—Purulent ophthalmia and otorrhœa; ozœna; sore, diphtheritic, and ulcerated throat (internally and as a gargle); salivation, with spongy swelling and bleeding of the gums; heart-burn, with sour eructations; chronic gastritis and cardialgia of drunkards; chronic violent laryngeal cough, dry, with stinging or smarting sensation on one side, as if a small ulcer were there; hooping-cough; chronic liver-disease; chronic diarrhœa and dysentery; fistula and fissure of the anus; prolapsus ani; torpid hæmorrhoids, the tissues having lost their contractile power; enuresis, with fœtid purulent urine; chronic corrosive and fœtid leucorrhœa; soft chancre; condylomata; ulcers, with rapid destruction of tissue, soft edges, of grayish-green colour, and tendency to *fungoid growths* (proud flesh, etc.); chronic varicose veins, with tendency to ulceration. In the toxæmic fevers *Nitric Ac.* is frequently required, especially in typhoid or malignant scarlatina, small-pox, etc.

57.—Nux Vomica—*Strychnos Nux Vomica—Vomit-nut.*

This is the seed of a tree of considerable size, indigenous to the Indian Archipelago, Southern India, Ceylon, etc. The fruit is a smooth berry, of the size of a large apple, of a beautiful orange colour, containing several circular flat seeds, covered with fine hairs. For homœopathic purposes we use the seeds *(nuces vomicæ)*, from which, when pulverized, we prepare an intensely bitter tincture or trituration, which, like other bitters, excite an increased secretion of saliva.

General Uses.—*Spasmodic affections of the nervous system dyspepsia, with constipation;* intermittent fever, with predominance of dyspeptic symptoms, crampy pains, etc. It is

constipation, or uneven action of the bowels, ✕
up early in the morning with headache anc
ideas, falling again into a heavy, unrefresh
generally most benefited by the administr
Vomica. The symptoms generally occur, or a
early in the morning, and are aggravated by fo
exertion.

NERVOUS SYSTEM.—*Tetanus*, without loss of
tetanic spasms alternating with relaxation a
spasm, pain, and *weariness*, with sensation in t
bruised; trembling of the limbs as in drunka
the attacks being preceded by dizziness, and c
sensations, as from insects, *in the face*, which a
violent jerks of the arms, ending in loss of
convulsive movements excited by touch; *mor*
the senses: paralysis of drunkards; early sta
tremens; tendency to apoplexy; neuralgic af
spinal marrow, with tingling, hard aching,
aggravated by motion or contact, restless slee
ful dreams, night-mare, mental depression, h
and other nervous diseases, associated with indi

HEAD.—*Headache*, congestive, worse after
throbbing, giddiness, flushed face, aching a
would split, and stupefaction, often connected
vomiting, or constipation, and increased by
stooping, and especially when occurring in st

persons; hysteric hemicrania; headache following intoxication; severe headache beginning with dazzling of the sight; luminous vibrations and waverings seen a little distance from the eyes, confusing the sight.

RESPIRATORY SYSTEM.—"Stuffy" cold in the head; dry, racking, spasmodic cough, causing soreness in the pit of the stomach, and aching of the head as if it would split; cough associated with gastric or liver derangement; chronic bronchitis of old people, with profuse and difficult expectoration; *spasmodic asthma*, the muscles of the chest being rigid during the attack, the patient oppressed with anxiety, and complaining of a soreness or aching under the breast-bone, the paroxysm ending in copious vomiting of phlegm; shocks and palpitation of the heart during asthma; spasm of the heart.

DIGESTIVE SYSTEM.—Toothache, associated with indigestion or pregnancy; spasmodic hiccough and difficulty of swallowing; *dyspepsia*, "the fore half of the tongue being comparatively clean and the back part coated with a deep fur" *(Bayes)*; sour, foul, or bitter taste in the mouth; *flatulence*; heart-burn; rising of a sour and bitter fluid; *water-brash*; "eructation of food soon after it is swallowed, without retching or straining, the food tasting much as it did when swallowed;" *cardialgia*, oppression of the stomach after eating, with depression of the spirits, ill-humour; sense of weight or pressure in the stomach, with soreness and sensitiveness; *acute indigestion* from indigestible food, or after intoxication, with pain, retching, and vomiting; chronic indigestion, with contractive or crampy pains, or *spasms of the stomach or bowels*, *flatulence*, and constipation; gnawing and sinking at the stomach; pain after the least food; aching pain in the epigastrium and hypochondrium; spasmodic vomiting and retching; morning vomiting of pregnancy; *spasmodic and flatulent colic*, the bowels feeling sore; *constipation*, the action of the bowels being "inharmonious an spasmodic," the patient having *frequent ineffectual urging*; hernia; spasmodic dysenteric attacks; hernia of women and children; strangulated "diarrhœa of infants when artificial food disagrees with them;" *piles* (in alternation with *Sulphur*), with congestive headache, pressing in the bowels; prolapsus, or stricture, of the anus, with constipation; chronic liver-complaint, especially in old people.

Urinary System.—Spasms during the passage of urinary calculi; stranguary, from chronic irritation of the lower portion of the spine; incontinence of urine from paralysis of the sphincters.

Generative System.—Irritability of the male sexual organs, with emissions; spasmodic pains in the spermatic cord, with retraction of the testes. Spasmodic menstrual colic, with premature and scanty discharge, cerebral congestion, and chilliness, in persons with dyspepsia and other conditions as above; *morning-sickness*; continual dribbling of the menses; *prolapsus of the uterus and vagina*; *metritis*; leucorrhœa.

Strychnia—*Strychnine*—the chief alkaloid of *Strychnos Nux Vomica*—is largely used by the Allopaths, but much less by Homœopaths, since it has not so wide and varied a curative range as *Nux Vomica*. Our use of it is almost strictly limited to the paralytic and the more violent spasmodic and tetanic affections curable by the drug.

58.—Opium—*Papaver Somniferum*—*Poppy*.

This plant, and preparations from it, have been used for medical purposes from the remotest antiquity. The *Opium* we use is obtained from Turkey and Egypt. Opium-smoking and eating, when once the habit is formed, soon becomes an all-absorbing passion. Dr. Bayes says that when he resided on the borders of Lincolnshire, he saw a great deal of the opium-eating and laudanum-drinking which is still carried on there. "The chemists in those districts sell immense quantities of Opium, in its crude state, every market-day, rolled into little sticks, in pennyworths and two-pennyworths. I have seen fen-farmers who were in the habit of buying *Laudanum* by the half-pint or even more, on every visit to their market-town. The habit is first commenced to allay the feeling of extreme lowness of spirits and bodily depression which affects the ague-stricken where intermittent fever is fully developed." A cachectic state of the body, and derangement of most of its functions, is generally noticed in those who habitually use the drug; "and in them the slightest scratch often degenerates into a foul and ill-conditioned ulcer" *(Waring)*.

Besides its prejudical use by adults, we would strongly condemn its employment, in the form of *Paregoric* and *Laudanum*, as a means of quieting young children, in whom it produces most injurious, and very often, fatal results;* its use in such instances, is, moreover, wholly inexcusable now that the light of Homœopathy reveals such medicines as our *Acon.*, *Bell.*, *Cham.*, *Coff.*, etc., as safe and potent means of removing, *not stifling*, the conditions which give rise to infantile restlessness and cries.

General Uses.—*Apoplexy*, with slow, full pulse, snoring-expiration; certain cases of *delirum tremens; convulsions* of children caused by *fright;* "acute fevers characterized by a sopor bordering upon stupor, and by absence of any complaint, snoring with the mouth open, half-jerking of the limbs, and burning heat of the perspiring body" *(Hahnemann)*; typhus, with partial suppression of urine, and sleepiness; unconquerable *drowsiness*, followed by *sleeplessness*, headache, listlessness, chilliness, etc.; stupefying, unrefreshing sleep,

* See a paper on "Fatal Poisoning by Allopathic Medication" in *The Homœopathic World*, July, 1869.

with snoring, half-open eyes, stertorous, irregul headache, with heaviness, throbbing of the arter the face, sleepiness after meals, with *contraction* especially in persons predisposed to apoplexy, alcoholic liquors largely; dyspepsia of drur digestive organs seem to have lost all tone; *stipation*, from utter torpidity and inaction of t and "when little or no inconvenience is felt fro action;" *lead-colic* and constipation; incarcer paralytic retention of urine, especially in young old people; sudden retrocession of acute erupti brain-symptoms characteristic of the drug.

Persons to whom *Opium* is most suitable are t torpidity of both mental and physical faculties in these patients the usual medicines seem to *Opium* has aroused their dormant energies an their nervous system susceptible.

clammy sweats in the face, and emaciation; typhoid conditions in various diseases, with parched and cracked, or blackish glazed, tongue; consequences of sexual excesses; marasmus; disease of bone; hectic fever. In persons to whose constitutional condition *Phosphorus* is suitable, there is, generally, a pale, sickly, sallow, or bloated appearance of the face, prostration of the nervous system, pains in the joints, tendency to lung-disease, quiet lowness of spirits, and gradual wasting.

NERVOUS SYSTEM.—Functional paralysis, and epilepsy, from debilitating causes—sexual excesses, want, etc.; progressive spinal paralysis, the brain being undisturbed; hemiplegia in old people of a scrofulous constitution, with creepings in the paralyzed parts, thick urine; weakness of children who are late in walking; marasmus, trembling, general debility, and depression of spirits.

HEAD, EYES, EARS, ETC.—Arthritic hemicrania, with swelling, inflammation, and intense painfulness of the affected part; chronic conjunctivitis; amaurosis, with lancinating pains through the eye-balls, and deep-seated pains in the orbits; deafness in strumous females and children, with humming, whizzing, dryness, and occasional oozing of greenish mucus; chronic catarrh, with inflammation of the nose, fœtid discharge of greenish mucus.

RESPIRATORY SYSTEM.—Cough with irritation throughout the chest; hacking, wasting cough, the lungs feeling crowded and tight, expectoration of rusty-coloured or greenish, and sometimes fœtid, sputa; cough and chest-troubles, with similar symptoms, occurring in, or following, typhoid, typhus, and other fevers; sense of heat or sharp pain during inspiration; chronic cough, with tough, reddish-brown expectoration; chronic bronchitis, with much constitutional disturbance, soreness of the air-passages, frothy and bloody or purulent and bloody expectoration, emaciation, hectic fever, etc.; *simple*, *typhoid, and chronic pneumonia,* the cough causing mucous, expectoration of mucus and blood; broncho-pneumonia (*Phos.* in alternation with *Ant. Tart.*); pleuro-pneumonia (alternately with *Bry.*); phthisis pulmonalis, in the early stage, also during the course of the disease: it relieves congestion, quiets the cough, and moderates diarrhœa, etc.

Digestive System.—*Decay of teeth* in the lower jaw, especially when extending to, or arising from, the jaw itself, with inflammation of the gums, *tendency to gum-boils;* irregularities of teething in the lower jaw, especially in scrofulous children with chronic diarrhœa, tendency to mesenteric disease; cardialgia, with frequent vomiting, sense of heat in the stomach, diarrhœa, with straining; hunger, with emaciation, white-coated tongue, etc.; impaired digestion from sexual excesses, with great weakness; gastro-enteritis, and disease of the stomach involving emaciation of the patient, ulceration, etc.; chronic diarrhœa, watery or colliquative, in nervous patients and children; mild diarrhœa of phthisis; *diseases of the liver* in which the functions of the organ are suspended: acute atrophy of the liver, cirrhosis, obstructive jaundice, etc.; malignant jaundice, burning distress in the stomach, black vomit; acute fatty degeneration of the liver; chronic jaundice.

Urinary System.—Thick, turbid, and scanty urine in typhoid conditions; high-coloured and frothy urine; fatty pellicles floating on the urine; albuminuria; nephritis.

Generative System.—Emissions weakening the patient; erections with speedy emissions; spermatorrhœa; impotence; satyriasis. Amenorrhœa or scanty menses in females who are pale, sallow, and waxy-looking, inclined to chlorosis, and of strumous constitution; chronic inflammation of the breasts with fistulous openings.

Skin.—Diseases of the skin in the neighbourhood of the lower jaw; fistulous ulcers, with fever; chilblains, from which a fœtid watery secretion exudes, in scrofulous females.

60.—Phosphori Acidum—*Phosphoric Acid.*

This is a colourless inodorous liquid, of an agreeable acid taste. It is obtained by the mutual action of *Phosphorus* and *Nitric acid* in distilled water.

General Uses.—*Physical or nervous debility*, from any cause, with *cold clammy sweats or profuse perspiration;* exhaustion from loss of the fluids of the body, as in hæmorrhage, spermatorrhœa, excessive or prolonged diarrhœa, etc.; passive hæmorrhage, consequences of grief, care, too rapid growth, onanism, etc. Phthisis, with colliquative sweats, great exhaustion, diarrhœa, and general hectic condition. Spinal weakness, with great fatigue on exertion, and frequent inclination to pass water; curvatures of the spine; scrofulous caries of bone, and consequent hectic fever. Falling off of the hair after a severe illness, or as a sign of general debility. In old-school materia medica it is considered tonic, refrigerant, and aphrodisiac, and is administered in large doses (10 to 30 min.) of the dilute acid.

Head, etc.—Headache at the back and nape of the neck, with pale face, from nervous exhaustion; dull or confused intellect, weak memory, dejection of spirits, etc., from seminal or other losses, or exhausting disease. Weakness of sight, and deafness, during, or consequent on severe disease.

Respiratory System.—Chronic bronchitis with bloody, purulent expectoration, and night sweats; pneumonia, with hardness of hearing, excessive weakness, pale sunken face, diarrhœa, etc.

Urinary System.—Too *frequent desire to pass water*, especially in the morning; frequent involuntary emissions of urine with nervous symptoms; diabetes mellitus; semi-phosphatic deposits in the urine, or alkalinity from nervous depression; milky urine in children.

Generative System.—*Seminal emissions from self-abuse;*

impotence from too rapid escape of the semen after an erection or before it is complete; general debility from sexual excesses or spermatorrhœa. Thin, acrid, and chronic leucorrhœa, with pale face.

61.—Phytolacca Decandra—*Poke-weed.*

Another of the "New American Remedies," *poke* is a native of the United States, growing along hedges and road-sides, in neglected fields and meadows, in moist ground, and flowering from July to September. The plant contains a good deal of caustic potash—45 per cent.

General Uses.—*Periosteal, syphilitic,* and *chronic rheumatism; glandular enlargements;* affections of the *mouth and throat;* and scrofulous, syphilitic, and other diseases, characterized by *feebleness of the nervous system and weak action of the heart.* Scarlatina anginosa with glandular enlargements, ulcerated throat, hoarseness, etc. *Chronic rheumatism,* with heavy aching and coldness in the affected limb, the pain being worse in warmth and in damp weather—glandular enlargements co-existing; joints swollen and tender, red, and shining, with inability to move the parts without extreme pain, worse at night; rheumatism of the hip-joint; nightly pains in the tibia, with nodes; stiff-neck, lumbago, and rheumatic and neuralgic affections of the lower extremities. There is a remarkable similarity between the effects of *Phytolacca, and Kali Hydriodicum, Mercurius,* and *Mezereum.*

Head, Nose, etc.—*Dull, heavy headache* in the *forehead,* vertex, and occiput, with yawning; syphilitic headache; acute coryza; ozœna, and syphilitic ulceration of the nose.

Respiratory System.—*Hoarseness* and *aphonia,* with great dryness, and sense as of a lump in the throat; cough, day and night, with feeling as of an ulcerated spot in the wind-pipe, above the breast-bone.

Digestive System.—Mercurial ptyalism and pains in the teeth; toothache, with inflammation of the gums and mouth; difficult dentition: Dr. Merrill says that *Phytolacca* has acted in many cases in this affection "like magic," the following symptom in the pathogenesis of the drug having suggested its use to him: "irresistible inclination to bite the teeth together;" darkish-red inflammation of the fauces, swelling of the tonsils, with superficial ulcers, and thick white mucus; ulcerated and chronic sore throat, with slight inflammation; *diphtheritic inflammation of the throat*, with pains in the head, neck, and back, and high fever, large holes being left when the white patches come away: in all these mouth and throat affections, *Phytolacca* should also be used as a *wash* or a *gargle*—50 drops of the tincture to half-a-pint of water. Vomiting, coming on very slowly, preceded by nausea, prostration, yawning, etc.; soreness and pain in the hypochondrium during pregnancy; "*constipation* in the aged, or those of very weak constitutional powers, with weak heart's-action, intermittent pulse, and generally relaxed muscular frame" *(Bayes)*; ulceration of the rectum; fissure and prolapsus of the anus; etc.

Urinary System.—Urine diminished, afterwards increased, and becoming albuminous; albuminuria, as in scarlet fever, diphtheria, etc.

Generative System.—Loss of sexual desire, relaxation of the genitals, and impotence; obstinate gonorrhœa and gleet; second and tertiary syphilis. Metrorrhagia; inflammation, swelling, and hardness of the breasts; *abscess, and other affections of the breast*; morbid sensitiveness and tenderness of the breasts during menstruation or suckling.

Skin.—(Internal and external use): *Chronic ulcers* and eruptions; tinea capitis; whitlow, felon, and syphilitic cutaneous diseases. Dr. Burt has cured warts by applying the tincture to them.

62.—Platina—*Platina—Platinum.*

An elementary substance, of the colour and lustre of silver nearly as tenacious as iron, existing in its native state in combination with other metals. After being purified, we make triturations of it.

GENERAL USES.—*Depression of spirits* and *melancholy*, even to the fear of death, with anguish about the heart, in females who suffer from profuse or premature menstruation, and watery leucorrhœa, especially if they are dark complexioned, of spare habit, and subject to neuralgic headaches; neuralgia with numbness, hysteria; or melancholia religiosa, associated with the above conditions; chronic congestion of the ovaries; induration and prolapsus of the womb; condylomata.

63.—Plumbum—*Lead.*

We use either the metal itself—*P. Metallicum;* the Carbonate—*P. Carbonicum;* or the Acetate—*P. Aceticum:* their actions are similar.

GENERAL USES.—*Chronic dull headache*, with depressed spirits, weeping mood, tendency to paralysis, and constipation; *blue margins on the gums*, with sponginess and shrinking, as in some cases of *phthisis;* wasting of the body similar to that caused by lead-poisoning, with palsy, epilepsy, neuralgia, or anæsthesia; *melancholy; obstinate constipation*, the fæces being dry, shaped like balls, and when there is spasmodic constriction of the sphincter ani; *colic*, relieved by pressure on the abdomen, with constipation, like lead-colic; etc.

Lead-colic or *Painter's-colic* is best treated by Opi., Alum., or Plat., according to the symptoms.

Preparations of *Lead* form part of all the so-called *Hair-restorers* we have yet seen, even though they have been advertised as not containing *Lead.* For the means of detect ing the presence of the metal in these preparations, and some remarks on the results of their use, see *The Homœopathic World*, Vol. iv. p. 36.

64.—Podophyllum Peltatum—*May-Apple—Mandrake.*

This plant, of the genus *Mandragora*, is probably the same as the one we read of in Scripture: its fruit, which is round and yellow, like a small orange, is very fragrant and luscious, and is still eaten in the East by women desirous of offspring. Strange legends are on record concerning the plant: such as its resemblance to the human form, this resemblance suggesting, we presume, its utility as a means of promoting fertility.

Of late the drug has come into general use by the Allopathic school, who regard it as a kind of "vegetable mercury."

General Uses.—Affections of the *liver*: *biliousness*, with fulness in the right hypochondrium, nausea and giddiness, bitter taste, tendency to bilious vomiting, bilious diarrhœa, and dark urine; chronic liver-complaint with *costiveness*; affections of the *bowels*: inflammation of the jejunum and ileum; diarrhœa of typhoid fever; *morning diarrhœa*; simple relaxation of the bowels, the stools being too large and frequent, but otherwise natural; dysenteric diarrhœa (rectal), and *diarrhœa with prolapsus ani at each stool*, especially in children. Prolapsus uteri, with affections of the bowels; swelling of the labia during pregnancy; and many other affections involving the *uterus* and the *ovaries*.

65.—Pulsatilla Nigricans—*Wind-flower—Meadow Anemone.*

This perennial flower is indigenous to elevated places in the greater part of Europe, where the soil is dry and sandy;

and the situation exposed. It is called "wind-flower," because generally found in an exposed situation. It blooms in the spring and autumn.

GENERAL USES.—The main sphere of action of *Pulsatilla* is the *mucous membrane* of the *digestive canal*, the *sexual organs*, and the *eyes* and *ears*; it also exercises great influence upon the *veins*. "In all the best cases of *Pulsatilla-cure* I have met with, *venosity* has been the prevailing constitutional symptom" *(Bayes)*. In *measles*, *chicken-pox*, *remittent fever*, and other diseases of children, its use is undoubted; it helps to clean the tongue, moderates catarrh, and checks diarrhœa. In uncomplicated *measles* it is almost a specific, and is especially valuable after the fever has been modified by *Aconite*. *Puls.* is also preventive of measles during its prevalence, or, administered during the disease, it tends to prevent its after-consequences. In *rheumatism* it is only indicated when the symptoms are of a sub-acute character, with swelling of the affected (chiefly the small) joints, and but little or no inflammatory redness, and when there is a marked tendency of the pains to wander from one part to another, and characteristic dyspepsia; rheumatic gout in females.

Puls. is especially suited to the ailments of the female sex, and to persons of a gentle, good-naturedly mischievous disposition, easily excited to laughter or weeping, having pale face, blue eyes, blond hair, freckles, and a tendency to leucorrhœa or other kinds of blenorrhœa, with an inclination to a deposit of fat under the skin *(embonpoint)*, and a "marked tendency to shed tears when the patient is describing her sufferings." There is absence of thirst, frequent chilliness and the pains are worse with warmth and during rest; but abate in the open air, or during moderate exercise.

HEAD.—Gastric headache, from rich, fatty, indigestible food, severe pain on one side behind the ear, as if a nail were driven in; headache on the left side; nervous or sick headaches, particularly in hysteric females, or connected with the menses; hysteria, or dejection of spirits, from milk- or menstrual-suppression.

Eyes, Ears, etc.—Styes; subacute inflammation of the lining membrane of the eyelids, with profuse lachrymation, agglutination, etc., in persons of the temperament described; ophthalmia following measles; twitching of the eyelids, with dazzling of the sight. Ear-ache of children, with passive purulent discharge; noises in the ear or deafness following catarrh or measles; loss or perversion of smell.

Circulatory System.—Varicose veins of the legs, and embarrassed venous circulation generally, especially in females, and when caused by the pressure consequent upon pregnancy; phlebitis in the leg.

Respiratory System.—Catarrhal affections of the air-passages, with loss of taste or smell; excessive expectoration of mucus, as in old cases of bronchitis; "mild hæmoptysis, in bronchitis marked by expectoration of mucus having a disgusting fœtid taste and smell;" bronchial relaxation after hooping-cough; nocturnal cough; dry "stomach-cough."

Digestive System.—Viscid, whitish mucus, thickly covering the tongue; bitter, sour, or foul taste; diminished or altered taste, with the *Puls.* characteristics. Dyspepsia caused by the use of pork, pastry, or other fat or rich diet; eructations tasting of food; vomiting of mucus or bile; heartburn; a feeling of distension after a meal, necessitating the loosening or removal of the dress; passive venous congestion of the abdomen. *Pains in the left side* (see also *Cimicifuga*), in females, between the hip and the lower margin of the ribs or a little above, associated with some derangement of the monthly period, is generally amenable to *Puls.* Mucous diarrhœa with sensitiveness of the abdomen, especially from rich, indigestible food, or occurring at night.

milky leucorrhœa; difficulty in urinating during pregnancy; false, delayed, or deficient (Scanty) labour; retained *placenta*; excessive after-pains; suppression of lochia; painful tension of the breasts, and a deficient secretion of milk. Administered some time previously to labour, facilitates that process. We invariably prescribe this or other remedy, according to the nature of each case, in the latter months of pregnancy, with the happiest results, and have had too many evidences of the value of the treatment to admit of the explanation of their being coincidences.

66.—Rhus Toxicodendron—*Poison-oak—Sumach.*

This shrub is indigenous to North America and some parts of the world; it abounds on the borders of rivers and marshy districts, growing very tall in a congenial soil. In susceptible persons contact with the shrub produces an erythematous and vesicular eruption, with itching and burning, going on to more severe results. An interesting case of poisoning by *Rhus* in a man who went to gather the plant for a Homœopathic Chemist in Scotland, with a remarkable corresponding case of cure by the same drug, will be found in *The Homœopathic World*, Vol. iv. p. 149, *et. seq.*

GENERAL USES.—*Rheumatism, strains*, some *skin affections, paralyses*, and *fevers* of a *typhoid* character. Sub-acute and *chronic rheumatism* and *lumbago, rheumatic sciatica*, and rheu*matic stiffness* and *lameness**; the indications for the

* A number of instances of cure illustrative of the kind of cases to which *Rhus* is suitable, and in which the special indications are well marked, may be found in *The Homœopathic World*, Vol. iii. pp. 188—9.

Rhus in this class of diseases, as also in *strains*, being: *Increase of pain during rest*, at night when warm in bed, on *first moving* the parts, and on *waking up* in the morning; continued exercise relieves the pain. Indeed, these indications are valid in some other conditions, not rheumatic; and some physicians give *Rhus* in any affection in which these symptoms are present. Moreover, the *right side* of the body is chiefly acted upon by *Rhus*. *Paralysis*, cold and painless, of a *rheumatic* character; paralysis of the lower limbs *(paraplegia)* in young persons and children, from cold—sitting on cold stones, standing in the wet, etc.—with great pain in the paralyzed parts; paralysis of the feet, as from a fall on the back. Fevers of a typhoid character sometimes require *Rhus*; but in these cases it is now generally superseded by *Baptisia*; but when rheumatic symptoms develop themselves during scarlet, gastric, or other fever, *Rhus* is a prime remedy; also when the fever-patient is continually moving himself for change of position as a means of relieving the aching of his back and limbs.

HEAD, EYES, ETC.—Rheumatic or arthritic hemicrania, the brain seeming to shake in the skull, with burning pains, and swelling of the head and face. *Scrofulous ophthalmia*, with burning pains in the eyes, lachrymation, intolerance of light, swelling and inflammation of the lids. Vesicular erysipelas of the nose and face.

RESPIRATORY SYSTEM.—"Cough, as in the bronchial cough of old people, coming on when first waking or on first moving about, accompanied by the expectoration of small plugs of tough mucus" *(Bayes)*; acute stitches flying through the chest at night, waking out of sleep, with dyspnœa; typhoid pneumonia.

DIGESTIVE SYSTEM.—Dyspepsia, with flow of water, dryness of the mouth, capricious or lost appetite, pressure in the stomach, and sense as if it were swollen; diarrhœa of a typhoid character, or diarrhœa ushering in or accompanying the early stage of fever, the evacuations being mixed with jelly-like mucus, blood, etc.

SKIN.—*Vesicular erysipelas* and erythema, with much burning and itching: for these affections *Rhus* is one of the best remedies; chronic *shingles* and eczema, especially of the palms of the hands; tinea capitis, with fœtid yellow matter under the scabs; superficial burns. In skin diseases, a special indication for *Rhus* is: intolerable *burning and itching.*

EXTERNAL USE.—*Formula.*—Twenty drops of the strong tincture to a half-pint of water.

Rhus is an extremely efficacious remedy as an external application in *sprains, injuries to ligaments, tendons,* joints, and the membranes investing the joints, especially when the indications above pointed out are present. Extensive *superficial burns,* the *stings* of insects, old chilblains, and sometimes warts, are relieved or cured by the external use of *Rhus,* given also internally. Great *burning and itching* indicate its use.

67.—Ruta Graveolens—*Garden-rue.*

GENERAL USES.—Rheumatism, and strains, of the *wrist* and *ankle; bruised* pains in the bones, joints, and cartilages, worse during rest; *weakness of sight from over-exertion of the eyes,* as in reading or sewing; aching, gnawing gastralgia; worms of children, with vomiting and colic; menorrhagia, with hysteric spasms and head-symptoms; *ganglion of the wrist;* bunion; "laming pain in the tendo achilles."

EXTERNAL USE.—*Formula.*—Twenty drops of the strong tincture to half a tea-cupful of water.

It may be used as a lotion to *bruises* instead of *Arnica,* when the latter remedy produces erysipelas in the patient, and when the contusion is more of *bone* than of soft parts. It is also said to assist in the uniting of fracture when that process goes on tardily.

68.—Sepia Succus—*Inky Juice of the Cuttle-fish.*

The Sepiæ are molluscæ of the seas. In the abdominal cavity is a sac containing a dark-brown juicy substance, with which the animal darkens the water to elude an enemy, or to capture prey. This liquid, dried, is inert in its crude state; but powerful properties are developed by our process of trituration.

General Uses.—*Chronic* diseases of women, connected with the menstrual function. Periodic sick-headaches, with sticking, heavy pain, and sometimes nausea and vomiting; cough, with grayish-white and salty expectoration; *scanty menstruation*, *leucorrhœa*, and menorrhagia, from venous congestion; amenorrhœa, with gastric derangement, weariness, and palpitation; retroversion, etc., of the uterus; "constipation, prolapsus, and hæmorrhoidal fulness in uterine disease;" flushes of heat; hysteria; subacute stage of gonorrhœa in females; itching pimples, producing a roughness and cracking of the skin, principally affecting the joints; perspiration under the arms and on the soles of the feet, having a peculiar smell, in nervous women; ringworm. *Sepia* is best adapted to anæmic cachectic women of delicate organisation, torpid functional action, who are disposed to skin-affections, sensitive to cold air, apt to be chilly, suffer from uterine derangement, mental depression and physical exhaustion, and are of mild disposition, inclined to melancholy and tears.

69.—Silicea—*Silicious Earth—Flint.*

Silica, or as Hahnemann styled it, *Silicea Terra*, is the only known oxide of Silicon; and is the principal ingredient in common glass. It is insoluble in water, acids, and nearly all liquids; hence it is of no service to the physician till

Hahnemann's process of trituration has developed its latent curative virtues, which are very important.

GENERAL USES.—Organic changes in the cellular, mucous, *lymphatic*, and *osseous* systems. Sweat about the head only; general tenderness of the surface; rickets; caries, and exfoliation of bone; tabes dorsalis; cachectic conditions in which the glands not only enlarge, but go on to slow, tardy *suppuration*. Phthisis pulmonalis, and chronic bronchitis, with very profuse expectoration, and hectic fever. Decay of teeth, and toothache from that source, the pain being increased by warm food and by inhalation of cold air, and is most violent at night. Enlargement and *white swelling* of joints; enchondroma; ganglia; housemaid's knee; *whitlow* (probably the best remedy); *scrofulous abscesses and ulcers*, spongy and readily bleeding, or torpid, with callous edges, and secreting an unhealthy pus; eruptions from a [illegible] *condition of the sebaceous follicles*, characterized by a secretion of yellowish lymph forming incrustations; impetigo capitis; suppressed, or excessive, *perspiration of feet*; etc. In its influence over suppuration—promoting when necessary, and controling when excessive—*Silicea* is probably second to none. Teste says it is especially suited to fat people, of a lymphatico-sanguine temperament; and Hahnemann mentions sweat about the head only as an indication for the use of the drug.

70.—Spigelia Anthelmia—*Animal Worm-grass—Pink-root.*

This plant is a native of the West Indies and South America. It was named from Adrian Spigelius, and, in America, is collected and sold by the Cherokee Indians. It is much valued by the allopaths of the United States as an anthelmintic.

General Uses.—*Rheumatic inflammation of the heart*, either simple, or as a complication of acute rheumatism;* chronic rheumatic affections of the heart; angina pectoris; darting, stabbing, or lacerating pains in the heart or in the face—*tooth-ache* or *face-ache,—with palpitation;* similar pains down the arms; neuralgic hemicrania, the pain being increased by motion, noise, and stooping; *rheumatic* and gouty *inflammation of the eyes* (Sclerotitis), amblyopia, and amaurosis; *worm-affections*, with vertigo, forgetfulness, depressed spirits, palpitation, *pinching* colic, itching at the anus, enuresis, and lassitude.

71.—Spongia Marina Tosta—*Roasted Sponge*.

The medicinal product yielded by sponge is obtainable by roasting the best Turkey sponge, after cleansing from all foreign matter, in a coffee-roaster; this has to be done very carefully, as, by slightly over-roasting, the therapeutic virtues of the drug are in some measure destroyed. *Iodine* is a considerable ingredient in the composition of *spongia;* nevertheless, the two remedies may not be used indiscriminately; the former has a much wider range of action than the latter.

General Uses.—Affections of the larynx, trachea, testes, and ovaries. Dryness of the larynx with *dry, hard, barking cough*, worse at night, and excited by a tickling and burning sensation; *hoarseness*, with dry cough, and obstructed breathing; *laryngitis;* laryngeal phthisis; *catarrhal croup* (in alternation with *Acon.);* painful, dry, hoarse, and croupy

* In a case of cardiac inflammation which occurred recently in our own practice, the patient being an old man who was intensely rheumatic, *Spigelia* acted with marvellous rapidity and curative power, after we had almost despaired of the patient's recovery. The violent "thumping," painful oppression, dyspnœa, etc., declined most satisfactorily, and the patient now follows his out-door occupation as usual.

cough, such as frequently precedes, or follows, croup; bronchocele and *goitrous enlargements* in children and young girls not requiring *Iodium*. Orchitis, and *orchocele*, the swelling being painful, and aching much when pressed upon; menorrhagia in scrofulous females; etc.

72.—Staphysagria—*Staves-acre—Palmated Larkspur.*

The *Delphinium Staphysagria* is a biennial bush which grows in the south of Europe, etc., the seeds of which we use by making a tincture from them. The plant is also called *louse-wort*—the bruised seeds having been used to destroy lice.

General Uses.—Nervous headache, with constrictive, boring, or pressive pains in the forehead, and acute stitches in the temples; neuralgia of the face and forehead, on both sides; smarting pains in the eyes, coming on in the evening; some ophthalmic conditions; neuralgic pains of the shoulder-joints and arms; morning nausea, as in pregnancy; irritable bladder, and catarrh of the bladder; *nocturnal emissions* with sexual excitement; drawing sensation in the spermatic cord, and aching-pain in the testes from walking; *spermatorrhœa*; impotence.

73.—Sulphur—*Sulphur—Brimstone.*

Sulphur is an elementary substance, occurring in beds in many parts of the world; and also as a volcanic produce, in its native form, near to volcanoes. It is a constituent element of various organic substances, as the albumen of eggs, etc., in some plants, but most abundantly in minerals and mineral waters. The substance is of a pale-yellow colour, is insipid, inodorous, insoluble in water, slightly soluble in alcohol, but more freely soluble in ether. We use the *Flowers of Sulphur* of commerce, after washing and re-washing it in alcohol.

General Uses.—*Diseases of the skin* and *mucous membranes*; affections resulting from *constitutional cachexia—scrofula*, etc.; complications arising from the *non-development* or *retrocession of eruptive diseases*: on this point Mr. Nankivell thus writes us: "It is most valuable when the exanthem does not readily appear; I have noticed its brilliant effects in the incipient stage of small-pox, when the head was severely affected with intense pain, and in a state threatening coma;" *diseases alternating with, or following suppressed, eruptions*; *scabies*; chronic tendency to boils: Dr. Hughes gives a good proof of the homœopathicity of *Sulphur* to this condition, when he states that a patient of his who accompanied her husband to Harrogate, and, though in good heaalth, joined him in drinking the waters, returned home covered with boils; "the Harrogate waters, too, if drunk largely and incautiously, appear to be capable of bringing on apoplexy:" hence the homœopathicity of *Sulphur* to some cases of chronic congestive headache; "*excess of venosity*," and consequent diseases; chronic *gouty* (atonic) *and rheumatic affections*, with drawing, tearing, or boring pains, or pains as if the parts were sprained, and *itching about the painful parts*; tensive pains in the joints and muscles; rheumatoid pains, waking the patient early, and preventing sleep again; hot flashes over the back and down the spinal column; *chronic lumbago* or *sciatica*, in persons who suffer from constipation, piles, or varicose veins; nervous complaints—neuralgia, shooting-pains, chronic headache, trembling weakness, rigidity of the joints, etc.—arising from repelled itch or other cutaneous disease; ill-health of children and others without definite disease, especially when there is alternate diarrhœa and constipation, the diarrhœa being extremely fœtid, and accompanied by fœtid flatulence; nightmare with palpitation, in cachectic persons; etc.

Sulphur is very valuable (1) in *commencing the treatment* of many *chronic diseases;* (2) as an *intercurrent remedy*, during their course, as in scrofulous diseases of the joints, chronic hydrocephalus, glandular enlargements, chronic gout and rheumatism, phthisis, etc.; (3) when the organism fails to respond to the action of other remedies which are homœopathic to the condition: in such cases, a dose or two of *Sulphur* will often arouse the dormant energies, and render the system susceptible to the medicines indicated; and (4) *after acute disease* in any organ. "When the part is left gorged with venous blood, and the arterial has not recovered its due balance, *Sulphur completes the cure.*" In all deep-seated chronic maladies it is of essential service, either as the main remedy, or as an adjunct to others.

Sulphur is pre-eminently *indicated* in diseases affecting patients previously troubled with eruptions, ulcers, sores, and in diseases traceable to the scrofulous element. The *pains* are *worse at night*, and *in damp* and *changeable weather*.

HEAD, EYES, AND EARS.—Chronic headache, with congestion—aching fulness, and vertigo; chronic hydrocephalus. Scurfiness of the eyelids; stye; chronic inflammation of the eyes in the scrofulous; sub-acute conjunctivitis and ulceration of the cornea; catarrhal and strumous ophthalmia, and chronic sore eyes, with itching and smarting, in unhealthy individuals. Sores behind and about the ears, with itching; partial deafness, with roaring noises, and sweating or moisture and frequent itching in the ears.

FACE AND NOSE.—Pimples on the face—*acne* (internal and external use). Acute nasitis; erysipelatoid and chronic inflammation of the nose, with swelling and illusions of smell.

CIRCULATORY SYSTEM.—Increased pulsation of the aorta, from the heart to the clavicle, with purring noise; when lying on the back, pulsations are felt in the abdominal aorta; abnormal irritability of the heart, with palpitation, as in hysteric patients of an unhealthy or scrofulous constitution; incipient aneurism of the aorta in the scrofulous.

RESPIRATORY SYSTEM.—*Catarrh* with confusion of the head, weariness, and prostration of the limbs; catarrh of measles, etc.; *chronic catarrh*, and tendency thereto, attacks occurring from the least exposure to unfavourable change of weather, with sneezing, soreness of the nose, hoarseness, tightness of the chest, and acrid, mucous discharge from the nostrils; chronic cough, coming on in paroxysms, at night, with expectoration of thick phlegm, excited by tickling in the larynx; coughs following prolonged catarrh or acute fevers; chest-symptoms from suppressed eruptions; oppression and anxiety in the chest, with aching, sore spots, dull stitches, and weight and pressure in the chest; *scrofulous consumption*, and phthisis in patients with rough, unhealthy skin, or having itching vesicles; *excessive*, and *foul-smelling*, purulent *expectoration* (see *Sulphurous Acid*); mild *hæmoptysis* in bronchitis, with fœtid expectoration; chronic hæmoptysis, and *chronic pneumonia*, in scrofulous and phthisical persons; plastic pleurisy; asthma, alternating with eruptions on the skin, etc.

DIGESTIVE SYSTEM.—Soreness, swelling, and cracks of the lips and corners of the mouth; warty excrescences on the lower lip; sour, bitter, and clammy taste, with yellow coating on the tongue; painful swelling of the tongue; heartburn, sense of weight in the stomach, weariness after eating, and other symptoms of *chronic indigestion* in scrofulous persons; in the obstinate vomiting of hysteric girls, Mr. Nankivell informs us that *Sulphur* (30th potency) is often very useful; *chronic constipation* (in alternation with *Nux Vom.*), either with or without piles, the fæces being hard, dry, dark, expelled with straining, and sometimes streake[d] with blood; diarrhœa—fœtid, watery, with fœtid flatul[ence] and alternating with constipation, in the scrofulous, [in] enlargement of the mesenteric ganglion; *ascarides*, wit[h] and burning of the anus, in unhealthy children; bearing-down pain in the direction of the anus, and *piles*, dependent on abdominal plethora (in alternation with *Nux Vom.*), with burning at the anus, and tenesmus; *soreness, excoriation, itching,* or *exudations about the anus; bleeding piles,* with hæmorrhage of *dark venous blood*, and constipation; *suppressed piles*—hæmorrhoidal colic, backache, palpitation, cerebral or pulmonary congestion, vertigo, etc.

URINARY SYSTEM.—Frequent desire to pass water during the day, and enuresis at night (compare *Ferrum*), in scrofulous children.

GENERATIVE SYSTEM.—Weakness of the sexual organs, with excitement and swelling, in the scrofulous. Profuse menstrual discharge of black, clotted, and gluey blood; slimy, yellowish leucorrhœa; constitutional tendency to prolapsus, miscarriage, ulceration of the breasts, or sore breasts and nipples.

SKIN.—*Scabies, acne,* herpes circinnatus, and ringworm (internal and external use); *recent prurigo;* intertrigo, crustea serpiginosa, and *general eruptions in unhealthy children;* chronic erysipelatous inflammation of the skin on various parts—the arms, legs, etc.—with burning and itching, and desquamation; *boils* and *whitlows*, in persons in whom they are apt to recur; liver-spots; chronic ulcers, scrofulous or varicose, with much burning and itching, and discharge of fœtid pus; *corns and warts* which tend to inflame; icy-coldness of the feet, with burning of the face and hands.

In skin-affections, a prominent *indication* for the use of *Sulphur* is—*itching* with burning, *increased by warmth* and slight friction, but pleasantly *relieved* for a short time by vigorous rubbing or by scratching.

74.—Sulphurosum Acidum—*Sulphurous Acid.*

When sulphur or brimstone is burnt, a highly characteristic pungent and stifling odour is evolved, which is the odour, not of sulphur, but of its oxide—*Sulphurous Acid;* this gas, collected in water, forms the *Sulphurous* (a compound very different from the *Sulphuric*) *Acid* of the shops. Within the last few years, this acid has acquired considerable notoriety, chiefly through the publication of a pamphlet by Dr. Dewar, of Kirkaldy, that gentleman having used the drug largely, and obtained most satisfactory results by its administration in a variety of diseases. An article "On the Use of Sulphur Vapour—Remedial and Preventive," by Dr. Baikie, appeared in the January number of *The Homœopathic World* for 1868, in which the general sphere of the remedy is pointed out, together with suggestions on the method of its exhibition, and some useful cautionary hints. In other parts of the same journal (Vol. III.), are further remarks on the uses of *Sulphurous Acid*, both within and without the domain of medicine, which are worth perusal. Dr. Morrisson has also recently published a pamphlet "On Sulphurous Acid," with cases illustrative of its therapeutic sphere, especially as an external remedy, in conjunction with other Homœopathic measures. Its dynamic action is similar to that of *Sulphur*, but it is more generally convenient and applicable for local use than the ointment of its base; and for inhalation, the *spray-producer* enables anyone to use it with ease and perfect control, while its fumes are readily producible at any time.

General Uses.—*Throat and chest affections*—diphtheritic sore throat, chronic catarrh, cough, bronchitis, asthma, etc *neuralgia and toothache; cutaneous diseases*—ringworm o' surface, eczema, cracked and chapped hands, ulcers, etc.; *vegetable and animal parasites*—scabies, thiasis, etc. It is chiefly appropriate to chronic *affec*

abdomen, etc.; scarlet eruption on the skin, with gastric disorder, *from eating shell-fish.*

Caution.—The indiscriminate use of *Turpentine* as an external application in rheumatism, burns and scalds, wounds, etc., is frequently productive of most mischievous results.*

76.—Veratrum Album—*White Hellebore.*

This plant is indigenous to the mountainous districts of Europe, and is found in great abundance on the Swiss Alps. "The ancients employed this drug with a sort of barbarous inconsistency in the treatment of mental derangements. This 'Helleborism of the ancients' was chiefly conducted on the island of Anticyra, in the Greek Archipelago, upon the principle of kill or cure, consisting of a course of evacuations, by the mouth, bowels, and skin, which either drove all the devils out of the poor possessed, or else consigned him to the land of Stygian shadows" *(Hempel).*

General Uses.—*Asiatic cholera*, when violent vomiting and purging are more prominent symptoms than those of prostration or collapse; *choleraic diarrhœa*, with violent vomiting; ague, with extreme coldness; *cramps* of the *abdomen* or of the *calves*, whether or not occurring during cholera, the muscles being drawn up into knots: third stage of *hooping-cough.*

Special indications for the use of this drug are:—General *coldness*, with *blueness*, *debility*, sunken and pinched features, *cramps*, faintness and *faintings*, *feeble*, almost imperceptible *pulse*, *cold tongue* and breath, *cold sweats* and *great thirst;* also

* At the time of writing we have under treatment a patient, who, in alighting from a carriage, slipped, and slightly abraded the surface over the shin-bone; *turpentine* was promptly applied, the wound inflamed, and now the whole anterior aspect of the limb is in a sad ulcerated condition.

sun-stroke, alcoholic stimulants, *teething*, etc., or from suppressed discharges. The symptoms are:—A sense of fulness and weight, throbbing, sometimes with stupefaction; increased sensitiveness to sound, with buzzing and roaring; double, partial, dim, or otherwise disordered vision; nausea and vomiting; tingling and numbness in the limbs; mental confusion; etc. In general *gastric affections* it is superior to *Verat. Alb.*, especially if there be much *irritability* of the stomach—vomiting, *pyrosis*, etc., and when the last-named symptoms occur during pregnancy. *Puerperal fever*, *metritis*, and *mania*; hysterical convulsions. In *pneumonia*, Dr. Hale considers it better than *Acon.*, administered in alternation with *Phos.*; but the *Verat. Vir.* should be discontinued immediately the pulse falls to its normal rate. Cardiac debility, with fainting and collapse therefrom; palpitation with faintness, or dyspnœa. Piles, with neuralgic pains in the rectum and anus; acute nephritis and cystitis; orchitis; etc.

Its *local use*, in a diluted form, is said to have dispersed local inflammations, cured scabies, shingles, and chronic skin-affections; and Dr. Dalzell informs us that a compress saturated with a lotion of Keith's concentrated tincture—ʒj ad aq. destil. ℥vj—is valuable in inflammation of the cœcum; also that *inflamed corns*, *bunions*, etc., are greatly benefited by being touched with the tincture.

78.—Zincum—*Zinc*—*Spelter*.

We use either the metal itself—*Z. Metallicum*, its sulphate—*Z. Sulphuricum*, or its oxide—*Z. Oxydatum*.

General Uses.—*Chronic headache*, with violent, obstinate pain; with depression of spirits; *melancholia;* hysteria; palpitation, and "spasmodically-contracted pulse;" chronic atrophy of the brain; paralysis of the brain in scarlatina, or acute hydrocephalus; infantile convulsions; chorea; epilepsy;

aversion to labour, defective and even idiotic memory, dimness of sight, and weakness and heaviness, or jerking, of the limbs; neuralgic pains; dry atrophy, without hectic; somnambulism; etc. Ague, with repeated rigor, malaise, nausea, and constriction of the chest, followed by a short hot stage, and profuse sweating. Dry, spasmodic cough, and pneumonia, with violent stitches in the chest on taking an inspiration, and expectoration of blood-streaked tenacious mucus; convulsive asthma. Cardialgia, *chronic vomiting of food*, with little retching, and obstinate constipation, in delicate and nervous females. Chronic gleet; eruptions following suppressed gonorrhœa. Obstinate pimples, with soreness; chronic and ulcerated herpes; etc.

Antidotes.

In the event of a medicinal over-dose having been administered, two drops of the *Tincture of Camphor*, or a strong infusion of *Coffee*, will arrest any unpleasant consequences. For the general treatment of cases of poisoning, the chapter on "Poisons," in the larger edition of this work, may be consulted.

PART IV.

Accessories in the Treatment of Disease.

1.—Cod-Liver-Oil.

The value of this agent in the treatment of many constitutional diseases is amply confirmed by long experience. It should be regarded as food rather than medicine, although the minute amount of *iodine* it contains may account for its curative virtues in many cases in which Cod-liver-oil has been the only remedy given.

The complaints in which cod-liver-oil is of service need not be enumerated here, as it has already been prescribed in numerous instances in the preceding pages. We may, however, state that it is specially valuable in the various forms of *scrofula*—chronic discharge from the ears, strumous ophthalmia, enlargement of the glands, strumous disease of the bones, strumous abscesses, etc., and, in short, in all diseases which require fatty-substances as food, and *iodine* as a remedy.

In the treatment of *consumption* it stands, by almost universal consent, pre-eminent; when given in suitable cases, its power in checking emaciation, and raising the tone of the muscular structures is too well known to need confirmation now.

The value of cod-liver-oil is often very marked in the sequelæ of many acute diseases or inflammations occurring in middle-aged and in old persons, in whom the reparative powers are less active than in children; also in the after-effects of the acute fevers of children, who have suffered, previous to such attacks, from impoverished health, scrofula, etc., as chronic discharge from the ears and nose after scarlet-fever and measles; the after-stages of hooping-cough; rickets, chorea, etc., are generally controlled and complete restoration aided, by the administration of cod-liver-oil. Chronic rheumatism and gout, chronic bronchitis, chronic skin diseases, and the degenerative diseases of the aged, are all more or less benefited by the employment of this agent.

Cod-liver-oil should not, however, be administered indiscriminately. It is generally inadmissible during the persistence of acute febrile symptoms, congestion, hæmoptysis, or any active form of disease; digestion is then impaired, the mucous membrane irritable, and the oil is only likely to occasion disorder. The sphere of cod-liver-oil is to remove exhausting, and increase general tone; this is best accomplished when active morbid processes and local irritation have subsided, for then the system is in a condition to appropriate a larger amount of nourishment.

Some caution is necessary to be observed in the administration of oil to obviate nausea or eructations. Such effects generally result from the quantity or quality of the oil used. The large quantity of oil taken in some cases occasions disorder of the digestive mucous membrane, or it passes off with the evacuations. We generally recommend it, at first, in teaspoonful doses, twice a day, with, or immediately after food; if the stomach be intolerant of it, a tea-spoonful, or for young children, even a less quantity, once a day. If there be extreme difficulty in retaining the oil, we prescribe it at bed-time, just as the patient is lying down to sleep.

The disagreeable effects of oil, and the repugnance felt towards it, have often been created by inferior and disgusting preparations, and we fully endorse Dr. Chambers' remarks, who, writing on consumption, says, "To find the easiest assimilated oil, and to prepare the digestion for the absorption of the oil, are the main problems in the cure of consumption." The oil we invariably recommend for its easy assimilation, agreeableness, and high nutritive value, is *Möller's purest Norwegian Cod-liver-oil.* We have prescribed this variety exclusively for several years, and have found in numerous cases that patients who previously could not take oil on account of the unpalatableness, fishy, or rancid compounds they had attempted under that name, experienced no difficulty whatever in taking Möller's oil. Considering the value of cod-liver-oil, and its being so frequently prescribed in the foregoing pages, we are glad to be able to give our emphatic recommendation to so pure a preparation as the one above named.

As a vehicle, cod-liver-oil may be taken in *claret.* The oil should be poured upon the wine, so that it does not touch the glass, but be floated on it as a large globule. It may then be swallowed without taste. A few morsels of agreeable food may then be eaten. In this way the most capricious person may take the oil without any discomfort. Another plan to obviate taste and prevent nausea is to take a pinch of salt immediately before and after the oil.

2.—Food for Invalids,* Infants, etc.

Essence of Beef.

By the following method, excellent beef-tea, containing a large amount of nourishment, may be prepared:—"Mince, as fine as possible, a piece of lean beef; let it stand in its own weight of cold water (a pound to a

* While this sheet was passing through the press, a brief article on "Th[illegible] of Diet for Invalids" appeared in *The Homœopathic World* (October, 1[illegible] Mr. Nankivell condemns the administration to invalids of "such unw[illegible] Arrow-root, Tapioca, Sago, Corn-flour, Tous les mois, and so forth. I[illegible] it is far better to give well-boiled rice with a moderate quantity of m[illegible] recommends the use of oat-meal.

for six minutes; place on the fire till it boils; then let it simmer for fifteen or twenty minutes; strain, and add a little salt." But the following is a far cheaper, purer, and more effective preparation of beef-essence—LIEBIG'S EXTRACT OF MEAT (Tooth's manufacture, the consignees of which, are Messrs. W. J. Coleman and Co., 13, St. Mary-at-Hill, London*). From personal use, we can strongly recommend this preparation as containing all the nutritive properties of meat, and as much superior to many compounds sold as "Extract of Meat." It is agreeable to the palate and stomach, and is an admirable article of food for all cases of *physical debility*, and extreme emaciation, especially after profuse losses of blood; collapse from wounds; for patients suffering from severe and prolonged fevers; in the last stages of consumption; bad cases of indigestion, in which the stomach rejects any but fluid kinds of food; as an article of diet for nursing mothers; etc., etc. In extreme cases of exhaustion, the extract is mixed with wine, and has thus been used with striking success. Two advantages arising from the use of this article are its digestibility, and the facility and promptness of its preparation.

Beef-tea offers a *fluid* form of food just adapted to an imperfect condition of the digestive and general bodily functions, which being more or less suspended, require nourishment which only needs the slightest processes for its assimilation. It is from the ease with which it is digested and absorbed that its restorative effects may, at least in part, be attributed. Taken after fatigue it has a remarkable power of raising the vigorous action of the heart, and dissipating the sense of exhaustion following severe or prolonged exertion.

It can also be *readily* prepared for use. By the addition of a small quantity of the extract to a little hot water, according to the proportions directed on each jar, beef-tea is *immediately* prepared; an important consideration when an exhausted patient is waiting for food.

NEAVE'S FARINACEOUS FOOD.

Many years' experience in the use of Neave's Food seems to demand from us a distinctive notice, and to justify the recommendation of it as an excellent article of diet for the invalid, the dyspeptic, and others with feeble digestive power who cannot take food in a more solid form. Competent chemical analyses have found the preparation to contain every constituent necessary for the nourishment of the body; and this has been abundantly confirmed by what we have frequently observed as the result of its use. It should be prepared according to the directions supplied with the food, taking care not to make it too thick; and it may be seasoned to the patient's taste. It also makes a very agreeable *gruel*, being more easily prepared and answering the purpose better than that made from oatmeal, etc. In many cases a cupful of this food taken daily is highly beneficial; for suckling women it is far better than stout, porter, etc.; and for infants it is, in the majority of cases, the best substitute for the mother's milk. A great advantage in the adoption of this diet is that any inter-

* Tooth's preparation of Liebig's Extract may be obtained from any Homœopathic chemist.

ference in the action of the bowels is altogether unnecessary, as, by varying the quantity of milk mixed with the food, the most regular action is secured. In cases in which farinaceous food cannot be tolerated, *Sugar-of-Milk* may be substituted: generally, however, this intolerance is due to improper methods of preparation.

SUGAR-OF-MILK.

A still lighter food and one which may be used when the farinaceous food does not agree, is a preparation of cow's-milk and sugar-of-milk. The former should be reduced by slight dilution with water, as it contains too little sugar, but more oil *(cream)* than can be digested by weak stomachs. In cases in which it is necessary to bring up a child by hand from birth, *sugar-of-milk* is most suitable to commence with. *Formula.*—"Dissolve one ounce of the *sugar-of-milk* in three quarters of a pint of boiling water. Mix as wanted with an equal quantity of fresh cow's milk, and let the infant be fed with this from the feeding-bottle in the usual way. Always wash the bottle after feeding, and put the teat into cold water, letting it remain until wanted again."—*The late Mr. H. Turner.*

It is important to use only cow's milk of a good quality, and always to administer it at the same temperature as that of breast milk *(see Lady's Homœopathic Manual, p.p.* 180—1*)*. After the third or fourth month, *Neave's Farinaceous Food* is generally more suitable.

3.—Demulcent Beverages.

BARLEY-WATER.—Wash a table-spoonful of pearl-barley in cold water; then add to it two or three lumps of sugar, the rind of one lemon, and the juice of half a lemon; pour on the whole a quart of boiling water, and let it stand for two or three hours, and strain it. Instead of lemon, currant-jelly, orange-juice, or sliced liquorice may be used to flavour. Barley-water is a valuable demulcent in colds, affections of the chest, hectic fever, etc. It is also useful in *strangury* and other diseases of the bladder and urinary organs.

GUM-WATER.—Gum is a mild nutritive substance, less stimulating than most other forms of nourishment. On this account it is admirably adapted to inflammation of the mucous membranes generally, as in catarrh, bronchitis, etc. *Gum-Water* is prepared by adding one ounce of gum-arabic, and half-an-ounce, or less, of white loaf-sugar, to one pint of hot water.

LINSEED TEA.—This is often a useful beverage for soothing irritation in coughs, catarrh, consumption, pneumonia, diarrhœa, dysentery, inflammation of the bowels, leucorrhœa, difficult micturition, and other inflammatory diseases. It is prepared by adding one ounce of lin
and half-an-ounce of sliced liquorice root, to two pints of boiling
and macerating in a covered vessel near the fire for two or three
should then be strained through a piece of muslin, and one or
spoonfuls taken as often as necessary.

BARLEY-WATER, *Gum-Water, and Linseed Tea* are more or less useful in similar conditions, one being substituted for the other to suit the patient's taste.

LEMONADE.—Cut a lemon into slices, put them into a jug with several pieces of loaf sugar. Pour over it a pint of boiling water, cover it, and let it stand till cold. After straining, it is fit for use.

NITRIC LEMONADE.—Add twenty to thirty drops of *Acidum Nitricum dilutum* to eight ounces of pure cold water, and flavour with honey or loaf sugar; from a teaspoonful to a tablespoonful, according to age, two or three times daily. Useful for allaying sickness in hooping-cough, asthma, chronic bronchitis, consumption, loss of blood from the bowels, fœtid smell of the skin or urine, cold feet, night sweats, etc.

4.—Warm Baths.*

WARM BATH.—The temperature of the water must be raised to 98° F., or to what is agreeable to the back of the hand; then, if the patient be a child, immerse him up to his neck, and apply a cold wet towel to the head, or a large sponge, after dipping it in cold water; the cold towel or sponge may be applied for about three minutes, but the child kept in the bath for ten or fifteen minutes. If the sight of the water make the child afraid, a blanket should be spread over the bath, the child placed upon it and gently let down into the water, even with its dress on, if necessary to prevent fear. The temperature should be *fully maintained* by additions of fresh hot water carefully poured down the side of the bath, till the patient comes out. The bath should be given in front of a good fire, and a warm blanket be in readiness to wrap the patient in directly he leaves the bath.

The warm bath (92° to 98° F.), and the hot bath (98° to 112° F.), are therapeutic agents of great value in many affections. They are chiefly used to equalize the temperature of the whole body, to soothe the nervous system, to control the action of the heart, to promote perspiration, to relax the muscular and cutaneous system, and, especially, to equalize the distribution of blood throughout the body. In the latter instance a disproportionate quantity of blood in the internal organs is recalled to the surface.

The warm bath is often of signal benefit in the diseases of children—*Convulsions, Spasmodic Croup, Measles, Scarlatina, etc.;* also in *Dropsy after Scarlatina*, as well as in other dropsical affections. In the simple or inflammatory fevers of children, it calms the nervous excitement, and is often followed by refreshing sleep.

It is also highly soothing, and aids the cure in inflammatory diseases of the kidneys, bladder, and uterus; in spasmodic stricture of the urethra; the passage of renal and biliary calculi; in many spasmodic affections of the bowels—*colic, etc.;* in *prurigo, tetanus, diabetes, Bright's disease,* and in the *melancholy of insanity.*

* For the correct or safe administration of warm baths, a good bath-thermometer is indispensable.

THE VAPOUR BATH.—This has a similar action and is applicable to most of the cases mentioned under the "warm bath," but is more particularly useful for adults in some forms of rheumatism, and dry scaly diseases of the skin. The patient should sit upon a wooden-seated chair, undressed, and be enveloped, chair and all, in blankets closely secured at the neck, and extending down to the floor. A vessel containing about a gallon of boiling water should then be placed under the chair, the clothes well-secured in all directions to confine the vapour, and perspiration will soon follow. After the patient has been in the bath a few minutes, a thoroughly hot or red-heated brick or piece of iron should be added to the water, and the clothes again well closed in. During the bath one or two tumblers of cold water should be sipped. To prevent headache the forehead should be bathed with a sponge dipped in cold water, or a napkin wrung out of cold water laid on the head. If necessary, also, the feet should be put in a pan of moderately hot water, the heat of which should also be maintained by adding, after a few minutes, fresh hot water. After the patient has perspired for ten or fifteen minutes, he should be *quickly* washed with tepid water, dried, and at once retire to bed. Or he may sit in a *shallow bath* at a temperature from 60° to 80° F., the extremities and trunk being well rubbed by an assistant, and water gently poured over the head for three or four minutes, after which the patient should be dried and retire to bed.

THE HOT-AIR BATH.—In this bath a spirit-lamp or a saucer containing one or two ounces of spirits-of-wine or rectified spirits-of-naptha, after being set on fire, is substituted for the hot water of the vapour bath; but the blankets are used in the same manner. It may also be followed by the tepid wash or shallow bath. As the spirit burns, heat is generated around the patient, and perspiration produced. If spirits in a saucer be used, and it be necessary to prolong the perspiration, a larger quantity of spirit may be used, but none should have to be added after the spirits have been lit.

THE HOT FOOT-BATH.—Immediately before retiring to bed, the patient should be undressed, but well covered with one or two blankets, which should also cover the foot-bath, so that the steam may have access to the body generally; the feet and part of the legs should then be put in hot water (98° F.), and the temperature afterwards increased by fresh additions of hot water, for ten, fifteen, or twenty minutes, according to the strength of the patient, and until free perspiration breaks out on the face. He should then be rapidly washed with tepid water, rubbed dry, get into bed, be well covered with clothes, and perspiration be further encouraged by drinking cold water. On rising in the morning he should take a cold plunge, or shower-bath, or quickly sponge over the whole surface of the body, and afterwards the trunk and extremities should be vigorously dried by means of a sheet or large towel. This local warm bath is used for a variety of purposes, and, if adopted early and carried out according to the following directions, will promote general perspiration, and arrest or relieve *catarrhs*, *fevers*, etc., in their incipient stages.

The *hot foot-bath*, or the *hot sitz-bath* is also useful in sudden suppression of the menses from exposure to cold or wet; it relieves the distressing sensations of the patient, and aids the re-appearance of the function.

Headache, palpitation, the hysteric sensation of choking, etc., are likewise removed or relieved by a local warm bath.

THE BLANKET BATH.—This is an easy method of inducing perspiration. A blanket is wrung out of hot water, and wrapped round the patient. He is then packed in three or four dry blankets and allowed to repose for thirty minutes. The coverings may then be taken off, the surface of the body rubbed with warm towels, and the patient made comfortable in bed (*Tanner*).

THE WET-PACK.—A macintosh sheet, or stout blanket or quilt, should be spread on a mattress, and over it a thick linen sheet, *well* wrung out of *cold* water. In fevers, the colder the water is, the better; for very delicate persons with feeble reaction, water at 68° may be used. The patient is to be extended on his back naked on the wet sheet, so that the upper edge covers the back of the neck, but the lower one is to project beyond the feet; holding up the arms, one side of the sheet is to be thrown over the body and tucked in; the arms are now placed by the sides, and the other part of the wet sheet is thrown over all, and tucked rather tightly in, turning in the projecting ends under the feet. The macintosh or blanket is then to be brought over all the sheet, and well tucked in round the neck, at the sides, and over the feet, so as completely to exclude the air. A stout quilt or extra blanket is to be put over all. In a short time the patient will become warm; the sensation is most agreeable, especially in fevers. The patient may remain in the pack for thirty, forty-five, or sixty minutes, the duration being regulated by the effects produced. The patient should then be put into a shallow-bath at 68°, well washed, dried, and put to bed. It may be repeated once, twice, or thrice a day, according to circumstances and the violence of the attack. Perspiration may be encouraged by giving sips of cold water. If the head become congested, or the face flushed, while in the pack, a cold compress should be applied over the forehead. By attention to the above directions, any person can apply the wet-pack. The wet-pack is invaluable in the *early* stages of all fevers; and in *scarlatina, measles, small-pox, etc.*, it assists in bringing out the eruption.

*** For suggestions on Bathing as a hygienic measure, see Part I. p.p. 50–3. Also an article on the "Water-cure, or Hints on Bathing," in *The Homœopathic World*, September, 1869.

5.—Glycerine.*

Glycerine or the glycerine of starch, is of great use as an external application, when the lips or hands are chapped, or when the skin is hot, rough, and inelastic, as after eczema and other skin complaints. It quickly gives suppleness to the tissues, and removes burning, tingling, or smarting. It should be mixed with an equal quantity of water, or, still better, of eau-de-Cologne, as without such dilution the tissues may be inflamed and made to smart. The glycerine of starch may also be used

* Chiefly from Ringer's Therapeutics.

in xeroderma to make the skin soft and supple. A bath should also be taken each day, and the application applied after the body is wiped thoroughly dry. Glycerine is a good application to the meatus of the ear, when the tissues are dry, or when the tympanum is ruptured. In the latter instance it covers the opening, and so, for a time, supplies the place of the lost membrane. In acute diseases, when the lips, tongue, and gums become dry and coated with dried mucus, these parts should be washed quite clean, and kept moist by glycerine. This greatly improves the comfort and look of the patient. Glycerine sometimes answers best when diluted with an equal quantity of water.

In chronic diseases, as phthisis, at their last stage, the tongue and inside of the cheek become dry, red, and glazed, and usually with great thirst. These discomforts may be lessened, and often removed, by washing the mouth with glycerine and water. If the glycerine be used alone, it is liable to make the mouth clammy and sticky. If thrush have attacked the mucous membrane in the above-mentioned disease, this may be quite removed by the employment of the glycerine.

Glycerine of carbolic acid may be applied with advantage to fœtid sores, such as open cancers, whether on the surface of the body or in the uterus. It removes the offensive smell of the discharge, and also improves the condition of the sore. Probably this preparation would be of use in Lister's most admirable method of treating wounds.

Glycerine of borax is a good application to pityriasis of the scalp; it may also be employed in aphthæ and thrush of the mouth.

Glycerine, or glycerine cream, is one of the best preventatives of bed-sores. The part exposed to pressure should, if possible, be washed every morning and evening, with tepid water, and carefully wiped quite dry with a soft towel, and then a little glycerine, or glycerine cream, rubbed gently over the part with the hand. If the part be at all sore or tender, the latter is best. Glycerine should be used before any redness or tenderness occurs, as it is preventative rather than curative.

6.—Wet Compresses.

A cold compress consists of two or three folds of soft linen, wrung out of cold water, applied to the affected part, and covered by a piece of water-proof material—oiled-silk, gutta-percha, or india-rubber cloth—which should project a little beyond the wet cloth on all sides, so as to prevent the access of air and evaporation from the linen. In parts subject to considerable motion, as the throat and neck, the edges of the oiled-silk should be folded in over the wet linen so as to prevent its exposure to the air.

For cachectic persons with feeble reaction, the compress may be held for a minute in front of a fire before applying it.

In general, compresses are best applied at night, as it is impossible to keep them in nice apposition while moving about. After removing them in the morning, the parts should be sponged with cold water to restore the tone of the skin.

spread on warmed linen already cut to the required size and shape, or put into a bag and applied. Linseed-meal retains heat and moisture for a long time, but is liable to irritate skin of a fine delicate texture, or when it is inflamed with an eruption.

BREAD POULTICES.—Place slices of bread into a basin, pour over them boiling water, and place the whole by the fire for a few minutes, when the water should be poured off, replaced by fresh boiling water, and this again poured off and the bread pressed, beaten with a fork, and made into a poultice. Bread poultices are especially valuable for their non-irritating, bland properties.

CHARCOAL POULTICES.—Uniformly mix charcoal with bread, and just before the application of the poultice sprinkle the surface with a layer of charcoal. Or charcoal may be sprinkled on a wound, sore, or boil, and over it a simple bread poultice applied. Charcoal poultices are used to correct offensive smells from foul sores, and to favour a healthier action.

CARROT POULTICES.—Boil carrots quite soft, mash them with a fork, and apply in the ordinary way. They are said to make wounds cleaner and healthier.

Poultices are chiefly useful in the following complaints:—Pneumonia, pleurisy, bronchitis, pericarditis, peritonitis, acute rheumatism, lumbago, and to mature abscesses, boils, etc., and to facilitate the discharge of matter.

When used to mature abscesses or disperse inflammation, poultices should extend beyond the limits of the inflamed tissue; but afterwards, when the boil or abscess has discharged, the poultices should be very little larger than the opening through which the matter is escaping. A large poultice continued too long, soddens and irritates the part, and is liable to develop fresh boils around the old one.

In deep-seated inflammations—pneumonia, etc.—they should be renewed as soon as they become cool, and the former one not disturbed till the fresh one is ready to replace it. In bronchitis and pneumonia, a *jacket-poultice*, to go round the chest, with tapes to secure it in front and over each shoulder, is necessary to ensure efficient and uniform action.

To retain heat for a long time, poultices over a large surface should be covered with oiled silk, or with a layer of cotton wool. One of these methods is preferable to a very thick poultice, which might cause inconvenience or pain.

In acute lumbago they must be applied thick, hot, large enough to cover the affected part, and be renewed immediately they become cool. After continuing this treatment for one to three hours, the skin should be wiped dry and covered with flannel, and this again with oiled silk. Like the poultice, this last application promotes free secretion from the skin, to which the good results are mainly due.

As a substitute for a poultice, *spongio-piline* may sometimes be used. It is made of sponge and wool felted together in three layers, and coated on one of its surfaces with caoutchouc to render it impermeable. By moistening the soft inner surface with water, the warmth and moisture of the ordinary cataplasm are secured; or by sprinkling the same surface with lotions, it may be made the vehicle for various medicinal substances.

Spongio-piline is often valuable during the [illegible] of [illegible] irritable sores, and especially when required for persons [illegible] their usual occupations. But for the relief of severe pain, [illegible] poultice is the most soothing application. Poultices should be [illegible] till pain has subsided, or the sore begun to granulate; afterwards a [illegible] compress, covered with oiled-silk, should be applied as the best [illegible].

8.—Fomentations.

Fomentations, by means of flannel wrung out of hot or boiling water, are employed for similar purposes as poultices, but are lighter and [illegible] to increase the pain of sensitive parts. The hot flannel is placed in a towelling, and twisted round till as much water as possible is expressed. If well wrung, it may be applied very hot without any danger of [illegible] the skin.

Fomentations with hot water are useful in *relieving pain*, *arresting inflammation*, and checking the formation of matter, and are often [illegible] adjuncts to poultices. *Acne indurata* and similar inflamed [illegible] often be dispersed or reduced in size by hot fomentations. Combined with poultices, they expedite the passage of matter to the surface, and [illegible] subsequent expulsion. In such cases the value of fomentations and poultices depends upon the heat and moisture; water for the fomentation should therefore be used *hot*, and fresh additions of hot water [illegible] becomes cool. After well-fomenting, poultices should be applied [illegible] possible, and frequently renewed.

In inflammations, spasms, and pains affecting deeply-seated structures, as in the chest or abdomen, great and quick relief often follows fomentation.

Dry Fomentations.—When heat alone is required and it is desirable to avoid the relaxation of tissues which moisture would occasion, dry heated substances—flannel, bran, chamomile flowers, salt, sand, etc., are used. After thoroughly heating the substance, it should be placed in a bag made for the purpose, and which has also been previously heated. Sometimes, as in spasm and its accompanying pain, a thin piece of flat tile, heated in an oven, and wrapped in warmed flannel, may be employed. If more evanescent heat is required, flannel, strongly heated before the fire, may suffice.

9.—Enemata—*Injections*.

Enema is a liquid injected into the large intestines, through the anus, by means of a suitable instrument. Injections are used for various purposes, and consist of different substances, chiefly as follows:—

1.—*To relieve the bowels.*—Injections act, not simply by washing away the accumulated fæces, but by distending the rectum and promoting peristaltic action more or less through the whole intestinal canal. For this purpose a large quantity—one or two pints, or even more—should be injected. After the introduction of the fluid, the patient should lie down and retain the injection for ten or fifteen minutes. So large a quantity of fluid could scarcely be introduced or retained, except by patients who have previously used injections. As a general rule, the best fluid for injection is *cold* or *warm water*. Warm injections are sometimes useful to relieve pain or irritation, either in the bowel or in an adjacent organ—the bladder, the uterus, or even the kidneys—but should be used sparingly.

2.—*To restrain diarrhœa.*—For this purpose small injections only are necessary—one to two ounces; if copious enemata are used, the intestines are stimulated to contract and expel their contents.

Starch, tepid, is an excellent material for such a purpose; it should be made of the consistence of cream, and about two ounces used. In incurable cases, and when the diarrhœa resists other means, a few drops of opium should be added to the starch. Starch injections are especially useful in acute, excessive, and dangerous diarrhœa of typhoid fever, dysentery, phthisis, and the choleraic diarrhœa of children.

3.—*To remove thread-worms.*—For this purpose, half-a-pint to a pint of water, to which a dessert-spoonful of salt has been added, answers the purpose admirably (see page 394). In order that the water may be thrown as high up into the bowel as possible, a vaginal tube may be attached to the enema-syringe, and, after being well greased, gently pushed right up the bowel. Here, however, as in other cases, general treatment is necessary to correct the systemic condition on which the disease depends.

4.—*To convey nourishment.*—Injections are sometimes used to sustain the system, by introducing food up the rectum when it cannot be taken by the stomach, as in acute gastritis, obstinate vomiting, cancer, etc. Beef-tea, soup, milk, the brandy-and-egg mixture, etc., may be administered in this way. It is necessary that the rectum should be empty before injecting nourishment. Medicinal substances are also sometimes administered by enemata.

10.—Inhalation.

In its therapeutic sense, inhalation is the act of drawing air, impregnated with the watery vapour of medicinal substances, into the air-passages. It is an extremely useful mode of administering various remedies when their action is chiefly required on the mucous surfaces of the respiratory passages. *Iodine*, *Sulphurous Acid*, *Kreasote*, *Borax*, *Permanganate of Potash*, *Aconite*, *Hyoscyamus*, *Belladonna*, *Ipecacuanha*, *Carbolic Acid*, etc., may be well given by inhalation in certain diseases chiefly involving the throat and large bronchial tubes, or in irritative or convulsive cough, or when there is fœtid expectoration. Quinsy, catarrhal and ulcerated sore throat, chronic bronchitis, phthisis, etc., may be more or less benefited by inhalation. The method of inhaling is very simple, and is often done quite effectively, and with less effort, than with a special inhaler. All that is required is a jug of *hot* water, over which the face may be held, and a towel so arranged that it covers the face below the eyes and surrounds the top of the jug, so as to confine the vapour. A few drops of the drug to be inhaled being dropped into the hot water, the medicine finds ready access to the air-passages through both the mouth and the nose. This may be practised for five or ten minutes at bed-time, and if necessary, and the patient has not to be exposed to cold air during the day, it may be repeated once, twice, or oftener in the day. In acute inflammatory diseases of the throat, simple or medicated vapour may be administered as frequently as the patient's strength and other circumstances permit. A portion of the drug thus administered reaches the lungs and enters the general circulation; but the chief action of the medicated vapour is on the throat and bronchial mucous surface.

In grave prostrating diseases—diphtheria, croup, etc.—vapour may be inhaled by diffusing it through the apartment by the steam from a kettle with a long spout, kept constantly boiling, or by forming a tent over the bed and covering it with blankets and then bringing a pipe to convey the steam under it. In urgent cases where suffocation is threatened, the room may be quickly filled with vapour by hanging wet towels before a large fire. In ordinary cases, simply keeping water boiling in the centre of the room will moisten the atmosphere sufficiently.

Besides the administration of various remedies to the respiratory passages, the local application of the *steam of hot water* is very serviceable; it soothes the inflamed mucous membrane, aids expectoration from the lungs, and removes mucus from the crypts and follicles of the tonsils.

Inhalation can, however, be only a subordinate method of treatment in constitutional diseases, such as consumption, and is chiefly palliative rather than curative. A well-chosen Homœopathic remedy administered in the usual way, just as certainly reaches the seat of the disease as anything inhaled can do, and at the same time tends to correct the constitutional error on which the local symptoms depend.

When a patient has to be exposed to cold air after inhalation, the vapour should be *cold*, and formed and distributed by the spray-producer; this is an important precaution. In many cases in which it is desirable to use topical applications directly to a diseased part, this is the best method; the fluid may be injected or thrown as a fine spray, so as to be inhaled by the patient, by means of the *spray-producer*. By breaking up the fluid into a very small spray, substances can be inhaled without inconvenience, and brought into direct contact with the bronchial tubes, even as far as their small ramifications.

11.—Some Directions on Nursing.

* The services of an intelligent, experienced nurse, form a part of the treatment of the sick quite as essential as the administration of medicine. To aid her to some extent in the performance of this duty, the following *general* hints are offered. Particular instructions, suited to various diseased conditions, are given, when needful, throughout Part II., under "Accessory Treatment." Persons having the charge of patients should

always refer to this portion of the section in which the case of illness is described, and also be familiar with the various directions contained in this Part IV. Special directions concerning infectious fevers are given in the section on typhoid fever, pp. 120-125. In serious and difficult cases, the medical attendant alone can furnish instructions adapted to the peculiarity of each case; and it is the nurse's duty faithfully to carry out his directions, and to report to him at each visit the effects of the treatment.

1st.—*The Sick Room.*—The following points should be kept in view: (1.) The apartment should be *airy.* A spacious, well-ventilated room, allowing an uninterrupted admission of fresh air, and the free escape of tainted, is a valuable element in the management of the sick. Fresh air can only be ensured by an open window or door, or both. It is generally desirable to have a blazing fire kept burning night and day, both in summer and winter, as this assists in the efficient ventilation of the room; but the patient's head should be protected from its direct effects. This is more especially necessary in infectious diseases, for the poison is thus diluted with atmospheric air, and so, losing its power, becomes inoperative. To the same end, the room should be divested of all superfluous furniture—carpets, bed-hangings, etc. (2.) The room should be provided with a *second bed* or convenient couch, to which the patient should, if possible, be removed for a short time at least once in the twenty-four hours. This ensures a change of atmosphere around the patient's body, and at the same time allows the bed to be aired. (3.) The apartment should be *darkened;* not by excluding all light and air, by closed shutters, or closely-drawn bed-curtains, but by letting down the window-blinds, and securing a *subdued* light, and by protecting the patient's face from the glare of gas, lamps, etc. (4.) The sick room should be *quiet.* Silk dresses and creaky boots should not be worn; the crackling noise made by anyone reading a newspaper is often most distressing to invalids; the tones of the voice should be gentle and subdued, but whispering avoided; all unnecessary conversation and noise must be forbidden. (5.) The *temperature* of the room should be regulated by a *thermometer*, as the sensations of the nurse cannot be depended upon as a sufficient guide; but a thermometer, suspended out of a current of air and the direct heat of the fire, will correctly indicate the temperature of the room. The temperature may be varied according to the nature of the disease from which the patient suffers. In fevers, inflammation of the brain, etc., about 55° will be the proper warmth. In inflammation of the lungs, and bronchitis, a higher temperature is necessary—60° and upwards. In all inflammatory affections of the chest, the air to be breathed ought to be warm, and also moist (see "Inhalation"), so as not to irritate the inflamed delicate lining of the air-tubes. Cold air and too many bed-clothes are sure to increase the mischief. Under all circumstances it must be remembered that the temperature considered necessary is on no account to be maintained by excluding fresh air from the room, and making the patient breathe air over and over again which has already been made impure.

2nd.—*Cleanliness.*—Fears are often expressed that in washing the surface of a patient's body, or even in changing his linen, any eruption or rash should be driven in, or that cold should be taken. If done properly, there is not the least ground for any such fear. The patient should be sponged over as completely as possible at least once a day with warm or cold water, as may be most agreeable to his feelings, and then quickly dried with a soft towel. If the patient be much exhausted, a small part of the skin may be washed at one time; or instead, first a damp, and then a dry towel may be used under the bed-clothes, so as to disturb the patient as little as possible. The value of this application of water is stated page 120–1.

3rd.—*Beverages.*—In most cases of illness, especially at the commencement, cold water, barley-water, gum-water, raspberry-vinegar-and-water, apple-water, toast-and-water, lemonade, or soda-water (see "Demulcent Drinks"), is nearly all that is necessary. There is sometimes a foolish objection raised to allowing cold water to a patient; but it is not only most refreshing, but an agent of supreme importance, lowering excessive heat, giving vigour to the relaxed capillaries, and accelerating favourable changes. The quantity of cold water given at a time should be small—one to two table-spoonfuls—and repeated as often as desired. Sucking ice is also both useful and grateful to many patients.

4th.—*Food not to be kept in the sick-room.*—Miss Nightingale's suggestion on this point is so important, but, we regret to observe, so often disregarded, that we venture to repeat it here. It is this—do not keep the food, drink, or delicacies intended for the patient, in the sick-room or within his sight. The air of the apartment is liable to deteriorate them, and the continuous sight of them to excite disgust. Rather take up for him, at the fitting time, and by way of surprise, two or three teaspoonfuls of jelly, or as many fresh grapes as he may consume at once, or the segment of an orange. Or, if it be appropriate to his condition, a small cup of beef-tea, covered, with one or two narrow slips of toasted bread, just from the fire; this is very much preferable to attempting to swallow even a less quantity from a basinful that has been kept for many hours within the reach of the patient's hand and eye.

Watching patients, moderation in convalescence, change of air on recovery from illness, etc., are elsewhere enforced, and may be found by the index.

INDEX:

GENERAL AND GLOSSARIAL.

In which the significations of many words, not found in the common dictionaries, are given, when these words are not explained in the text.

Many Conditions and Symptoms, not specified in this Index, are referred to in the MATERIA MEDICA, *and, more particularly*, in the CLINICAL DIRECTORY, Part V.

See *Hints to the Reader*, pp. xii to xiv, and *Preface*.

AA, an abbreviation of the Greek word *ana*, used in pharmacy, and signifying *of each*
Abdomen, compress for, 408-9, 642; dropsy of, *see* Ascites; enlarged, *see under* Ascites, Worms, etc.
Abscess, 493-7; acute, 493-4; from diseased bone, 494; mammary, 494-5; thecal, 478; opening of, 496
Accessories in disease, 634-48
Accidents, *see* Injuries
Acetic acid *(vinegar)*, 150, 181, 190, 378
Aching and stiffness from exertion, 522
Acne, 466-8
Aconite-lotion, 269; vapour, 337, 645
Aconitum Napellus, 525-9; therapeutic value, 525-6; uses, 526-7
Actæa, *see* Cimicifuga Racemosa
Acute rheumatism, 165-71; flannel in, 171; healthy action of the skin, 184; well-chosen diet in, 184
Administration of remedies, 69-71
Adynamic (*with debility of vital power*)
Ægophony, 343
Æsculus Hippocastanum *(Horse-chestnut)*, 407, 414
Agaricus Muscarius *(Fly-agaric)*, 259, 261, 422, 468, 470
Age, old, and senile decay, 499-508
Aged, treatment of, 505
Ague, *see* Intermittent fever
Ague-cake, *see* Enlarged spleen
Air, pure, 36-40; impure, 148; spoiled by breathing, 36
Airy sleeping-rooms, 37-9
Albuminuria, 430-3
Alcohol, in snake-bite, 490-1; food-character of, 121-2; drinking, *see* Stimulants
Alcoholic stimulants in fevers, 121-3
Aloes, *see* Aloe Socotrina, 529
Alopecia areata, 484; *see also* Baldness
Alternation of medicines, 71
Alumina (*Oxide of Aluminium*), 407
Amateur practitioners, 524
Amaurosis, 281-6; symptoms, 281-2; causes, 282; treatment, 282-4; on preservation of sight, 284-6
Amblyopia, 281
Ammonia in hydrophobia, 491
Ammonium Carbonicum, 307, 330
Anacardium Orientiale, 455
Anæmia *(poverty of blood)*, 227-9
Anæsthesia, 265
Anasarca *(general dropsy)*, 100, 229-33
Aneurism, 311
Anger, effects of, *see under* Cham., etc.
Angina faucium, *see* Throat, sore
,, pectoris, 265, 305-6, 561
,, trachealis, 319
Ankles, swelling of, *see* Œdema
Ankylosis, 493
Anorexia *(loss of appetite)*, 368-9
Anthelmintics *(worm-destroyers)*, 392
Anthrax *(carbuncle)*, 476-7
Antidotes, 633
Antimonium Crudum, 529-30
,, Tartaricum, 530-1
Antiseptics — Sulphurous Acid, 627-8; Carbolic Acid, etc.
Anus *(the termination or orifice of the rectum or lower bowel)*; prolapsus, 418-9; itching of the, 417-8
Anxiety, effects of, *see under* Ignatia, Acon., China, Nux Vom., etc.
Aperients during sickness, 404
Aphonia *(loss of voice)*, 327
Aphthæ, *see* Thrush

Apis Mellifica, 531-2
Apnœa *(suspended respiration)*, from drowning, 509-10
Apocynum Androsemifolium, 457
Apocynum Cannabinum, 203, 231
Apoplexy, 236-43; warnings, 237; symptoms, 238; predispositions, 238-9; how to distinguish from epilepsy and drunkenness, 240-1; treatment, 241; accessory and preventive measures, 242-3; *see also* 534
Appetite, loss of, 368-9; voracious or depraved, 369
Argentum Nitricum *(nitrate of silver)*, 276, 277, 335, 358, 444
Arnica-bath, 522, 534
Arnica Montana, 532-5; external use of, 534-5; caution, 535
Arsenic-poisoning, *see* Poisons; *also* 552
" " in ague, 134-5
Arsenicum Album, 535-8
Arterial bleeding, 517
Arthritis, *see* Gout
Articular (*pertaining to joints*)
Asafœtida *(assafœtida)*, 264
Ascaris lumbricoides *(long or round worms)*, 388
Ascites *(abdominal dropsy)*, 230-1
Asiatic cholera, *see* Malignant cholera
Asphyxia, 509-10
Asthenic *(applied to diseases characterized by want of vigour)*, *see* Sthenic
Asthma, 333-8; prevention of, 337-8
Ataxy, locomotor, 248
Athletic sports, 44, 448
Atmospheric influences and diarrhœa, 396-7
Atrophy *(non-nourishment; wasting)*
Auscultation, 211
Aurum Metallicum, 538-9
Axilla *(the armpit)*

Bacon-fat to the skin, 83-4
Back, pains in the, *see under* Crick-in-the-back, Lumbago, Piles, Rheumatism, Muscular fatigue, Urine, etc.
Baker's itch, 458-9
Baldness, 484, 550, 609
Ball-room, 44
Banting-dietary, 498-9
Baptisia Tinctoria, 539-40
Barber's itch, 469
Bark, *see* China
Barley-water, 637
Baryta Carbonica, 540
Bath, cold, 51, 327; temperature of, 51; sponge, 50; sea, 50; sea-salt in, 52; shower, 52, 264, 338; Turkish, 53; warm and hot, 638-40
Bathing, 50-3; cautions, 51, 201, 216, 270
Beard, cultivation of, 333, 359-60; use of, 469
Bedrooms, airy, importance of, 37-9
Bed-sores, 121
Beef, essence of, 477, 635-6
Beef-tea, 636
Bee-stings, 485, 487
Belladonna, 540-4, vapour of, 645
Benzoic Acid, 438
Beverages, demulcent, 637-8, 648; for dyspeptics, 375; in fevers, 121
Biliousness, 421-5
Bilious-fever, *see* Remittent-fever
Bismuthum *(Nitrate of bismuth)*, 371, 37
Bites and stings, 487-9; venomous and poisoned, 489-91
Black eye, 515, 534
Bladder, catarrh or inflammation of, 433-4, 437; irritability of, 436, 438; spasm of, 436
Blanket-bath, 640
Blankets in rheumatism, 171
Blear-eyes, 291
Bleeding, how to arrest, 516-7; from the nose, 301-2; varicose vein, 314-5
Blindness, *see* Amaurosis; *also* Cataract
Blinds and curtains, 40
Blistering-fly, 549; *see also* Cantharis
Blisters, 550
Blood diseases, 75-164, xiii
Blood-shot eye, 273
Blood, spitting of, and vomiting of, 365
Blood-vessels in the aged, 502-3
Bloody flux, *see* Dysentery
Boil, 474-5
Bone, broken, 519-21; disease of, 494
Bones, in old age, 501
Boots, thin-soled, 49; tight-fitting, 479-80
Borax, 346, 468, 645
Bowels, confined, 403-9; consumption of, 218-9; relaxed, 395; falling of, 418-9
Brain, concussion of, 511-2; fever, *see* Typhus; inflammation of, 234-6
Branny tetter, 459-60
Bread, brown, its value, 28-31, 406, 408; poultice, 643
Breakfast, 25-6
Breast, abscess of the, 494-5
Breast-pang, *see* Angina pectoris
Breath, shortness of, *see* Asthma, Bronchitis, Phthisis, etc.; odour of, 64; offensive, *see under* Aurum, Merc., Carbo Veg., etc.
Breathing, 63-4; to restore suspended, 509
Bright's disease, 430-3
Broken bone—arm, leg, rib, etc.—519-21
Bromium *(Bromine)*, 321-2
Bronchitis, acute, 328-33; chronic, 329-33; increased mortality from, 329-30; prevention of, 332-3

Bronchocele, *see* Goitre
Brow-ague, *see* Neuralgia
Brown bread, 28-31, 408
Bruise, 514-5
Bruit *(a sound heard on auscultation)*
Bryonia Alba, 544-6
Bubo, sympathetic, 442
Bug-bites, 485, 488-9
Bunion, 481-2
Burnett's disinfecting fluid, 301
Burns and scalds, 512-4
Business, influence of, 54, 304

Cachexia *(bad habit of body)*
Cactus Grandiflorus, 546
Calcarea Carbonica, 554-5
„ Phosphorata, 556
„ Sulphurata, *see* Hepar Sulphuris
Calcareous degeneration, 242
Calculus, 434-6
Calendula, 556
Calomel, 404
Camphor, 547-9, 633
Cancer, 188-91; varieties, 188; operative measures in, 191
Cancrum Oris, 347-8
Canker of the mouth, 347-8
Cannabis Sativa, 549
Cantharidine pomade, 550
Cantharis Vesicatoria, 549-50
Capsicum Annuum *(Cayenne pepper)*, 371, 398, 415
Carbolic acid, 110, 641, 645
Carbo Vegetabilis, 551-2; animalis, 468
Carbuncle, 476-7
Carcinoma, *see* Cancer
Cardiac *(pertaining to the heart)*
Cardialgia mordens, *see* Heartburn
Caries of teeth, 352
Carrot poultices, 643
Cataract, 287-9
Catarrh 323-7; summer *(Hay asthma)*, 318; epidemic, *see* Influenza; bronchial, 323; of bladder, *see* Cystitis
Catheter, 440
Causticum, 552
Cedron, 135, 136
Cerebral *(pertaining to the brain or cerebrum)*
Chafing of infants, 452-3
Chalk-stones, 177, 185-6
Chamomilla Matricaria, 552-4
Change of air, 124, 377
Chapped hands, 470
Charcoal poultices, 643
Chelidonium Majus *(Greater celandine)*, 341, 422, 424, 427
Chemosis, 276-7
Chest compress, 642
„ for medicines, 69

Chicken-pox, 87-8
Chigoe, 485
Chilblains, 470-1
Child-bed fever, *see* Puerperal
Child-crowing, *see* Croup
Chimaphila Umbellata *(Pipsissiwa)*, 434
China, 557-9
Chink-cough, *see* Hooping-cough
Chin-whelk, 469
Chinese feet, 480
Chloasma, 485
Chlorate of potash, *see* Kali Chloratum
Chloric ether, 306
Chloride of lime, 124; of zinc, 124, 301
Chloroform liniment, 269
Chlorosis, 229
Cholera, English, 140
„ malignant, 140-5; sanitary and hygienic measures, 145
Choleraic diarrhœa, 140-5
Chordee, 442
Chorea, 261-2
Churches, badly ventilated, 39-40
Cicuta Virosa *(Water hemlock)*, 259
Cimicifuga Racemosa, 559-63
Cina Anthelmintica, 563-4
Cinchona, *see* China
Cinnabaris, 600
Circulation, to restore, 509-10
Circulatory system, diseases of, 304-17
Cirrhosis, 423
Cistus Canadensis *(Rock rose)*, 463
Clap, *see* Gonorrhœa
Cleanliness, 50, 647-8; in fevers, 120
Clematis Erecta, 280, 291, 440
Clergyman's sore throat, 357-60
Clergymen, longevity of, 54
Clinical Directory, vi
Clinical thermometer, 61-3
Clothing, 46-50; colour of, 48; change of, 48; materials for, 49, 201, 216; scanty, 329-30
Cocculus Indicus, 564-5
Cocoa, 26, 375
Cod-liver oil, 634-5; how to take, 635; in scrofula, 201; in consumption, 215; neuralgia, 269
Coffea Cruda, 565-6, 633
Coffee-drinking, 370, 438, 566
Colchicum, 566-7
Cold bath, *see* Bath
Cold in the head, 323-7; excessive sensibility to cold, 326-7
Colic, 268, 401-3
Collapse *(prostration, or interruption of the powers and actions of life)*, 143
Collinsonia Canadensis, 567
Colliquative diarrhœa, 397
Collodion in erysipelas, 163
Colocynthis, 568

Coma *(lethargic sleep)*; coma-vigil, 105
Comocladia Dentata *(Guao)*, 463
Compresses, wet, 641-2
Concussion of the brain, 511-2
Condylomata *(warty excrescences of a syphilitic character)*
Condy's fluid, 359; *see also* Kali Permanganicum
Confined bowels, 403-9
Congestion, in typhoid fever, 115; of the liver, 421
Conium, 568-9
Conjunctivitis, 203, 273-4
Constipation, 403-9; injections in, 644; in the aged, 406
Constitutional diseases, 165-283, xiii
Consumption, pulmonary, 206-18; symptoms, 206; diagnosis, 211; causes, 211; general measures, 214-8; climate, 217; of the bowels, 218-9
Contagion *(transmission of a poisonous principle by contact)*
Contusion, 514-5
Convalescence, cautions in, 124
Conviviality and gout, 179
Convulsions, infantile, 254-5; hysteric, 262-4; epileptic, 255-61
Cooking, 31-3; animal food, 31-3
Copaiba, 444
Copper-pennies, 570
Corks, 69
Corns, hard, soft, and inflamed, 479-80
Corpulence, 497-9
Coryza, 323-7
Costiveness, *see* Constipation
Cotton-wool, in burns, 513
Cough, *see under* Catarrh, Bronchitis, Pneumonia, Phthisis, etc.; *also* the Materia Medica; hooping, 152-6
Coup-de-Soleil, 243-4
Cow-pox and vaccination, 84-7
Cracks in the skin, 471
Cream, 215, 269
Creosotum, *see* Kreasotum
Cretinism, 315
Cricket, 44
Crick-in-the-back, 563; neck, 172-3, 174
Cross-bar swing, 217, 222
Croup, 319-23; inflammatory, 319; dangers of, 320; spasmodic, 319-23; treatment, 321-2; accessory measures, 322; prophylaxis, 323
Crusta lactea, *(milk-crust)*, 463, 466
Cuprum Aceticum, 570
" Metallicum, 569-70
Cutaneous system, diseases of, 451-91
Cuts, 517; *see also* Wounds, lacerated
Cyanosis, 571
Cynanche tonsillaris, 360-3

Damp, affections from, [illegible]
Dandriff, [illegible]; [illegible]
Darkening the [illegible], [illegible]
Dead, how to restore the [illegible], *see under* Asphyxia
Deaf-dumbness, [illegible]
Deafness, [illegible]; not stupidity, [illegible]
Death, painless, [illegible]
Debility, [illegible], [illegible]; and [illegible], [illegible]; *see also* Emaciation
Decay, senile, [illegible]
Degeneration, [illegible]; [illegible], [illegible]
Delirium tremens, [illegible]; *see also under* Bell., Hyos., Opi., etc.
Demulcent beverages, [illegible]
Dentition, *see* Teething, [illegible]
Depression of spirits, *see under* [illegible], [illegible], Merc., Plat., etc.; *also* Hypochondriasis, Liver-complaint, etc.
Derbyshire-neck, 315-7
Desquamation *(scaling off of the skin)*
Diabetes, 282-5
Diagnosis *(distinguishment, by signs and symptoms, of one disease from another)*
Diarrhoea, 395-401; injections in, [illegible]
Diathesis *(constitutional disposition)*
Dietary, plan of, [illegible]; [illegible], [illegible]
Diet, etc., in fever, 121-3
Difficult breathing, *see* Dyspnoea
Digestion, physiology of, [illegible]
Digestive system, diseases of, [illegible]
Digitalis, 570-1
Dinner, 26; late, 27-8
Dioscorea Villosa *(wild yam-root)*, [illegible]
Diphtheria, 146-52
Diphtheritic paralysis, 148, [illegible]
Directions about medicines, [illegible]
Directory, Clinical, vi.
Disease, signs and symptoms of, [illegible]
Diseases of heart and membranes, [illegible]
Diseased animal food, [illegible]
Disinfectants—Sulphurous Acid, [illegible]; Carbolic Acid, Chloride of Lime, Condy's Fluid, Burnett's Fluid, etc.
Disinfection, 110, 117, 124
Disorders of teething, 349-50
Disposition in which to eat, [illegible]
Division of nerve in neuralgia, [illegible]
Dizziness, *see* Vertigo
Dogs and tape-worms, [illegible]
Dose, 70-1; repetition, 71; over-dose, [illegible]
Drainage, imperfect, 14[illegible]
Draining of houses, etc., [illegible]
Drinking-water, 390-1; [illegible], [illegible]
Drinks, demulcent, 637-8
Dropsy, 229-33; of the abdomen, [illegible]; brain, 245; after scarlet-fever, [illegible]

Drosera Rotundifolia, 571
Drowning, apparent death from, 509-10
Drugs hurtful, 403-6
Drunkenness differs from apoplexy, 240
Dry tetter, 460-1
Dulcamara, 571-2
Dumb ague, 133-4
Dwellings, 42-3; and epidemics, 43
Dynamic *(pertaining to strength, power, or force; applied to the influence of agents on the organism not explicable by mechanical or chemical causes)*
Dysentery, 382-5; chronic, 385
Dyspepsia, 366-77
Dyspnœa, 63; *see* Breath, shortness of

Ear-ache, 293-4
Ear, boxing the, 298; discharge from, 294-6; diseases of, 293-9; foreign bodies in, 518-9; general hints on, 298-9; inflammation of, 293-4; pain in, 293-4; wet or damp, 298
Eating, reasons for, 366-7; too quickly and frequently, 370; disposition suitable for, 376
Ecchymosis, 515, 579
Ectosoa, 387, 484
Ectropium, 290
Eczema, 463-6
Effluvia *(exhalations, vapours, etc.)*
Egyptian or contagious ophthalmia, 275
Electricity, 248
Emaciation, 206, 208-9; *see also under* Ars., Iod., China, Merc., etc.
Emissions, *see* Spermatorrhœa
Emotional disturbances, *see under* Acon., Bry., Cham., Chin., Ign., Nux V., etc.
Employments, why unhealthy, 54-8; posture in, 56-7
Emprosthotonus, 249
Empyema, 342
Encephalitis, 234-6
Encephaloma, 188
Endemic *(applied to diseases peculiar to the inhabitants of particular countries)*; *see also* Epidemic
Endocarditis, 167
Enemata, 644-5
English cholera, 140, 395
Enlargement of the glands, *see* Glandular enlargements; of the heart, *see* Heart-diseases; of the liver, 421; of the spleen, 133
Enteralgia, *see* Neuralgia of the bowel
Enteric-fever, 110-25; diagnosis from typhus-fever, 101-2; prevention of, 117; sequelæ, 119
Enteritis *(inflammation of the bowels)*, 401; *see also under* Ars., Merc. Cor., Tereb., etc.
Entophyta, 388
Entozoa, 387
Entropium, 290
Enuresis, *see* Urine, incontinence of
Epidemic *(applied to diseases which are prevalent, but not native, and due to a temporary cause)*; *see* Endemic
Epigastric *(pertaining to the epigastrium or region of the stomach)*
Epilepsy, 255-61; distinguished from apoplexy, 240; from hysteria, 263
Epistaxis, 301-2
Eructations, *see* Dyspepsia, Pyrosis, Flatulence, etc.
Eruptions, *see* Skin-diseases
Eruptive fevers, 76; course of, 76
Erysipelas, 160-4
Erythema, 451-2
Essence-of-beef, 635-6
Etiology *(the science which treats of the causes of diseases)*
Euphrasia Officinalis, 572-3
Evening parties and ventilation, 39-40
Exanthemata *(eruptive diseases)*, 76
Excess in the pleasures of the table, 395
Excesses, sexual, *see* Sexual excesses
Excoriations, *see* Chafing
Excrescences *(preternatural growths)*, 475
Exercise, 44-5, 201, 216; times for taking, 44-5; gymnastic, 44, 217
Exertion, excessive, *see* Exhaustion
Exhaustion, muscular, from over-exertion, 522; *see also under* Arnica
Exophthalmic bronchocele, 317
External remedies for medicine-chest, 73
Extract of meat, Liebig's, 636
Eye, diseases of, 273-92; black, 515; douche for, 286; foreign bodies in, 518; shade for, 286; spots before, 286-7; waters for, 277
Eyes, of the aged, 504; over-use of, 283, 284, 287; sore, *see* Ophthalmia; *see also* Sight
Eyelids, eversion of, 290; granular, 291; inflammation of, 289; inversion, 290; sore, 289; stye on, 289-90

Face-ache, *see* Neuralgia, *and* Toothache
Face, swelling of, œdematous, 231
Facial neuralgia, *see* Neuralgia; paralysis, 247-9
Fainting-fit, 307
Falling of the bowel, 418-9
Falling-sickness, *see* Epilepsy
Falls and stuns, *see* Contusion, *and* Concussion
False measles, 453; pleurisy, *see* Pleurodynia
Famine-fever, see Relapsing-fever

Farinaceous food, 636-7
Fatigue, muscular, 622, *see also under* Arnica; mental, *see under* Nux Vom., Phos. Ac., etc.
Favus, *see* Parasitic diseases of the skin
Feather-beds, 376
Febricula, 127-9
Feeding of infants, 349, 350
Feet, aching and soreness of, 584; perspiration of, 630; swelling of, *see* Œdema
Felon, 478
Females, diseases of, vii
Femoral *(pertaining to the femur—thigh-bone or thigh)*
Ferrum, 573-4
Ferrum Iodidum *(Iodide of Iron)*, 199, 247
Feverishness, *see under* Acon., Cham., Gels., *and* Verat. Vir.
Fever, Brain, *see* Typhus; Enteric, 110-26; Eruptive, 76; Famine, *see* Relapsing; Gastric, *see* Enteric; Hay, 318; Hectic, 209; Intermittent, 130-8; Low, *see* Typhus; Remittent, 138-9; Rheumatic, 165-73; Scarlet, 94-100; Simple, 127-9; Typhoid, *see* Enteric; Typhus, 100-10; Yellow, 129-30
Filix Mas *(male-fern)*, 392-3
Finger, gathered, see Whitlow
Fistula in ano, 410-2
Fits, *see* Ague, Apoplexy, Convulsions, Epilepsy, Hysteria
Fits of infants, 254-5
Flannel, 47-8, 171, 201, 215, 226, 244, 270, 433, 455
Flatulence, 369
Flea-bites, etc., 486
Flesh, proud, 475
Fluoric acid, 314
Flux, bloody-, *see* Dysentery
Fœtid breath, *see* Breath
Fomentations, 644
Fomites *(clothing, etc., imbued with contagion)*
Fontanelles *(the spaces left in the head of an infant, where the frontal and occipital bones join the parietal,*

Habits, 376-7
Hæmatemesis, 365-6
Hæmoptysis, 367
Hæmorrhage, how to arrest, 516-7; from the lungs, 365; from the stomach, 365; from a varicose vein, 314-5; vicarious, 366
Hæmorrhoids, 412-7
Hair-washes and restorers, 612; falling off, 550, 609; *see also* Alopecia *and* Baldness
Hamamelis Virginica, 578-9
Hands, chapped or cracked, *see* Chilblains
Hand-feeding of infants, *see* Infants
Harvest-bug bites, 485, 488-9
Hay-asthma, 318-9 [*Sabadilla* is a good remedy]
„ -fever, *see* Hay-asthma
Head affections, *see under* Dyspepsia, Neuralgia, Catarrh, etc.; *also* the Materia Medica, *especially under* Acon., Bell., Bry, Glon., *and* Nux Vom.
Health and occupations, 54-8; observations pertaining to, 25-6
Healthy dwellings, 42-3
Heartburn, 369
Heart complications in rheumatism, 167
„ diseases, causes of, 304; difference between functional and organic, 309; palpitation of, 307-8; organic and functional disease of, 309-11, 534; weakness in the aged, 502, 504
Heat spots, 464
Hectic fever, 209, 212
Height and weight as aids to diagnosis, 211
Helleborus Niger, 579
Hemicrania, *see* Neuralgia
Hemiopia, 281
Hemiplegia, 247
Hepar Sulphuris, 580-1
Hepatalgia, 422
Hepatitis, 420-1
Hepatic (*pertaining to the liver*), congestion, 421-5; dropsy, 230; neuralgia, 265; spots, 435
Hepatization, 340
Hernia, 386-7, 401
Herpes, 461-3
Hiccough, 369
Hints on nursing, *see* Nursing
Hints to the reader, xii-xiv
Hip-joint, disease of, 492-3
Hoarseness, 327; in young children and croup, 323
Hobbies, 260
Hobnailed liver, *see* Cirrhosis
Homœopathic (*according to the law of similars; pertaining to Homœopathy*)
Homœopathy (*curing disease by drugs which, given to healthy persons in sufficient doses, are capable of producing conditions or symptoms similar to those of the disease to be cured*); not a mere system of dietetics, 25; novice in, xiv
Hooping-cough, 153-6
Hordeolum, 289-90
Hornet stings, 487
Horseback exercise, 44
Hot-air bath, 639
Hot baths and fomentations, 638-40, 644
Housemaid's knee, 481
Hunger, excessive after typhoid fever, 119 *see* Appetite
Hunger-pest, *see* Relapsing fever
Hunting-field, 533
Hydatids, 389
Hydrastis Canadensis, 581
Hydrocyanic (*Prussic*) acid, 250, 269, 306, 318, 335
Hydropathic applications, 638-40, 641-2; in typhoid fever, 121
Hydrophobia, 250-3; precaution in, 253
Hydrocele, 230
Hydrocephalus, acute, *see* Tubercular meningitis
Hydrocephalus, chronic, 245-7
Hydrochloric acid, *see* Muriatic acidum
Hydrothorax, 230, 342
Hygiene, 46-58
Hydro-pericardium, 230
Hydrops articulorum, 230
Hyoscyamus Niger, 582, 645
Hyperæmia (*local excess of blood*)
Hyperæsthesia (*excessive or morbid sensibility*)
Hypertrophy (*applied to tissues and organs having an excess of nutrition, indicated by increase of size, and sometimes of consistence*); *see also* Atrophy
Hypochondriasis, 270-2
Hysteria, 228, 262-4; fit of, 263-4

Ice in diphtheria, 151
Icterus, *see* Jaundice
Idiocy and cretinism, 315
Ignatia Amara, 583
Impetigo, 466
Impotence, 445
Impure water, 390-1, 396
Incontinence of urine, 437-9
Incubation (*period of development, as that of hatching eggs*)
Indigestible kinds of food, 396
Indigestion, *see* Dyspepsia
Idiopathic (*the original disease*)
Indiscretions, social, 389

stomach, 363
Influenza, 158-9
Ingrowing of nail, 479
Inguinal *(pertaining to the groin)*
Inhalation, 645-6; of Kreasote, 332
Injections, 644-5; in constipation, 409; piles, 416-7; worms, 394
Injuries, 509-23
Insanity, 271; of the muscles, 261
Insects, stings of, 487-9
Insolation, 243-4
Inspection, 210
Intercostal neuralgia, *see* Neuralgia
Intermittent fever, 130-8; prevention of, 138; sequelæ of, 139
Intermittent pulse, 60, 307-8
Intertrigo, 452-3
Intestinal worms, *see* Worms
Intoxication distinguished from apoplexy, 240
Invalids, food, etc., for, 635-8
Iodide of Potash, *see* Kali Hydriodicum
Iodine, *see* Iodium, 584-6, 621, 634, 645
Ipecacuanha, 586-7, 645
Iris Versicolor, 588-9
Iritis, 279-81
Iron, *see* Ferrum
Irritation of the skin, 485
Itch, 486-7, 570; barber's, 469
Itching of the anus, 417-8; of the skin, 456-8

Jacket-poultice, 643
Jalap, 404
Jaundice, 425-7

Kali Bichromicum, 176, 589-90
,, Chloratum *(chlorate of potash)*, 149, 345
,, Hydriodicum, 175, 176, 591
,, Iodidum, *see* Kali Hydriodicum
,, Permanganicum *(permanganate of potash)*, 645
Kidney, inflammation of, *see* Nephritis
Kink-cough, *see* Hooping-cough
Kitchens, subterraneous, 298
Kreasote inhalations, 332

Lemon-juice, in scurvy, [illegible]
Lepra, 460-1
Leucorrhœa and Scrofula, [illegible]
Lice, *see* Pediculi
Lichen, 468-9
Liebig's Extract of Meat, [illegible]
Lienteria, *see* Diarrhœa [illegible]
Ligatures, 517
Light, 40-1
Limestone and Goitre, 316
Lime-water, 444; and milk, [illegible]
Liniments, 173
Linseed-meal poultices, [illegible]
Linseed tea, 637
List of medicines, 73-3
Liver, diseases of, 420-5; [illegible]; complaint, 421; [illegible]; deranged, after ague, [illegible]; [illegible] ment of, 421; [illegible]
Liver spots, 485
Lobelia Inflata *(Indian [illegible])*, [illegible]
Lockjaw, 249-50
Locomotor ataxy, 248
Loss of blood, [illegible]; of voice, [illegible]
Low fever, *see* Typhus
Lumbago, 171-2, 173
Luncheon, 27
Lungs, bleeding from, [illegible]; inflammation of, 338-41; *see also* Consumption
Lupus, 191-2
Lycopodium Clavatum, [illegible]
Lymphatic glands, disease of, [illegible]

Maceration *(the process of almost dissolving a solid ingredient by steeping it in a fluid)*
Maggot-pimple, 467
Malaria *(bad air: applied to certain effluvia from marshy ground)*, [illegible], 287
Malignant cholera, 140-5; disease, *see* Cancer; tumour, [illegible]
Mammæ *(the breasts)*
Mammary *(pertaining to the breasts)* abscess, 494-6
Mandrake, *see* Podophyllum
Manganum *(manganese)*, [illegible]

Market-garden vegetables, and Worms, 390
Marsh-miasm, *see* Miasma
Mastication, 370, 373-4
Masturbation, *see* Self-abuse
Materia Medica *(medical materials: the branch of medical science which relates to medicines; it embraces both pharmacology and therapeutics)*, xiii., 524-633
Materies morbi *(diseased matter)*
Measles, 88-94; diagnosis from scarlet-fever, 90; false, *see* Roseola; sequelæ, 92; and consumption, 93
Meat, baked, boiled, or roasted, 31-3; diseased, 396; Liebig's Extract of, 636
Medicines, the, 68-74; alternation of, 71; directions for taking, 69; genuine, 74; list of, for medicine-chest, 72-3; proper dose, 70
Medicine-chest, 69
Mediæval epidemics, 43
Meibomian glands, swelling of, 291
Melancholic depression, *see* Hypochondriasis
Meningitis, 234-6; tubercular, 202-3
Mensuration, 211
Mentagra, 469
Mental emotions and diarrhœa, 397
Mental and physical training, 448
Mercurius and its preparations, 594-600
Mesenteric disease, *see* Tabes mesenterica
Metastasis *(the transference of local symptoms of disease from one part of the body to another)*
Mezereum *(spurge-olive)*, 457, 610
Miasma *(minute particles of an infectious substance floating in the air; as, the emanations from swampy grounds, marsh-miasm, etc.)*
Micturition *(urination)*, *see* Urine
Milk-crust, 463-6
Milk in fevers, 122
Milk-leg, *see* Phlegmasia dolens
Milk-sugar, 637
Miner's-elbow, 481
Miscellaneous diseases, 492-508
Moderation in convalescence, 124
Mole, 482
Morbus coxæ, 492-3
Morphia *(morphine: an alkaloid of opium, the narcotic principle of that drug)*, 270
Mortification, *see* Gangrene
Moschus *(musk)*, 264, 307, 310
Mother's mark, 482
Mouth, canker of, 347-8; inflammation of, 345; sore, 345-7
Mumps, 156-8
Muriatis Acidum, 600
Muscæ volitantes, 113, 286-7
Muscles, exhaustion of, 522; formation of, 45; of the aged, 501-2
Muscular fatigue, 552; rheumatism, 171-3
Musquito-stings, 487-9

Nævus, 482-3
Nail, ingrowing of, 479
Naja Tripudians *(virus of the Cobra di Capello)* 306
Natrum Muriaticum
Natural decay, 499-506
Nausea, *see* Dyspepsia, Vomiting, etc.
Nausea marina, 380-1
Neave's Farinaceous Food, 347, 350, 364, 400, 636-7
Nephritis, *(inflammation of the kidneys)* desquamative, 430, 434
Nerve, division of, 270
Nervous symptoms in typhus, 105
Nervous system, diseases of, 234-72
Nettle-rash, 453-5
Nettle-stings, 487-9
Neuralgia, 264-70; varieties, 264; symptoms, 265-6; causes, 266; treatment, 267-9; protection from cold, 270: division of the nerve, 270
Nightmare, 369-70
Night-sweats, 212
Nitre in Asthma, 337
Nitric lemonade, 638
Nitricum Acidum, 601
Nitro-Glycerine, *see* Glonoine
Noises in the ears, 298
Nomenclature, new, of diseases, v., xii.
Normal *(that in which there is no deviation from the general rule)*
Nose, diseases of, 300-3; foul discharge from *(ozæna)*, 300-1; bleeding from, 301-2; polypus in, 302-3; loss of smell, 303
Nostrils, plugging the, 301-2
Novice in Homœopathy, xiv.
Nursing, hints on, 646-7, *see also* 520-5
Nux Moschata *(nutmeg)*, 264
Nux Vomica, 601-4

Oat-meal, 635; porridge, 170
Obesity, 497-9
Occipital *(pertaining to the occiput, the back part of the head)*
Occupations and health, 54-8, 448
Odontalgia, *see* Toothache
Œdema *(local dropsical swelling)*, 230-2
Offensive breath, *see* Breath
Old age and senile decay, 499-506
,, premature, 506
Oleum Crotonis *(Croton-oil)*, 465
Onanism, *see* Self-abuse

Onion in stings, 488
Onychia, 479
Opacity in the crystalline lens, see Cataract
Ophthalmia, medicines for, 277-9; scrofulous, 203-5; catarrhal, 273-4; neonatorum, 274-5; purulent, 274-5; of infants, 275-6; gonorrhœal, 276-7; tarsal, 291
Ophthalmic medicines, 277-8
Opisthotonus, 249
Opium, 604-6
Orchitis, 442
Otorrhœa, 294-6
Ovarian dropsy, see Dropsy
" neuralgia, see Neuralgia
Over-dose of medicine, 633
Over-exertion, 622
Overloading the stomach, 374
Oxyuris vermicularis, 388-9
Ozæna, 300-1

Pack, wet, 640; in rheumatism, 170-1; in typhus fever, 109
Pain, its indications, 65
Painter's colic, 612; paralysis, 248
Palpitation, 307-8
Palsy, see Paralysis
Paralysis, 247-9; facial, 247-9
Parasitic disease of the intestines, 387-94, 626
Parasitic diseases of the skin, 484-6, 626
Paregoric, 605
Pariplegia, 248-9
Passions, the, and industry, 66-7, 448
Pathology (*the doctrine or investigation of the nature of diseases*)
Peas, 30
Pediculi (*lice*), 456, 485
Percussion, 211
Pericarditis, 167
Peripneumonia, see Pneumonia
Peritonitis, 427-9
Permanganate of Potash, see Kali Permanganicum
Peruvian bark, see China
Petroleum (*rock-oil*), 380, 384, 444
Pharyngitis, 357-60
Phenic acid, see Carbolic acid
Phimosis, 442
Phlebitis, 312
Phlegmasia dolens, 312
Phlegmatic (*cold; sluggish; not easily excited into action or passion*)
Phosphate of lime, see Calcarea Phosphorata
Phosphori Acidum, 609-10
Phosphorus, 606-8
Photophobia (*intolerance or dread of light*), 203-4, 236; see also Ophthalmia, etc.
Phthiriasis, [illegible]
Phthisis pulmonalis, [illegible]
Physicians, [illegible]
Physicking children, [illegible]
Physiology (*the science which treats of the healthy action or functions peculiar to living beings*)
Phytolacca Decandra, [illegible]
Pigeon breast, 319; cure of, [illegible]
Piles, 312, 413-7
Pilules, [illegible]
Pimples, 466-8
Pityriasis, 459-60; versicolor, 485
Platina, 612
Pleurisy, 341-4
Pleurodynia, 174, 341, 463
Pleuro-pneumonia, 339
Plugging the nostrils, 301-2
Plumbum, 612-3
Pneumonia, 338-41
Pneumo-pleuritis, 339
Podagra, see Gout
Podophyllum Peltatum, 613
Poisons, 522-3, vi.
Poisoned wounds, 489-91
Polycrests, 534
Polypus, 302-3; of the nose, 302-3
Pomade, Cantharidine, 590
Poppy, see Opium
Porridge, oatmeal, 170, 625
Porrigo capitis, 485; decalvans, [illegible]; larvalis, 486; favosa, 484
Port-wine stain, 482-3
Posture and health, 56
Poultices, 642-4
Power of the mind over sea-sickness, [illegible]
Precautionary measures in fevers, [illegible]
Pregnancy, vomiting during, [illegible]; see also under Nux Vom., etc.
Premature old age, 606
Prickly heat, [illegible]
Professional treatment, advantages of, [illegible]
Professions and health, 54-8
Prognosis (*the art of judging beforehand the course of disease*)
Prolapsus ani, 418-9
Prolonged nursing, 283
Prophylactics (*preserving or defending from disease*)
Prophylaxis (*the art of preventing disease*)
Proud flesh, 476
Prurigo, 456-8
Pruritus ani, 417-8
Psoriasis, 460-1
Ptosis, 247-8
Ptyalism (*salivation*)
Puerperal ephemera, 164; fever, 164; peritonitis, 428
Pulmonary, see Phthisis

Pulsatilla Nigricans, 613-6
Pulse, in health and disease, 58-60; intermittent, 307-8
Pure air, 36-9; in scrofula, 195
Purgatives, 403-4; 405-6
Purging, *see* Diarrhœa
Purpura, 225-6
Purulent ophthalmia, 274-6
Pyrosis, 378

Quinine, 557; poisoning in ague, 134-5, 137
Quinsy, 360-3

Rabies, *see* Hydrophobia
Rachitis, 219-23
Ranunculus Bulbosus (*butter-cup*), 169, 176, 267, 463
Rash, *see* Nettle-rash, Prurigo, and other skin-diseases
Reader, hints to the, xii.-xiv.
Red-gum, *see* Strophulus
Relapsing fever, 125-6
Relaxed bowels, *see* Diarrhœa
,, throat, 357-60
Remedies, *see* Medicines
Remittent fever, 138-9
Renal dropsy, 230; *see also* Bright's disease
Repetition of doses, 71
Residence, healthy, 42-3, 217
Respirator, the natural, 333, 359-60
Respiratory system, diseases of, 318-44
Rest for the aged, 506; for the fever-patient, 120
Retching, *see* Vomiting
Retention of urine, 439-41
Rheumatic fever, *see* Rheumatism, acute; gout, 169; paralysis, 248
Rheumatism, acute, 165-71; heart-complications in, 167; how it differs from gout, 181; hydropathic treatment in, 170-1; blankets in, 171; muscular, 171; chronic, 173-6; muscular weakness, 172
Rhododendron Chrysanthum (*Siberian rose*), 169, 174, 231, 268
Rhus Toxicodendron, 616-8
Ribs, beading of, 220
Rickets, *see* Rachitis
Rigor, 102, 111, 125, 131, 146
Ringworm, of the surface (common), 484; vesicular, 462
Risus Sardonicus, 249
Room, sick-, darkening, 41
Roseola, 453
Rose-rash, 453
Rose, *see* Erysipelas
Round-worm, 388
Rowing, 44, 217
Rubini's treatment of cholera, 143
Running from the ears, 294-6
Rupture, 386-7
Ruta Graveolens, 618

Sabadilla (*Indian barley*), *see under* Hay-asthma
Salts, nutritive, contained in food, 29-31
Sambucus nigra (*Black elder*), 306, 335
Sanguinaria Canadensis (*Blood-root*), 301, 303
Sanitary measures in cholera, 145; in typhus, 106
Sarracenia purpurea (*Huntsman's cup*), 82
Sausages and pork, *see* Dyspepsia; *also* 394
Scabies, 484
Scalds and burns, 512-4
Scalled-head, 463-6
Scarlatina, } 94-100; diagnosis from
Scarlet-fever } measles, 90, 97; inhalation in, 99; prevention, 97; sequelæ, 100
Scars after vaccination, 86
Sciatica, 173-4, 265
Scillæ maritima (*squills*), 438
Scirrhus, 188
Scorbutus, *see* Scurvy
Scratching, 457-8
Scrofula, 192-219
Scrofulous disease of the glands, 205; of the hip-joint, 492; ophthalmia, 203-5
Scurvy, 226-7; land scurvy, 225-6
Scutellaria Lateriflora (*skull-cap*), 252
Scybala, 383
Sea-bathing, 50; salt-baths, 52; voyage, 217
Sea-sickness, 380-1; power of the mind over, 381; prevention of, 381
Sea-voyage, 217
Sebaceous tumour, 483
Secale Cornutum (*ergot of rye*), 301, 379
Seat, itching of, *see* Itching of the anus
Secondary diseases, *see* Sequelæ
Self-abuse, 258, 445-50; *see also* Sexual Excesses
Seminal emissions, *see* Spermatorrhœa
Seminium (*seed or germ; as that of typhus-fever*) 107
Senega (*snake root*) 231, 330
Senile decay, 499-508
Sensibility to cold, how to diminish, 326
Sensitiveness to light, *see* Photophobia; sound, 298; *see also under* Cham., China, Ign., etc.
Sepia succus, 619
Sequelæ (*morbid affections following others; secondary diseases*) of diphtheria, 148; Enteric-fever, 119; I-

Sugar-of-milk, 347, 637
Sulphur, 622-6
Sulphuric acid, 259, 371, 378
,, ether, 306
Sulphurous acid, 486, 627-8, 645
Summer-catarrh, *see* Hay-asthma; diarrhœa, 395, 397-9
Sunlight, importance of, 40-1
Sunstroke, 243-4
Suppers, *see* Nightmare, 369-70
Sweating, *see under* Mercurius, China, etc.
Swelling of the glands, *see* Glands, Goitre, etc.; of the extremities, *see* Œdema; white, of the joints, 493
Swellings, dropsical, 231
Swing, cross-bar, 217
Swooning, 307
Sycosis, 469; *see also* Condylomata
Symptoms and signs of disease, 58-68
Syncope, 307
Syphilis, 187-8

Tabacum *(tobacco)*, 380
Tabes mesenterica, 218-9
Tænia solium, 389
Tamus communis, 470
Tannin, 303, 444
Tape-worm, 388
Taraxacum (*dandelion*), 422
Tarsal ophthalmia, 291
Tartaricum Emeticum, *see* Antim. Tart.
Tea, 27, 310, 370, 406, 438
Teeth, stopping carious, 352; extraction of, 353; preservation of, 353-4; decay of, 591
Teething, 349-50; disorders of, 349-50
Tellurium, 463
Temperature in health and disease, and the clinical thermometer, 61-3
Temperature of bath, 51
Tenesmus, 383
Terebinthina, 628-9
Testicles, neuralgia of, 265; inflammation of, 442
Tetanus, 249-50
Tetter, *see* Herpes
Teucrium Marum Verum, (*cat-thyme*) 303, 392-3
Thecal abscess, 478
Thermometry, clinical, value of, 61-3, 211
Thin boots, 49
Thorns, stings, etc., how to extract, 489, 518-9
Thread-worms, 388
Throat compress, 359, 642; deafness, 296-7; sore, 356-7; *see also* Catarrh, Quinsey, Aphonia, etc.
Thrush, 345-7
Thuja Occidentalis (*Arbor Vitæ, tree of life*), 303, 444, 482, 483
Thyroid glands, enlargement of, 315
Tic-douloureux, *see* Neuralgia
Tight-lacing a cause of piles, 414
Tinctures, 69; how to drop, 70; for external use, 73
Tinea, *see* Parasitic diseases of the skin
Tinnitus Aurum, 298
Tobacco smoking, 282, 337, 354, 370; and scrofula, 197
Tongue, in health and disease, 64-5; inflammation of, 355; cracked or fissured, 356; ulcer on, 356
Tonic spasms, 249
Tonsils, enlarged and inflamed, 357-60, 361
Toothache, 351-4
Tooth-rash, 459
Tormina, 383
Toxæmic (*a poisoned state of blood*)
Toxicology (*an account of poisons*)
Tracheotomy, 150, 322-3
Training, mental and physical, 448
Traumatic (*caused by wounds*)
Treatment of the aged, 505
Trees and woods, influence of, 43
Trichina Spiralis, 388
Trismus, *see* Tetanus
Triturations, 69
Tubercle, *see* Scrofula
Tubercular Meningitis, 202-3
Tuberculosis (*degeneration of tissue into tubercular matter*)
Tumour sebaceous, 483
Tumours, malignant and non-malignant, 189
Turkish bath, 53
Turpentine, 628
Typhoid (*applied to diseases marked by, or in which occur great prostration, cerebral disturbance, and "low" symptoms; resembling typhus*)
Typhoid-fever, *see* Enteric-fever, 110-25
Typhus-fever, 100-10; diagnosis from typhoid, 101-2; prevention of, 110

Ulcer, 471-4; in the stomach, 364; on the tongue, 356; varicose, 314-5
Umbilical (*pertaining to the navel*)
Unhealthy employments, 55, 196
Uræmia, 431
Urethra, stricture of, 440
Urinary system, diseases of, 430-50
Urine, in health and disease, 66-8; difficulty in passing, 436-7; inability to pass, 439; incontinence of, 437-9; retention of, 439-41; sediment in, 435, 437; suppression of, 439
Urticaria, 453-5
Urtica Urens (*stinging nettle*), 455, 513
Uva Ursi (*bear berry*), 440

Lightning Source UK Ltd.
Milton Keynes UK
UKHW020915211118
332624UK00010B/1389/P

9 780266 856016